Physiological Measures

of the

Audio-Vestibular System

Edited by

Larry J. Bradford

Children's Division of the Menninger Clinic
The Menninger Foundation
Topeka, Kansas

With a Foreword by

S. Richard Silverman

Central Institute for the Deaf
St. Louis, Missouri

ACADEMIC PRESS New York San Francisco London 1975
A Subsidiary of Harcourt Brace Jovanovich, Publishers

ACADEMIC PRESS, INC.
111 Fifth Avenue, New York, New York 10003

United Kingdom Edition published by
ACADEMIC PRESS, INC. (LONDON) LTD.
24/28 Oval Road, London NW1

Library of Congress Cataloging in Publication Data

Bradford, Larry J
    Physiological measures of the audio-vestibular sys-
tem.
    Includes bibliographies and index.
    1.   Ear–Diseases–Diagnosis.   2.   Audiometry.
3.   Vestibular function tests.   I.   Title.
[DNLM: 1.   Vestibular function tests.   WV272 B799p]
RF123.B7   617.8′075   74-10211
ISBN 0–12–123650–1

Contents

List of Contributors

Numbers in parentheses indicate the pages on which authors' contributions begin.

Larry J. Bradford, Children's Division of the Menninger Clinic, The Menninger Foundation, Topeka, Kansas (1, 249)

Werner D. Chasin, Otolaryngology Division, Tufts University School of Medicine, Boston, Massachusetts (13)

Alfred C. Coats,* Departments of Physiology and Otorhinolaryngology and Communicative Sciences, Baylor College of Medicine, Texas Medical Center, and the Audio-Vestibular Laboratory and Neurophysiology Service, The Methodist Hospital, Houston, Texas (37)

Rita B. Eisenberg, Bioacoustic Laboratory Research Institute, St. Joseph Hospital, Lancaster, Pennsylvania (319)

Alan S. Feldman, Department of Otolaryngology, State University of New York College of Medicine, Upstate Medical Center, Syracuse, New York (87)

Theodore J. Glattke, Division of Otolaryngology, Stanford University School of Medicine, Stanford, California (147)

William G. Hardy, The Johns Hopkins University School of Hygiene and Public Health, The Johns Hopkins School of Medicine, The Johns Hopkins Hospital, Baltimore, Maryland (177)

Donald C. Hood, Department of Otolaryngology, The Hospital for Sick Children, Toronto, Ontario, Canada (349)

Song Ping Lee, Department of Otolaryngology, Topeka Medical Center, Topeka, Kansas (13)

F. Blair Simmons, Division of Otolaryngology, Stanford University School of Medicine, Stanford, California (147)

Ira M. Ventry, Department of Speech Pathology and Audiology, Teachers College, Columbia University, New York, New York (215)

* Present address: Physiology Department, Baylor College of Medicine, Texas Medical Center, Houston, Texas.

Foreword

When I began my professional career, the terms *coin click, watch tick, whisper,* and *conversational voice, Politzer Lärmapparat, Schwabach, Rinne,* and *Weber* tests were more than items out of the conventional historical chapter in textbooks. They were the "audiometric" implements and methods of the day. Although we cannot deny the occasional usefulness of intelligent application of some of these tests even now, there is no doubt that the subsequent evolution of a variety of audiometers constituted the major audiological development of the time. We see that audiology is no exception to the well-known principle of the history of science that the emergence of new and valuable instruments attracts people to their constructive use. The methods and techniques associated with audiometry have generally been those of classical psychophysics, such as the methods of limits, adjustment, and paired comparisons requiring active participation in the test by the subject. These methods are obviously not suited to young children or to "difficult-to-test" subjects, particularly where clear understanding of test instructions is required of the subject.

I believe that this book points to a next significant step in the progress of audiology as important as the advent of the conventional audiometer. The methods described and documented herein are potentially and, in many instances, demonstrably applicable to patients heretofore inaccessible to conventional audiometry. Furthermore, they may add to the specificity with which we can associate test results with particular conditions and elements in the audio-vestibular system, whether it is the determination by impedance audiometry of the nature of a lesion in the middle ear, or the lesion is in the base or apex of the cochlea as determined by evoked cortical response audiometry.

Furthermore, we are aware that nature produces lesions that we cannot reproduce in the laboratory. Perhaps, it may not be too optimistic to predict that astute clinical observations by physiological methods may add to our understanding of the way in which the normal audio-vestibular system functions. Of course, we need to be cautious in our promises and expectations, and we must constantly appeal to scientific rigor to avoid indiscriminate, unwarranted, and extravagant claims for the value of any method. This, I believe, the contributors to this volume have done.

S. Richard Silverman
Central Institute for the Deaf
St. Louis, Missouri

Preface

Procedures utilizing voluntary responses have been found to be quite satisfactory for the assessment of most persons with audio-vestibular system impairments. However, such voluntary response tests are not satisfactory for the assessment of all persons, as some percentage of patients require utilization of indirect procedures to assess the integrity of the system. Obtaining an accurate assessment of the audio-vestibular system of many children and adults, including the mentally retarded, emotionally disturbed, and neuromuscularly impaired, has necessitated the development of indirect procedures that do not depend upon voluntary responses. A variety of these indirect procedures are available to professionals responsible for such assessments. Information about these procedures is scattered among works in medicine, psychology, and audiology, but has not been presented systematically in a single volume for students and professionals of otolaryngology, neurology, pediatrics, and audiology.

It is the purpose of this book to present a comprehensive view of currently available principles and methods for indirectly assessing the audio-vestibular system. In order to allow the book to serve as a single, self-contained reference, a chapter is included on ear pathologies and the otologic examination. Each chapter is intended to be complete in itself, and no attempt has been made to integrate the various procedures. The book is addressed to those persons who wish to acquaint themselves with the physiological and electrophysiological measures for the solution of old problems of accurately determining the status of the audio-vestibular system. Although voluntary test procedures "indirectly" measure the physiologic functioning of the audio-vestibular system, these tests have not been included here because they are discussed thoroughly in other books. As new research appears so rapidly, the contents of this book can be taken only as the current state of the art, with the hope that some readers will be challenged to expand the frontiers with further research.

Acknowledgments

This book is dependent upon the cooperation of many people, the most important being our patients, to whom we owe a great debt for teaching us so much. My special appreciation is extended to William G. Hardy, Professor of Communicative Sciences, The Johns Hopkins University, to Murray Goldstein, Associate Director, National Institute of Neurological Diseases and Stroke, and to my colleague at The Menninger Foundation, Clyde L. Rousey, for their encouragement, support, and assistance in the planning of the book. It has been a pleasure and privilege to share with the contributors the evolution of their final manuscripts. Their cooperation and personal sacrifice to meet the deadlines while maintaining active teaching, clinical, and research activities has made them admired friends and respected colleagues. The compilation of the book was greatly facilitated by Karen Newmann who typed and retyped manuscripts. Finally, I gratefully acknowledge my wife, Mary Ann, for her editorial assistance, help with the laborious task of checking citations and references, and moral support without which I would have faltered many times.

Chapter One

Audio-Vestibular System: Yesterday, Today, and Tomorrow

Larry J. Bradford [1]

The history of science is marked by a slow but steady progress from the unknown to the known. The tower of knowledge about the ear has been built from bricks laboriously fashioned over the years—even centuries. Each new finding provides an immediate solution for some problem, but for others it suggests still another question. All too often these one-time advancements have become fused into the facts we know, while the names of their creators and their struggles have been forgotten. The tower of physiological measures available to examine the audio-vestibular system is well-based, but it should never be considered as completed. Today's edifice is the result of yesterday's efforts and is the structure on which to build tomorrow's achievements—an edifice not built for the sake of knowledge alone, but also for the sake of better care and treatment for people with audio-vestibular impairments.

I. YESTERDAY

The flesh is heir to numerous misfortunes including deafness, which has been referred to in documents dating from the beginnings of written history. The *Nei Ching Su Wên* (ca. 2697 B.C.) is reportedly the oldest known medical book and is considered to be a classic treatise on internal

---

[1] Children's Division of the Menninger Clinic, The Menninger Foundation, Topeka, Kansas.

medicine. This document is attributed to Huang Ti, or The Yellow Emperor, and contains references to the causes and cures of deafness, including the use of acupuncture (Veith, 1966). Two Egyptian medical papyri from the XVIIIth Dynasty, the Ebers and the Hearst (ca. 1550 B.C.), presented "prescriptions" for ear diseases and deafness (Leake, 1952). These papyri are considered to be compilations of medical writings dating from around 3000 B.C. This assumption is not without support, as the practice of medicine was flourishing during the early Egyptian dynasties. The great pyramids built in the IIIrd and IVth Dynasties were designed by Imhotep who, as a skilled physician, was elevated to the "God of Egyptian Medicine" after his death. Otitis media was described by the Babylonians as fire extending into the ear, dulling hearing, and producing pus which exudes with "offensive fetor" (Sigerist, 1951). Sigerist also reported that the Navaho Indians in the United States have age-old "Nite Chants" or ceremonials for curing various injuries and diseases of the head, including deafness. Deafness and its cure are referred to in the New Testament of the Bible in Matthew 11:5 and Mark 7:11. Hearing impairments appear to be one of the oldest known afflictions of man, but the understanding of the anatomy and physiology of the ear, the assessment of its functioning, and the accurate knowledge of its diseases and treatments advanced slowly.

Anatomical writings on the ear appeared in the sixteenth and seventeenth centuries. Andreas Vesalius, the Belgian anatomist, provided a description of the middle ear in his 1543 treatise, *De Fabrica Humani Corporis*. Although he did not describe the stapes because of its smallness, this omission was soon corrected by Giovanni Filippo Ingrassia of the University of Naples (Garrison, 1961). The inner ear was discovered by Empedocles (490–435 B.C.), and Galen (A.D. 138–201) named it the "labyrinth" (Boring, 1942). But Gabriele Falloppio, a pupil of Vesalius, discovered and described in 1561 the chorda tympani, auditory nerve, and semicircular canals. He felt, as did the early Greeks, that the cochlea was air-filled, and that the air amplified sound and stimulated the auditory nerve. This position was maintained until 1742 when Theodor Pyl noted, and Domenico Cotugno and Philipp Meckel confirmed, the existence of fluid in the labyrinth and its role in the transmission of sound in 1744 and 1777. Bartolommeo Eustachi, an Italian anatomist, described in 1562 the tube between the mouth and the middle ear in a monograph entitled *De Auditu Organis*. However, Boring (1942) reported that this tube was originally discovered by one Alcmaeon in the sixth century B.C. The first book on otology, "Traité de l'Organe de l'Ouie," was written in 1683 by Joseph-Guichard Duverney, a Paris professor of anatomy and physician to King Louis XIV. Albrecht von Haller synthesized and systematized the known facts about the ear in his 1763 publication, *De Auditu*, which appeared as one of his eight volumes on human physiology. His description of the auditory meatus, cone-shaped tympanic membrane, Eustachian tube, three ossicles, oval and round windows to the labyrinth, the vestibule, the cochlea with its two-and-one-half turns and spiral plate, vestibular and tympanic canals, and the semicircular canals remains accurate today.

After a fashion, otology has been practiced for centuries, but it was not until the nineteenth century that it became a medical specialty. It is a curious historical fact that diseases of the ear were late in receiving the attention of the medical profession and until the 1800s were relegated to quacks. That the treatment of eye and ear diseases was replete with quackery is demonstrated by the following advertisement placed by a "Doctor" James Graham in the July 19, 1773, issue of the *New York Gazette and the Weekly Mercury*:

> Doctor Graham, Oculist and Aurist, is arrived in this City, from Philadelphia, and may be consulted at his apartments at Capt. Fenton's opposite Trinity Church, in the disorders of the Eye and its appendages; and in every species of deafness, hardness of hearing, ulcerations, noise in the Ears, etc. Persons born Deaf and Dumb, and those labouring under any impediment in their Speech, by applying personally, will probably be assisted. The Doctor intends to sail for England in a few months; those, therefore, who have occasion for his assistance, must apply immediately [Packard, 1963, p. 1161].

Otology has no definite beginning, although Jean–Marc–Gaspard Itard of France may be considered the modern pioneer of ear physiology, rehabilitation, and clinical otology. His book, *Traité des Maladies de l'Oreille et de l'Audition*, published in 1821, is considered to be the first formal treatise on diseases of the ear. Guthrie (1937) attributes the renaissance of otology in England to the work of James Hinton, Joseph Toynbee, and William Wilde (fathers of the distinguished historian Arnold Toynbee and writer Oscar Wilde). Wilde's contributions in establishing otology on a scientific basis were so numerous that Guthrie considers him to be the father of otology as a modern medical specialty. Wilde wrote in the introduction to his book, *Aural Surgery*, published in 1853:

> I have labored to divest this branch of medicine of that shroud of quackery with which it has been encompassed. . . . The practitioner of Aural Surgery or Aurist ought to be a well educated surgeon or physician who applies the recognized principles of medicine to diseases of the organ of hearing [Guthrie, 1937, p. 175].

The American Otological Society, as an offshoot of the American Ophthalmological Society, was founded in 1868 (Packard, 1963). Papers read before that society appeared in *Transactions*, which was first published in 1869.

The advancement of hearing testing, beyond listening to a watch placed next to the ear and taking the whispered voice test, occurred in the nineteenth century, starting with tuning forks and acuity meters and culminating in the twentieth century with electronic audiometers. Although John Shore invented the tuning fork in 1711 (Garrison, 1961), its wide usage for auditory testing did not occur until after Chladni (1802) assessed the range of human hearing and studied bone conduction. The tuning fork tests developed by Weber (1834), Rinné (1855), and Schwabach (1885) are still used today by otologists. The "acuity meter" constructed by Wolke (1802) is the first device made specifically for the purpose of testing hearing. This instrument consisted of a stick attached to an upright board. The stick was dropped onto the board from various heights, the distance of which could be read from a scale. Various devices of this type appeared throughout the 1800s, such as the "acumeter" of Itard (1821) and Politzer (1878). An "electric tuning fork" was constructed by Helmholtz (1862). Following the invention of the telephone receiver by Alexander Graham Bell in 1876, Hartmann (1878) connected the receiver to Helmholtz's electric tuning fork. This advancement resulted in the "electric sonometer" of Hughes (1879). It was Richardson (1879) who first used the term "audiometer" when discussing Hughes' sonometer. He wrote that "the world of science in general and the world of medicine in particular, is under a deep debt of gratitude to Professor Hughes for his simple and beautiful instrument which I have christened the audimeter, or less accurately, but more euphoniously, the audiometer [Feldmann, 1970, p. 42]." Electronic audiometers appeared in the early 1900s. The continuous frequency instrument of Schaefer and Gruschke (1921) employed a back-feed oscillator, and the "Otaudion" of Schwarz (1927) employed a beat frequency oscillator. These two methods of audiofrequency generation were employed in the design of audiometers until after World War II.

Audiology, as a nonmedical specialty, developed in the United States from the auditory testing and rehabilitative programs for World War II veterans. The word "audiology" is both unusual (a word formed from the Latin *audire* and the Greek *logos*)[2] and of uncertain origin. The term

---

[2] The words *audiometer* and *audiogram* also combine the Latin *audire* with the Latinized Greek words *metron* and *gramma*. There are, however, other words in the English language which display a similar etymology from both Latin and Greek elements, such as *television, automobile, fluoroscope,* and *antitoxin.*

simultaneously and independently appeared in 1946 by Carhart and Canfield (Canfield, 1972). However, Canfield has reported that claims for coining the term have been made by Mayer B. Schier in 1935, by the National Auricular Foundation in 1938, and by Stanley Novak in 1939. In 1949, Canfield stated that audiology encompasses the entire field of hearing by these words:

> Gradually being recognized as a developing professional specialty, Audiology—the science of hearing—is a newly integrated concept of human hearing. Including more than the medical aspects of ear disease, it embraces every concept of art and science which can contribute to, or form a part of, the propagation of sound, its transmission to the ear, its fate within the human organism, the psychological process based upon the interpretation of the perceived sound, and the consequent reaction of the person to the mental concept engendered. Audiology considers everything that can be of aid or detriment to the life from sounds which can or should be heard [pp. 3–4].

Audiology is the most recent specialty to join in the detection of impaired functions of the ear. A thorough assessment of the audio-vestibular system of many patients requires the combined and coordinated efforts of an otologist, otoneurologist, and audiologist. These professions have differing ages and have come from varying backgrounds. The combined contributions of these specialists are necessary today if the auditorially disabled are to receive the best evaluations and treatments.

II. TODAY

This book represents the cooperative efforts of many people because the complexity of the audio-vestibular system requires expertise in different fields of knowledge. The contributors were selected because of their pioneering work or their extensive knowledge about and research with a particular technique. An attempt has been made to present information about each technique in sufficient depth to permit an understanding of the procedure, its purpose, limitations, and needs for additional research. The current state of knowledge of each procedure is presented (1) to be used as it has been developed and refined at the time of writing and (2) to be heuristic for those wanting to fashion even better methods for understanding the audio-vestibular system.

A. Otologic Assessment

Doctors Lee and Chasin discuss the advances that have been made in otology and emphasize the various assessments of the audio-vestibular system made by otologists. They present information obtained from a complete history, and the procedures for arriving at an otological diagnosis which is necessary for planning treatment and management of persons with a hearing impairment. They underscore the importance of viewing a hearing impairment as only one part of the patient's total medical condition. Then, focusing on the ear, they discuss vestibular and radiological assessments and conclude with information about hearing disorders in special conditions affecting the ear and acoustic nerve.

B.　Electronystagmography

The observation of eye movements to determine central nervous system functioning was pioneered by Johannes Purkinjie (1820), who described visual nystagmus, and Marie–Jean–Pierre Flourens (1828), who located cerebellar and labyrinthine vertigo. Robert Bárány, who devised the caloric test and did extensive research on the physiology of the inner ear, received the 1915 Nobel prize in physiology and medicine (Sourkes, 1966). Doctor Coats discusses the principles and techniques of recording eye movements by electronystagmography. He presents information about the neuro-otologic examination routinely administered in his clinic, which includes the ocular-dysmetria, gaze, sinusoidal tracking, optokinetic, paroxysmal nystagmus, position, and bithermal caloric tests. An interpretation of the abnormal findings from these tests is presented to illustrate their diagnostic importance for differentiating between peripheral vestibular system and central nervous system impairments.

C.　Impedance–Admittance Measurements

The assessment of middle-ear function by impedance measurements dates from 1867, when Lucae measured the tension of the tympanic membrane from a model of the ear and from human subjects. In his studies, he used the "acoustic interference tube" designed by Quincke (1866), which was also the prototype of the acoustic bridge designed by Schuster in 1934. Doctor Feldmann discusses the development of impedance measurement reintroduced for clinical use by Metz (1946) and the current status of the acoustic impedance battery of tests available to evaluate the function of the middle ear and some aspects of sensorineural function. The principles and functioning of mechanical acoustic bridges and electroacoustic instruments are presented. After outlining the preliminary steps for making the measurements, he discusses the clinical application of static acoustic impedance, tympanometry, intra-aural muscle reflex evaluations, and tests for determining the functioning of the Eustachian tube.

D. Electrocochleography

The electrical responses at the round window have been known since the first reports on cochlear potentials by Forbes *et al.* (1927) and Weaver and Bray (1930a,b,c) and on the VIIIth nerve action potentials by Derbyshire and Davis in 1935. Doctors Simmons and Glattke discuss the use of an electrophysiological procedure for assessing the integrity of the cochlea. They present information about the characteristics of the cochlear potential, summating potential and compound action potential which can be detected by electrodes placed near the cochlea. They discuss the instrumentation and stimuli used for eliciting and recording these responses, illustrate their findings, and discuss ways that the procedure may be used clinically and for research.

E. Reflex and Conditioning Audiometry

The cochleopalpebral reflex has been known since Johannes Müller discussed the reflex as a test of hearing in his classic treatise, *Handbuch der Physiologies des Menschen für Vorlesungen,* first published in 1834. Doctor Hardy discusses the various reflex and conditioning procedures developed by other researchers for testing of neonates and infants. He offers a new perspective on these widely used procedures and challenges users to assess their opinions and procedures in light of what information early testing can provide.

F. Conditioned Galvanic Skin Response Audiometry

Although Féré (1888) is considered to be the first person to demonstrate the psychogalvanic reflex, credit for this discovery rightfully belongs to Vigouroux (1879a,b). This reflex has been used extensively in psychological research, but it was Albrecht (1918) who first employed the reflex as a test of hearing. Doctor Ventry presents information about the rise and decline of GSR audiometry. He attributes the reason for the resultant disillusionment with the procedure as a diagnostic test of hearing to failures to employ adequate methodology for administration of the test. He presents an extensive discussion and illustration of the procedural steps that are necessary to obtain valid and reliable GSR responses to auditory stimuli. Although he points out that conditioned galvanic skin audiometry may not be used successfully with difficult-to-test children, he demonstrates that the procedure does have value when properly administered, to test older children, adults, and persons suspected of having a functional hearing loss.

G. Respiration Audiometry

Kymographic tracings of respiration cycles were first recorded by Vierordt and Ludwig in 1855. Following the development of the pneumograph by Marey in 1876, continuous breathing patterns could be traced with ease. The Marey pneumograph was used for studying respiration by physiologists for many years. Doctor Bradford discusses the history of respiratory alterations to sound, and the development of and research with respiration audiometry. This research has been directed toward determining a valid respiration alteration at or near the threshold of pure-tone stimuli. The research compared thresholds obtained by standard procedures to thresholds determined from respiration changes with normal hearing and hearing-impaired persons of varying ages. Clinical illustrations are presented with dogs and difficult-to-test persons for whom voluntary responses could not be obtained. Particular emphasis is given to psychogenic hearing losses by discussing the influence of psychic factors on hearing sensitivity.

H. Cardiotachometry

Although the ancient Egyptians and Greeks may have entertained the idea that blood moved through the body, it was not until 1628 that William Harvey described the heart as a muscular pump and demonstrated the circuitry of blood in the body. Instrumentation for recording cardiac activity has included the hemodynometer (Poiseuille, 1828), the sphygmomanometer (Marey, 1876), and the electrocardiograph (Waller, 1890). Albrecht (1918) was the first to record blood pressure changes in response to sound. Since the development of the cardiotachometer by Boas in 1928, measurement of cardiac alterations from auditory stimuli have been made possible. However, this instrument has been used only in a limited way for examining auditory system function. Doctor Eisenberg has devoted her research efforts to developing and refining cardiotachometric procedures for determining cardiac responses to the synthetic vowel "ah." She discusses the equipment and procedures used in her laboratory and illustrates how cardiotachometry can be used for assessing the auditory system of infants and difficult-to-test persons.

I. Evoked Cortical Response Audiometry

Caton detected electrical currents directly from the brain of animals and reported the finding to the British Medical Society in 1875. Hans Berger (1929) demonstrated that the alpha and beta waves found in dogs could be detected from the scalp in man. It remained for Davis (1939) to record evoked cortical responses to auditory, visual, and tactile stimuli. Of all the indirect procedures used to determine auditory functioning, evoked cortical responses have undoubtedly been researched the most extensively. Doctor Hood discusses the characteristics of the four known components of the auditory evoked cortical response—the brain-stem or early response, the fast or middle response, the late or slow response, and the contingent negative variation or very late response. He gives information about the nature of the response, measurement and analysis, effect of stimuli and subject state, and purposes for testing for each of the responses.

III. TOMORROW

An over-the-shoulder look at the past may cause some readers to be discouraged by the slowness of scientific progress and to dim their aspirations of ever being meaningful contributors to better detection procedures for the audio-vestibular system. Voltaire considered history as a depiction of the "follies of mankind." Oliver Wendell Holmes advanced the view that science is a "topography of ignorance." Resistances to scientific discoveries from religious and ideological sources as well as from scientists themselves (Barber, 1961) lend some support to this cynicism. Progress toward a better understanding of the unknown must start from the known. The slowness, the stumbling, and the delays should not be considered as impediments of progress. Simon (1957) offers a perspective for our understanding of the apparent slowness of man's achievements, with these words:

> If we were to compress the million years of man's existence to one twenty-four-hour day, our total range of written history represents 10 minutes; Christ was born less than 3 minutes ago. With our present time set at noon, David was King of Israel at 11:55; Julius Caesar conquered the then known world at 11:57; Columbus discovered the New World at 11:59, and the United States is 15 seconds old [p. 23].

Using this model, it could be said that the significant advances and development of instrumentation for making physiological measures of the audio-vestibular system have been available for only the past 10 seconds. The words of George Santayana (1957) may be considered good counsel for, and a challenge to, the disheartened clinician or researcher: "We must welcome the future, remembering that soon it will be the past; and we must respect the past, remembering that once it was all that was humanly possible."

The purposes of this book will be achieved to the extent that we have generated or renewed an interest for some persons in the physiological measures presently available for determining audio-vestibular system impairments, and to the extent that we have sparked an interest in others to reach for a better tomorrow with new physiological research on the audio-vestibular system.

REFERENCES

Albrecht, W. (1918). *Arch. Ohren Nasen Kehlkopfheilk.* **101**, 1.

Barber, B. (1961). *Science* **134**, 596.

Berger, H. (1929). *Arch. Psychiat. Nervenkr.* **87**, 527.

Boas, E. P. (1928). *Arch. Intern. Med.* **41**, 403.

Boring, E. G. (1942). "Sensation and Perception in the History of Experimental Psychology." Appleton, New York.

Canfield, N. (1949). "Audiology: The Science of Hearing." Thomas, Springfield, Illinois.

Canfield, N. (1972). *In* "Otitis Media" (A. Glorig and K. S. Gerwin, eds.), pp. 238–245. Thomas, Springfield, Illinois.

Caton, R. (1875). *Brit. Med. J.* **2**, 278.

Chladni, E. F. F. (1802). "Die Akustick." Breitkopf and Hártel, Leipzig.

Davis, P. A. (1939). *J. Neurophysiol.* **2**, 494.

Derbyshire, A. J., and Davis, H. (1935). *Amer. J. Physiol.* **113**, 476.

Feldmann, H. (1970). *Trans. Beltone Inst. Hearing Res. No. 22.*

Féré, C. (1888). *C. R. Soc. Biol. (Paris)* **5**, 28; 217.

Flourens, M.-J.-P. (1828). *Mém. Acad. Sci. (Paris)* **9**, 455.

Forbes, A., Miller, R. H., and O'Connor, J. (1927). *Amer. J. Physiol.* **80**, 363.

Garrison, F. H. (1961). "An Introduction to the History of Medicine," 4th ed. (reprinted). Saunders, Philadelphia, Pennsylvania.

Guichard, J.-P. (1863). "Traité de l'Organe de l'Ouie." E. Michallet, Paris.

Guthrie, D. (1937). *J. Laryngol. Otol.* **52**, 163.

Haller, A. von (1763). "Elementa Physiologiae Corpus Humani," Vol. 5, Book 15, pp. 186–305. Sumpt. Francisi Grasset & Sociorum, Lausanne.

Hartmann, A. (1878). *Arch. Ohrenheilk.* **13**, 297.

Helmholtz, H. von (1862). "Die Lehre von den Tonempfindungen als Physiologische Grundlage für die Theorie der Musik." Viewegg, Braunschweig.

Hughes, D. E. (1879). *Nature (London)* **77**, 102.

Itard, J.-M.-G. (1821). "Traité des Maladies de l'Oreille et de l'Audition." Meguignon-Marvis, Paris.

Leake, C. D. (1952). "The Old Egyptian Medical Papyri." Univ. of Kansas Press, Lawrence, Kansas.

Lucae, A. (1867). *Arch. Ohren Nasen Kehlkopfheilk.* 3, 186.

Marey, E.-J.-M. (1876). "Physiologie Expérimentale," Vol. 2. Libraire de l'Académie de Médecine, Paris.

Metz, O. (1946). *Acta Otolaryngol. (Stockholm) Suppl.* 63, 1.

Müller, J. (1834). "Handbuch der Physiologies des Menschen für Vorlesungen." Hölscher, Coblenz.

Packard, F. R. (1963). "History of Medicine in the United States," Vol. II. Hafner Publ., NewYork.

Poiseuille, J.-L.-M. (1828). Recherches sur la Force du Coeur Aortique. Graduating dissertation, Univ. of Paris.

Politzer, A. (1878). "Lehrbuch der Ohrenheilkunde." Enke, Stuttgart.

Purkinjie, J. E. (1820). *Med. Jahrb. (Vienna)* 6, 79.

Quincke, G. (1866). *Ann. Phys. Chem.* 128, 177.

Richardson, B. W. (1879). *Proc. Roy. Soc. Med.* 29, 65.

Rinné, H. A. (1855). *Prager Vierteljahrschr. Prakt. Med.* 1, 71; 2, 45.

Santayana, G. (1957). *In* "Book of Unusual Quotations" (R. Flesch, ed.). Harper, New York.

Schaefer, K. L., and Gruschke, G. (1921). *Passow-Schaefers Beitr. Hals. Nas. Ohrenheilk.* 16, 56.

Schuster, K. (1934). *Elekt. Nachr. Techn.* 13, 408.

Schwabach, D. (1885). *Z. Ohrenheilk.* 14, 61.

Schwarz, W. (1927). *Z. Hals. Nas. Ohrenheilk.* 18, 436.

Sigerist, H. E. (1951). "A History of Medicine." Oxford Univ. Press, London and New York.

Simon, C. T. (1957). *In* "Handbook of Speech Pathology" (L. Travis, ed.), pp. 3–43. Appleton, New York.

Sourkes, T. L. (1966). "Nobel Prize Winners in Medicine and Physiology" (Revised ed.). Abelard-Schuman, London.

Veith, I. (1966). "Huang Ti Nei Ching Su Wên: The Yellow Emperor's Classic of Internal Medicine" (New ed.). Univ. of California Press, Berkeley and Los Angeles.

Vierordt, K. von, and Ludwig, G. (1855). *Arch. Physiol. Heilk.* 14, 255.

Vigouroux, R. (1879a). *Gazette Med. Paris* 1, 657.

Vigouroux, R. (1879b). *C. R. Soc. Biol. (Paris)* 31, 336.

Waller, A. (1890). *Phil. Trans. (London)* 180, 169.

Weaver, E. G., and Bray, C. W. (1930a). *Proc. Nat. Acad. Sci. U.S.* 16, 344.

Weaver, E. G., and Bray, C. W. (1930b). *Science* 71, 215.

Weaver, E. G., and Bray, C. W. (1930c). *J. Exp. Psychol.* 13, 373.

Weber, E. H. (1834). "De Pulsu, Resorptione, Audita et Tactau: Annotations Anatomicae et Physiologicae." Köhler, Leipzig.

Wolke, C. H. (1802). "Nachricht von den zu Jever durch die Galvani-Voltaische Gehör-Gebe-Kunst beglückten Taubstummen und vor Sprengels Method sie auszuüben." Schulze, Oldenburg.

Chapter Two

Otologic Assessments

Song Ping Lee[1] and Werner D. Chasin[2]

I. INTRODUCTION

The ability to hear normally is a complex function which requires not only a healthy receptor, the ear, but also an intact nervous system. Similarly, in order to have a normal spatial equilibrium the body requires not only an intact vestibular organ, but also an intact neuromuscular system. Although in this chapter we are discussing otologic assessment, it is not proper to consider the ear as divorced from the remainder of the patient. Congenital disorders of the ear often coexist with anomalies affecting other parts of the body. Hearing and vestibular disorders can be caused by systemic diseases such as peripheral vascular problems, diabetes, or infections. Functional hearing losses may be due to emotional disturbances. Deafness may represent one manifestation of central nervous system (CNS) disease. A thorough otologic assessment, therefore, should look beyond the ear to the entire patient—his history, general medical examination, and psychosocial adjustment.

Disorders of hearing are divided into five categories according to the localization of the problem:

1. Purely conductive hearing losses are due to problems of the external auditory canal and/or the middle ear, the sound conducting apparatus.

---

[1] Department of Otolaryngology, Topeka Medical Center, Topeka, Kansas.
[2] Otolaryngology Division, Tufts University School of Medicine, Boston, Massachusetts.

Examples include any obstruction of the external auditory canal, drumhead perforations, and discontinuity of the ossicular chain from whatever cause.

2. Sensorineural hearing losses are those in which the problem lies in the cochlea (sensory), auditory nerve (neural), or both. Examples include losses from ototoxic drugs, acoustic trauma, presbycusis, and acoustic neuroma. By additional studies, including radiological and special audiological tests, the sensorineural losses can then be differentiated into sensory (cochlear) and neural (auditory nerve) lesions. In some instances, of course, there exists a combined sensory and neural lesion.

3. Mixed or combined hearing losses are ones in which the problem lies both in the sound conducting apparatus and in the cochlea, and/or the auditory nerve. Examples include congenital aural atresia with cochlear degeneration in addition to stapedial fixation, and posttraumatic deafness with both ossicular and cochlear damage.

4. Central hearing losses are due to a congenital or acquired lesion affecting the auditory pathways central to the cochlear nuclei. Such hearing impairments may be caused by trauma, tumors, and vascular infarcts.

5. Functional hearing losses, although nonorganic and due to emotional factors, may occur alone or may coexist with a lesser degree of organic hearing loss.

In order to arrive at an accurate diagnosis of the type, degree, and cause of the hearing loss, a clinician must proceed with the following steps: (1) extensive history-taking, (2) otologic examination, which might require a careful medical and neurological evaluation, (3) audiological evaluation, and (4) radiological studies. By following these steps, a site-of-lesion diagnosis can usually be made, and the subsequent management of the patient proceeds rationally according to the diagnosis.

II. HISTORY

As in all of medicine, the patient's history is essential and often the single most decisive factor in arriving at a diagnosis. The complete history must include the general medical, family, prenatal, perinatal and neonatal, and developmental histories. A very careful history of deafness in the family must be obtained. The history, of course, must give a clear account of otologic problems and a search for exposure to ototoxic factors such as drugs, noise, and trauma.

A. General Medical History

The clinician must obtain an accurate assessment of the general health of the patient and what diseases he has had throughout his lifetime. Rather than trying to elicit a history only of those illnesses which clearly affect hearing, it is wiser to list all known past disorders, both congenital and acquired. New syndromes are continually being described which link hitherto unrelated problems to disorders of hearing or vestibular function. In the case of suspected congenital deafness, it is especially important to learn of anomalies of other parts of the body. With acquired childhood deafness, it is important to obtain a history relevant to previous CNS infections and injuries, and of severe viral infections, especially mumps. In the event that the audiologist represents the first clinical contact with a child, it is essential that the audiologist refer the child to a pediatrician for an intensive general evaluation. The child may require further evaluations by appropriate specialists in neurology, neuropsychology, or psychiatry. In the case of hearing losses occurring in the post-pediatric age group, the possibility of congenital or hereditary etiologies must still be entertained, and a history relevant to these possibilities should be obtained. Not all hereditary deafness is congenital, a child with a genetically determined deafness may pass through the early years of life with normal or near-normal hearing. The hearing loss may not be clearly manifested until the second, or as late as the fourth, decade of life.

The concept of a high-risk register for deafness is useful in that it identifies those patients who should be observed with more than the usual caution for evidence of congenital deafness (Black *et al.*, 1971). A child who belongs to this register must be reevaluated at appropriate intervals before being cleared as having normal hearing.

B. Family History

A carefully obtained family history is the most important element in the diagnosis of the presence and type of hereditary deafness. The inquiry must extend beyond parents and siblings to aunts, uncles, cousins, grandparents, and if possible even beyond this to other relatives (Konigsmark, 1969; Proctor and Proctor, 1967). Larrsen (1960), as an example, found an incidence of hereditary factors in 80% of patients with otosclerosis. Not only does a positive family history aid in diagnosis, but it also enables the genetic counselor to prognosticate the likelihood that other progeny will develop deafness.

C. Prenatal History

In trying to arrive at an etiology for a case of deafness, the prenatal history must search for factors which occurred during the mother's pregnancy and are known to cause deafness. The audio-vestibular apparatus is most sensitive to damage or faulty development during the first trimester of fetal development. If the mother had a febrile illness with a skin eruption during pregnancy, it should arouse the suspicion of rubella or syphilis as a cause of deafness in the infant. Appropriate blood tests obtained on both child and mother can help in the diagnosis. Ototoxic drugs given to the mother during pregnancy can result in deafness in the child. Pregnancy complications such as uterine bleeding, toxemia of pregnancy, and threatened abortion can adversely affect the audio-vestibular apparatus of the fetus.

D. Perinatal and Neonatal History

Perinatal and neonatal problems are responsible for many cases of central hearing loss. The history should include accounts of distressful labor and delivery, birth injury, anoxia, prematurity, neonatal jaundice, and neonatal respiratory distress. Babies born prematurely (birth weight below 2500 gm) have a high incidence of deafness. The kernicterus of erythroblastosis fetalis (Rh incompatibility) is another cause of deafness.

E. Developmental History

A carefully obtained developmental history includes a description of motor, speech, and language development (Hughes, 1971). The latter in turn depends on an intact neurologic system as well as intact special senses, including hearing. A failure of speech and language development might be due to mental retardation or other CNS abnormalities. It follows, therefore, that a thorough evaluation of failure of speech and language development takes into account not only the child's hearing but also the integrity of his neurological system.

The clinician must inquire also about a regression in speech development. Such regression is seen in patients with hereditary deafness of delayed onset and with deafness that is due to acquired factors such as otitic meningitis and the administration of ototoxic drugs.

F. Ototoxic History

Ototoxic antibiotics and certain other medications, mechanical trauma, barotrauma, and intensive noise exposure can damage the auditory as well as the vestibular sense organs. Antibiotics that can damage the cochlea include streptomycin and dihydrostreptomycin (McGee, 1962), kanamycin (Jorgensen and Schmidt, 1962), and neomycin (Hawkins, 1967). Nonantibiotic cochleotoxic drugs include salicylates (aspirin), quinine, ethacrynic acid, and chloroquine (Mathog, 1970). Streptomycin and gentamycin are preferentially toxic to the vestibular sense organs, although hearing loss has also been ascribed to these medications. Simultaneous administration of two ototoxic drugs can be more damaging than administration of one drug. The deafness caused by the antibiotics is always permanent, whereas that caused by the other drugs tends to be temporary and reversible upon discontinuation of the medication.

G. Otologic History

The otologic history should inquire about the following factors: (1) probable cause of acquired deafness, (2) progressive or static deafness, (3) bilateral simultaneous or bilateral sequential deafness, (4) age of apparent onset of deafness, (5) constant or fluctuating hearing loss, (6) associated aural symptoms, (7) history of ear infections and trauma, (8) previous ear surgery, (9) other cranial nerve involvement, (10) history of aural pain, and (11) history of dizziness or imbalance.

Often the parent or the patient can cite the actual cause of the hearing loss, and the clinician should ask this obvious question. It is surprising how often one can save time and avoid circuitous maneuvers to arrive at a diagnosis that is readily available from the patient.

A static hearing loss is generally either congenital or caused by a single ototoxic insult. A progressive hearing loss is characteristic of certain types of hereditary deafness, otosclerosis, Meniere's disease, repetitive exposure to intense noise, or acoustic neuroma. Simultaneous progressive involvement of both ears occurs in repetitive exposure to noise, presbycusis, syphilis, allergic endolymphatic hydrops, some cases of otosclerosis and hereditary deafness. Sequential and progressive involvement of both ears occurs in most cases of otosclerosis, in some cases of chronic bilateral otitis media and in some cases of Meniere's disease. The age of onset can rule in certain causes and exclude other causes of deafness in a given patient. For instance, a 5-year-old child with a bilateral severe conductive hearing loss does not have otosclerosis, but is more likely to have a middle-ear malformation such as congenital fixation of the stapedes in the oval windows.

A fluctuating hearing loss is one which changes from day to day or week to week. A fluctuating hearing loss is characteristic of the endolymphatic hydrops which occurs in Meniere's disease or in syphilis, chronic or recurrent Eustachian-tube obstruction, and salicylate-induced hearing loss. The deafness which is caused by injuries, otosclerosis, hereditary factors, and by most other conditions does not tend to fluctuate, though it may very well progress in a uniformly downward direction over a period of months or years.

Associated aural symptoms that should be sought in the history include a feeling of fullness or blockage of the ears, tinnitus, noise intolerance, autophony, paracusis Willisiana, and diplacusis. A sensation of fullness is characteristic of endolymphatic hydrops, Eustachian-tube obstruction with or without a middle-ear effusion, and, paradoxically, in the condition of the patulous or overly patent Eustachian tube. Patients with most other forms of hearing loss, and peculiarly children with blocked Eustachian tubes, do not experience a feeling of blockage of the ears. Tinnitus can be present in almost all types of hearing impairments and is usually not a helpful clue in arriving at a diagnosis. One clear exception is the pronounced tinnitus coupled with a progressive unilateral deafness which characterizes the early stages of an acoustic neuroma. Noise intolerance is characteristic of endolymphatic hydrops and stapedius muscle paralysis resulting from Bell's palsy or stapedius muscle absence occurring after a stapedectomy. Autophony usually suggests a conductive hearing loss due either to a middle-ear effusion or to an overly patent Eustachian tube. Paracusis Willisiana, the paradoxical ability to hear conversation better in a noisy environment, is characteristic of conductive hearing losses, especially otosclerosis. Diplacusis, the perception of unequal pitches between the two ears, is characteristic of endolymphatic hydrops.

Precise information about previous ear surgery can be most helpful in making a determination of the cause of a hearing loss. Not only should the clinician ask what type of surgery was performed, but also he should make note of the patient's symptoms and clinical course after the surgery. It must be remembered that not only diseases cause a hearing loss, sometimes surgery can make a hearing loss worse. For example, a patient whose only symptom prior to mastoid–tympanoplasty was aural discharge, and who postoperatively had severe dizziness, may well demonstrate a severe or even total deafness in the affected ear as a result of intraoperative damage to the inner ear. The clinician should always inquire about a previous myringotomy, mastoidectomy, fenestration, stapedectomy or stapes mobilization, and tympanoplasty. Similarly, a careful history should be obtained about ear trauma, head trauma, and bleeding from the ear associated with an injury.

In acquiring a complete history about the hearing-impaired patient, information should be sought about involvement of cranial nerves other than the VIIIth—the cochlear and vestibular nerves. Such information may shed light on the nature of the disease process which is causing the deafness. A patient with nasopharyngeal cancer, for instance, may seek medical assistance because of a blocked and deafened ear. This patient may also have developed diplopia (double vision) as a result of the cancer, but he may not volunteer this information because he does not connect the two symptoms. Another patient may complain of unilateral hearing loss with tinnitus, but fail to mention that the side of his face is weak and that he can no longer pucker his lips to whistle. An acoustic neuroma not uncommonly will effect such a hearing loss and facial paralysis. Some of these causes can endanger the life of the patient if they are not discovered and treated in time.

Aural pain has numerous causes, but not every earache signifies ear disease. The earaches which have significance in audio-vestibular diagnosis are those associated with middle-ear and mastoid infections, tumors of the middle ear and mastoid, herpes zoster oticus, acoustic neuroma, and cancer of the nasopharynx. Other causes of aural pain include dental disease, tumors of the pharynx, disorders of the temporomandibular joint, infections of the pharynx, external ear and sinuses, and arthritis of the cervical vertebrae. When such pain occurs as an isolated symptom without any other aural accompaniments such as discharge, hearing loss, vertigo, tinnitus, or periauricular tenderness, it very likely represents a referred pain rather than one that is being produced by disease of the ear.

It is necessary to elicit a thorough history relevant to symptoms of dizziness (a disturbed sense of relationship to space), vertigo (a sensation of true whirling or turning), and imbalance. There are several reasons for this portion of the history. When the main problem is an auditory one, the presence or absence of and the nature of the dysequilibrium may help the clinician in arriving at a diagnosis of the hearing loss. When the chief complaint is one of imbalance, the audiological evaluation may shed light on the nature of the vestibular problem. Finally, the dysequilibrium may not be an otologic problem; it may signify a more remote general medical or neurological disorder. An excellent guide to the evaluation of the patient with dizziness can be found in Busis (1965) and Drachman and Hart (1972).

Dysequilibrium (vertigo, dizziness, feeling of imbalance) can be caused by diseases of the aural end-organ, neurological disorders, and systemic problems. End-organ dysequilibrium may be associated with auditory symptoms and findings. Examples of dysequilibrium due to combined audio-vestibular lesions include Meniere's disease, chronic otitis media with labyrinthine complications, and viral labyrinthitis. Examples of isolated vestibular end-organ problems include benign paroxysmal positional vertigo, vestibular neuronitis, and postgentamycin and streptomycin imbalance. Neurological causes of dysequilibrium include multiple sclerosis, epilepsy, brain tumor, and vertebrobasilar vascular insufficiency. Finally, examples of systemic disorders which cause imbalance include hypoglycemia, severe anemia, cardiac arrhythmias, and hyperventilation caused by anxiety.

In summary, it is to be emphasized that in evaluating the patient with audio-vestibular problems, the history must be a complete one which takes into account the entire patient, and not merely his aural problem. Having discussed the importance and nature of a thoroughly taken history, information concerning the otologic examination will be presented.

III. OTOLOGIC ASSESSMENT: HEARING

At the conclusion of the otologic examination, the clinician, in most instances, should be able to answer the following questions before he refers the patient to the audiologist:

1. whether or not the patient has at least some hearing in each ear;
2. whether one or both ears is totally deaf;
3. whether the patient can be classified as mildly, moderately, severely, or profoundly deaf;
4. whether the hearing loss is purely conductive, purely sensorineural, or combined, in each of the patient's ears;
5. what is the probable etiology of the patient's hearing loss.

The only exceptions to deriving this information from the history and otologic examination include the case of the very young child, the malingerer, or those patients with complicated neurological problems involving more than just audition.

The otologic examination begins by carefully listening to the patient's speech. The loud, clear speech of an adult suggests that the hearing impairment was acquired after the learning of speech and language. Unintelligible grunts and utterances suggest a severe congenital deafness, or deafness acquired in early childhood. The soft but articulate speech of an adult with a moderately severe hearing impairment suggests a conductive hearing loss, such as otosclerosis, with probable normal inner-ear functioning. Denasal speech with mispronunciation of consonants suggests a profound sensorineural hearing loss, as is seen in some forms of hereditary deafness. Slurred and hesitant speech may occur in patients with neurological disorders such as multiple sclerosis and vertebrobasilar vascular insufficiency.

The examination then proceeds with a search for visible abnormalities of the ear, head, face, and other parts of the body. Otologic anomalies often are part of a constellation of anomalies, that is, part of a syndrome. If the otologist does not feel competent to perform a thorough medical examination, he should have a child evaluated by a pediatrician, preferably one who is experienced in congenital disorders. Adults also must be examined for other abnormalities; the older man with the large head and bowed legs may have Paget's disease, with its attendant deafness.

Having formed some idea of the degree of normalcy of the remainder of the body, the otologist now focuses on the ears. Any cerumen, epithelial debris, and foreign matter must be removed from the external auditory canal so that the tympanic membrane, the mirror of the middle ear, can be visualized. Otoscopy can be performed with a variety of techniques, but magnification greater than that afforded by the ordinary otoscope is often required. The Hallpike–Blackmore monocular or the Zeiss binocular microscopes are admirably suited for this purpose. The otologist searches for signs of middle-ear inflammation, fluid in the tympanic cavity, perforations of the drumhead, anomalous appearing ossicles, and absence of ossicles. The pneumatic otoscope and the impedance bridge are helpful in diagnosing the conditions prevailing in the middle ear. Impedance measurements are discussed thoroughly in Chapter 5. Having completed the examination of the morphology of the ears, nose, and throat, the otologist then performs the evaluation of function.

While the otologist was taking the history, he has already had the opportunity to classify the patient's hearing as being mildly, moderately, severely, or profoundly impaired. The clinician must be sure to base this observation on how the patient hears without the benefit of visual clues; that is, he must speak to the patient from the side or with his back turned toward the patient. The hearing ability of each ear is evaluated by speaking from one side of the patient, while masking the opposite ear with a Barany noise apparatus. During this qualitative evaluation, the otologist can classify each ear as to its degree of hearing loss. At the same time, he can obtain a fairly accurate though qualitative idea of the discrimination ability of each ear by reciting a list of phonetically balanced words and asking the patient to repeat them. If the patient has a severe impairment, this test can be performed with the amplification provided by a speaking tube or Holmgren's ear trumpet.

The next step involves a determination of whether the hearing loss is conductive, sensorineural, or mixed. The Rinne test with tuning forks requires that the patient indicate whether he perceives air- or bone-conducted sound as being louder. The test must be performed with a series of forks beginning with the 64-Hz, and proceeding to the 4096-Hz fork, if necessary. The nontest ear is masked with the Barany apparatus. If the lowest frequency fork is heard louder by air than by bone conduction, the loss is sensorineural, and it is not necessary to use the other forks. If the lower frequency forks are heard louder by bone conduction, the series of forks is used until the point of conversion is reached. The conversion point is that frequency at which air- and bone-conducted sounds are heard with approximately equal loudness. The next octave fork is almost invariably heard louder by air conduction. For each octave that is heard louder by bone conduction than by air conduction, the air–bone gap increases about 10 dB on audiometric testing. Thus, an ear that converts at 256 Hz has a maximum air–bone gap of about 30 dB. An ear that converts at 128 Hz has not more than a 10-dB air–bone gap. When only the 64-Hz fork is heard louder by bone conduction, the air–bone gap turns out to be between 5 and 10 dB.

In performing the Weber test, the patient is asked to indicate whether or not a vibrating tuning fork (256 or 512 Hz), which the examiner holds on the midline of the skull or face, is heard louder in one ear than in the other. The patient with a unilateral conductive or combined hearing loss will hear the vibrations of the fork louder in the involved ear. If, upon repetition, the lateralization changes, then the patient either has bilateral conductive (or combined) hearing impairment or has misunderstood the test directions. In young children, the test may be unreliable. In the case of a recently acquired unilateral sensorineural hearing loss, the fork will be heard louder in the unimpaired ear. In the case of a long-standing profound unilateral hearing loss, the patient usually does not lateralize the tuning fork. In general, the chief value of the Weber test is the identification of a unilateral hearing loss as conductive or sensorineural.

There are various methods of testing Eustachian-tube function. These include use of the gas transducer test (Miller, 1965), impedance measurements, clearance of radio-opaque fluid from the middle ear down through the Eustachian tube (Compere, 1958), and reflux or fluid from the nasopharynx retrograde up the Eustachian tube (Bluestone et al., 1972). Although testing of Eustachian-tube function is important in evaluating patients with various types of chronic otitis media for clinical response to treatment and before surgery, it is not of great importance in audio-vestibular diagnosis.

At the conclusion of this portion of the otologic evaluation, the otologist should have a fairly accurate idea of the degree of hearing impairment in each ear and, in many cases, the probable etiology. Rarely should the experienced otologist receive from the audiologist a quantitative assessment that differs markedly from his own preliminary qualitative conclusions. Any significant discrepancy of this type calls for a thorough re-evaluation of the patient by both examiners. Failure to reassess the discrepant findings may lead to mismanagement or to ill-advised surgery.

IV. OTOLOGIC ASSESSMENT: VESTIBULAR

The vestibular end-organs (semicircular canal cristae and the utricular maculae) are embryologically and anatomically part of the peripheral auditory system. A complete evaluation of these organs must, therefore, be part of a total otologic examination. Although many disorders affect only the cochlea and its central connections, so many other diseases are known to affect the vestibular and cochlear systems that only by examining both systems can precise conclusions be made about the etiology and prognosis of certain auditory impairments. Examples of combined cochlear and vestibular disorders include Meniere's disease, acoustic neuroma, certain drug toxicities, temporal bone injuries, syphilis, viral labyrinthitis, multiple sclerosis, chronic otitis media with labyrinthine insult, some cases of severe otosclerosis, and certain congenital anomalies.

The vestibular examination is actually part of a more comprehensive investigation referred to as the "otoneurological evaluation"; that is, a general neurological evaluation of the peripheral audio-vestibular organs, their central projections, and their connections in the CNS. It leads the otologist centrally to an evaluation of the neurological ramifications of the audio-vestibular system. For example, consider a patient who presents a unilateral hearing loss and an ipsilateral facial paralysis. A number of peripheral conditions, such as cholesteatoma, tumor of the ear, or Bell's palsy with preexisting deafness, could account for this combination of symptoms. On the other hand, a large acoustic neuroma pressing on the brain stem, a pontine tumor, or a facial nerve sheath tumor can also produce these symptoms. Moreover, the patient may exhibit additional neurological abnormalities when a complete examination is carried out. The patient with an acoustic neuroma may also have involvement of the trigeminal nerve and of the cerebellum. The patient with a cholesteatoma may have a silent brain abscess. The patient with a middle-ear tumor may have involvement of the glossopharyngeal, spinal accessory, and vagus nerves. It must be understood that the audio-vestibular organs can react only in a limited number of ways to a large variety of disorders. They exhibit either decreased function (hearing loss, diminished caloric responses) or, sometimes, increased or perverted function (auditory recruitment noise intolerance and increased caloric responses, as in multiple sclerosis). It is only by being prepared to evaluate central as well as peripheral functions that the otologist can hope to make an accurate diagnosis of most cases of vestibular and audio-vestibular disorders.

The vestibular examination utilizes nystagmus, gait, and past-pointing as indicators of vestibular response to stimulation. Before the vestibular stimulation tests are begun, the otologist examines the patient for spontaneous manifestations of vestibular abnormalities. Gait testing is performed by having the patient, in comfortable shoes, walk with eyes open and eyes closed, first in normal and then in tandem fashion. The patient with poor bilateral vestibular function, as in that caused by streptomycin ototoxicity, will demonstrate a broad-based gait with eyes open, and severe difficulty in walking with eyes closed. When an uncompensated unilateral vestibular suppression is present, as in the case of a recent Meniere's spell or a posttraumatic destruction of one labyrinth, the patient will tend to drift toward the diseased side—especially when attempting to walk with eyes closed. Identical gait disturbances can be produced by nonvestibular lesions located in the CNS. For example, a patient with syphillitic tabes dorsalis also demonstrates a broad-based gait. It is, therefore, necessary to interpret gait disturbances in the context of the complete otoneurological evaluation.

In testing for past-pointing, the otoneurologist asks the patient to touch his own nose with the index finger and then reach out to touch the examiner's finger. He is asked to perform this maneuver rapidly several times, first with eyes open and then with eyes closed. Past-pointing consists of a tendency to overshoot the examiner's finger consistently to one side. This can result from vestibular stimulation and vestibular hypofunctioning, as well as from disorders of the CNS.

The Romberg test is performed by having the patient stand upright with feet together and eyes closed. A variation, the tandem Romberg test, has the patient stand with one foot before the other with eyes closed. An inability to maintain these postures because of a tendency to fall sideways or backward is seen in vestibular as well as in some CNS disorders.

Nystagmus is a rhythmical jerking of the eyes rapidly in one direction and slowly in the opposite direction. Nystagmus can be associated with ocular diseases and CNS disorders, as well as with vestibular disorders. The presence and direction of spontaneous nystagmus is noted, but as in the case of gait disorders, it must be interpreted in the context of the complete otoneurological evaluation.

In order to stimulate the semicircular canals for purposes of testing, the endolymph must be made to flow so as to deflect the cupula in which the hairs of the sensory organ, the crista, are embedded. In a clinical setting, the most practical method of causing such hair cell deflection is to irrigate each ear with water above and/or below body temperature.

The patient is seated with his neck extended backward 60° from the normal upright position. This places the lateral semicircular canal in a vertical plane, so that with the aid of gravity the caloric irrigation creates a maximum convection current in the endolymph, thereby producing maximum deflection of the hairs of the crista ampullaris. Each ear is irrigated with 5 ml of water at 0° with a 5-min interval between the tests on the two ears. After a 20-sec latent period, the patient with a normally responsive labyrinth will exhibit nystagmus, past-pointing, and a falling tendency when asked to stand. The nystagmus, the direction of which is named by the direction of the fast eye jerks, is directed toward the nontest side; past-pointing and falling are toward the test side. Nausea, vomiting, and sweating are normal accompaniments of such vestibular responses, although they do not occur in all patients. The otologist notes the following about the patient's responses:

1. whether stimulation of each ear does or does not produce a response;
2. the relative magnitude of the responses from each side (This magnitude can be measured in duration of nystagmus or in the number of beats occurring in a 10-sec interval.) The duration of nystagmus, the most commonly employed parameter, normally lies between 90 to 180 sec;
3. whether or not the subjective sensation of vertigo produced by the test is similar to the spontaneous dysequilibrium that caused the patient to seek medical attention.

The other practical method of producing a flow of endolymph for clinical testing purposes, the Barany rotation test, consists of turning the patient, who is seated on a rotating chair. After spinning the patient, for example, 12 times in a 20-sec period, the examiner stops the chair abruptly and observes the eyes of the patient for nystagmus. Such postrotatory nystagmus results from the inertia of the endolymph, which tends to continue to rotate in the lumen of the semicircular canals even though the patient and the walls of the canals have ceased to rotate. To test each ear, the patient is rotated first clockwise and then, after a suitable rest period, counterclockwise. The disadvantage of the Barany rotation test is that both ears are stimulated simultaneously, whereas in the caloric test, stimulation can be limited to one ear at a time. However, the rotation test might be the only vestibular stimulation test that can be performed on an infant or young child. In such a case, the patient is held in the appropriate position on the lap of the parent and both are rotated.

The evaluation of nystagmus as an indicator of labyrinthine function and response to stimulation has been greatly refined by the introduction of electronystagmography (ENG). An ENG apparatus records the move-

ments of the eyes on paper in a manner comparable to the familiar electrocardiograph. With the aid of ENG, it has become possible to detect
nystagmus which is not visible to ordinary observation, to quantitate the
speed of the nystagmus, to correct for spontaneous nystagmus, and to
perform positioning labyrinthine stimulation tests while recording the resulting nystagmus. Electronystagmography is described and discussed in
Chapter 4.

V. AUDIOLOGICAL ASSESSMENT

No attempt will be made here to enter into the details of the audiological evaluation, since this forms the substance of several chapters of
this book. A few remarks are in order, however, to relate the audiological
evaluation to the content of the otologic assessment.

The audiologist is a member of a team, which also includes the otologist, pediatrician or internist, neurologist, and neuropsychologist. The
audiologist cannot be placed in the position of making the diagnosis and
prognosis of a hearing loss or other audio-vestibular disorder. The audiologist quantifies a hearing loss, performs and interprets tests to localize
the site of a lesion, and plays a major role in the habilitation or rehabilitation of the patient with a communication handicap due to hearing impairment. The audiological evaluation assumes full significance only when
it is collated with the complete medical history, a thorough otologic
examination, and, when indicated, with the findings of other medical
examinations.

VI. RADIOLOGICAL ASSESSMENT

Radiological studies of the ear are useful in certain types of otologic
problems, but they are not required in all cases. Because of the additional
new information which can be obtained by the technique of hypocycloidal
polytomography, more patients with otologic disorders now, undergo
X-ray examination than previously. It is emphasized at the outset that
routine X-rays of the skull rarely render useful information about audio-
vestibular disorders.

A. Plain X-rays

Plain X-rays of the mastoids are of value in the assessment of middle-
ear and mastoid infections, in determining the extent of pneumatization

of the temporal bone in congenital aural atresia, in checking for suspected fractures of the temporal bone, and in the evaluation of tumors. Plain films provide the radiologist with an overall view of the temporal bone, but they often limit precise evaluation because so many different bone shadows are superimposed on the radiograph.

B. Tomograms

The various techniques of tomography, especially hypocycloidal poly-tomography, in effect slice the temporal bone into thin sequential layers, so that only a small depth (1–2 mm) of bone and tissue is in focus on the film plane. By virtue of this precision, it has become possible to recognize ossicular anomalies, bony closure of the oval and round windows, minute fractures of the labyrinthine walls, anomalous morphology of the laby-rinthine cavities, and subtle abnormalities of the internal auditory canal in cases of acoustic neuroma. Hypocycloidal polytomography can be help-ful in evaluating developmental as well as some acquired disorders of the ear, whether they involve the middle ear, the cochlea, the labyrinth, or all three.

C. Posterior Fossa Cisternography

In the evaluation of patients with suspected lesions in the internal auditory canal, especially acoustic neuroma, posterior fossa cisternography is of extreme importance. Many patients, who have symptoms and oto-logic and audiological findings suggesting a lesion of the VIIIth cranial nerve, must undergo this study which, if positive, might indicate the need for surgical removal of the tumor.

For this procedure, the patient is admitted to the hospital. It involves a lumbar puncture and the instillation of a small amount of contrast fluid into the lumbar subarachnoid space, which is continuous with the cerebro-spinal fluid spaces in the cranial cavity. The patient is then tilted into an appropriate position so that the radio-opaque fluid rises into the pos-terior cranial cavity, enters the pontine cistern, and flows into the internal auditory canal. The canal is occupied by the cochlear, vestibular, and facial nerves, which normally occupy only a portion of the diameter of its lumen. Failure of the fluid to enter the canal around the nerves sug-gests an obstruction, the most common cause of which is a neuroma of the vestibular nerve. At the conclusion of this radiological study, as much as possible of the contrast fluid is removed by lumbar puncture.

D. Angiography

A patient is ordinarily hospitalized for an angiographic study. The technique of angiography or arteriography involves the injection of a radioopaque fluid into the main artery of the area under study. In the case of otologic diagnosis, the vessels which are filled are the vertebral and, occasionally, the carotid arteries. From the main vessel, the fluid is carried in the circulating blood to the branches of these vessels. The neuroradiologist looks for displacement of vessels from their normal positions, and for areas of increased or reduced vascular filling by the contrast fluid. This gives him information about the presence, location, probable nature, and size of tumors.

E. Pneumoencephalography

A patient is hospitalized for this examination. By means of a lumbar puncture, spinal fluid is withdrawn and air is injected and allowed to rise into the cerebrospinal fluid spaces within and surrounding the brain. The air acts as a contrast medium and is readily distinguishable from brain and nerve tissues on the X-ray film. By this technique, the neuroradiologist can reach further conclusions about the presence and size of tumors. Pneumoencephalography, for example, is helpful in evaluating acoustic neuromas, which are so large that they have mushroomed out of the internal auditory canal and are growing into the cerebellopontine angle, causing not only auditory but also other neurological abnormalities by pressure on the brain and other cranial nerves.

F. Isotope Scans

Certain brain tumors concentrate radioactive (gamma-emitting) isotopes more heavily than does the surrounding normal brain tissue. This radioactivity can be detected and recorded on a photograph. In this test, the radioactive material in liquid form is injected into a vein in the arm. As it circulates throughout the body, it enters various tissues; but it tends to concentrate in the tumor, making the tumor visible on the scintiscan, as the recorded image is called (Chusid and McDonald, 1970).

VII. HEARING DISORDERS IN SPECIFIC CONDITIONS

In this section, those disorders commonly encountered in an otologic clinic will be categorized and described briefly.

A. External Ear

1. Obstruction of the external auditory canal by cerumen, epithelial debris, and foreign objects can cause as much as a 25- or 30-dB conductive hearing loss. This is easily correctable by removal of the occluding material. Obstruction of the external auditory canal is noticed more readily by a patient with a preexisting hearing impairment than by a person with basically normal hearing.

2. An external auditory meatus, which is artificially collapsed by test earphones, can present a pseudoconductive hearing loss which is detected only during audiometry, and which does not cause any actual hearing loss. The alert otologist or audiologist recognizes this condition, and has the hearing test performed after inserting a small straw or plastic tube in the meatus before applying the earphones.

3. Osteomata are small, skin-covered, bony excrescences which can be present in the inner half of the external auditory canal, especially in persons accustomed to swimming in cold water. These growths narrow the canal to such an extent that the remaining small space is easily occluded by small amounts of cerumen, hairs, and epithelial debris. By themselves, osteomata rarely cause a hearing loss. Occasionally, these growths must be removed surgically if they predispose the patient to frequent or chronic obstruction with its attendant mild to moderate hearing loss.

4. Congenital aural atresia can be unilateral or bilateral, and implies a failure of formation of the external auditory canal. The condition is associated with a 50- to 60-dB conductive- or mixed-type hearing loss, depending upon whether or not the cochlea has developed normally. Aural atresia may not only be associated with an abnormal auricle, but can signify serious abnormalities of the cochlea as well as maldevelopment of the brain. These children must undergo thorough pediatric and neurologic evaluation, so that all concerned are not frustrated when the child fails to develop normally once he is fitted with a proper hearing aid. Congenital aural atresia can be corrected surgically to a limited extent, although rarely does the surgery improve the hearing to a completely normal level. Surgery is indicated for this condition only when it is bilateral (Nager, 1973).

B. Middle Ear

1. The most common cause of mild to moderate hearing impairment in children is the condition known variously as "secretory otitis media," "serous otitis media," "glue ear," "catarrhal otitis media," "chronic tubotympanitis," or "fluid-filled middle ear." Because of poor Eustachian-tube

function, the middle ear is not adequately ventilated and, as a result, the middle ear fills with a fluid that originates from its mucous membrane lining. This condition can be corrected by myringostomy with an indwelling plastic or metal aeration tube. Most children eventually outgrow the condition by puberty. It is seen with exceptional frequency in children born with palatal clefts.

2. Serous otitis media in adults may have the same cause as in children, especially if the patient has a history of recurrent or chronic ear problems since childhood. In some adults, however, the underlying cause is a malignant tumor arising in the nasopharynx and occluding the Eustachian tube. An adult with a conductive hearing loss should be examined by an otolaryngologist to determine whether or not there is a serous effusion in the middle ear, and whether or not the patient is harboring a nasopharyngeal tumor.

3. Chronic otitis media causes a conductive or mixed hearing impairment. The condition implies the presence of a perforation or deep retraction pocket of the tympanic membrane, accompanied by either constant or recurrent aural discharge. Some, but not all, such ears have a cholesteatoma. This is a sac of skin which grows into the middle ear and mastoid, and can be associated with erosion of bony structures in the ear. Patients with chronic otitis media often require a mastoidectomy and tympanoplasty to rid the ear of chronically infected tissue, and to rebuild the sound-conducting mechanism of the middle ear which has been damaged by the chronic infection.

4. Otosclerosis is a common bony disorder which is often familial, and which causes the stapes footplate to become slowly and progressively fixed in the oval window (Lindsay, 1973). Although sometimes seen in children, otosclerosis more commonly begins to cause a hearing loss in the third and fourth decades of life. Otosclerosis usually affects both ears, although not always at the same time or to the same extent. The disorder affects females twice as frequently as males. It causes at first a purely conductive hearing loss and then a mixed deafness. Patients with otosclerotic deafness can be managed either with a hearing aid or by surgery. The latter is rarely mandatory, except in those few patients whose hearing loss is so advanced that they are not helped sufficiently by amplification alone. These patients gain more useful hearing with amplification from a hearing aid after having their air-conduction threshold lowered by a stapedectomy.

5. Congenital anomalies of the middle ear imply the abnormal formation or fixation of the tympanic ossicles. Any or all of the three ossicles may be involved. Patients with such anomalies may have a purely conductive or a mixed deafness, which may be unilateral or, more often, bi-

lateral. The tympanic anomaly may be isolated, but more often it is part of a constellation of anomalies. The condition is seen, for instance, in the syndromes of Treacher–Collins, Klippel–Feil, and Morquio. Deafness due to middle-ear anomalies can be managed either with amplification or by surgery.

6. Skull and ear trauma can cause dislocations or other disruptions of the ossicular chain, resulting in a purely conductive or mixed hearing loss. The resulting deafness can be managed by amplification or by surgery.

C. Inner Ear

Most of the disorders affecting the cochlea and auditory nerve are irreversible, and the deafness resulting from them can be managed only by auditory habilitation or rehabilitation.

1. Various forms of hereditary deafness have been described, some occurring as an isolated defect and some as part of a syndrome. In some cases, genetically determined deafness is present at birth; in others, it is manifested progressively during the first three decades of life. Excellent descriptions of the various forms of genetic deafness can be found in the writings of Konigsmark (1969) and of Proctor and Proctor (1967).

2. Congenital-acquired deafness is a nongenetically determined hearing impairment which is due to otonoxious events in the pre-, peri-, or neonatal developmental periods. Examples of prenatal insults include maternal rubella, maternal syphilis, and the treatment of the pregnant mother with ototoxic drugs. Perinatal events injurious to the ears of the baby include anoxia, kernicterus caused by erythroblastosis fetalis, prematurity, and birth injury. Neonatal factors which can result in hearing impairments include apnea, cyanosis, and cerebral birth injury.

3. Deafness can be caused by a viral or bacterial labyrinthitis. Viral labyrinthitis occurs in rubella, mumps, measles, cytomegalic inclusion virus, and in other diseases. It is usually a complication of a generalized viral infection. Bacterial labyrinthitis, by contrast, is usually a complication of a contiguous middle-ear infection, and can be caused by any of the bacteria which cause acute or chronic otitis media. A viral labyrinthitis may cause either partial or total deafness, whereas bacterial labyrinthitis usually results in severe or total hearing loss.

4. Postmeningitic deafness is the sequel of a bacterial labyrinthitis. The original infection may have spread from the middle ear to the brain via the inner ear. Less commonly, the infection reaches the meninges from other portions of the respiratory tract, and the labyrinth is involved as a peripheral complication. The otolaryngologist and audiologist

should insist that all children who have recovered from meningitis have an otologic and audiologic evaluation. In this way, patients may have postmeningitic deafness diagnosed as early as possible, so that rehabilitative measures may be instituted.

5. Congenital syphilis causes a hearing loss which is usually bilateral, and which behaves clinically and audiometrically much like the cochlear hydrops of Meniere's disease. These patients also have vertigo in some cases. If the cause of the hearing loss is discovered early, treatment with penicillin and steroids might save the patient's hearing.

6. Ototoxic drugs include those which are damaging principally to the cochlea, and those which injure mainly the vestibular end-organs. The cochleotoxic substances include neomycin, kanamycin, dihydrostreptomycin, vancomycin, and ethacrynic acid, all of which produce a permanent sensorineural hearing impairment. Salicylate and furosemide are unusual in that they cause a sensorineural hearing loss that is reversible upon discontinuance of the medication. Streptomycin and gentamycin damage the vestibular organs preferentially, although cases of deafness have been reported with these antibiotics. Recently, it has been found that ethacrynic acid potentiates the cochleotoxic effects of kanamycin.

The ototoxic drugs are usually administered by injection rather than orally. They are used only for serious infections. Their toxic effects are especially frequent in patients who have kidney failure, because the blood concentration of these drugs rises sharply when the kidneys fail to filter them from the circulation. Salicylates cause hearing loss only when they are taken in large amounts, as is most commonly the case in patients who are under treatment for severe arthritis.

7. Meniere's disease is characterized by hearing loss—often fluctuating—tinnitus, and recurrent episodes of vertigo. The disorder is caused by a distention of the endolymphatic spaces of the inner ear by an excessive accumulation of endolymphatic fluid. A fairly common variant of Meniere's disease, known as "cochlear hydrops," has all the auditory symptoms and audiological characteristics of this disorder, but the patient has little or no vertigo. The symptoms of endolymphatic hydrops are similar to those caused by Eustachian-tube blockage, but the audiologist finds a sensorineural loss in the former and a conductive loss in the latter. The hearing handicap in Meniere's disease is due not so much to the elevation in hearing threshold, as it is to the distortion of speech and recruitment of the affected ear, which tends to have a distracting effect even upon the uninvolved ear. After a destructive labyrinthectomy for incapacitating vertigo, patients usually volunteer the observation that their overall hearing has been improved by the procedure that has destroyed their hearing in the diseased ear. Reports vary that Meniere's disease involves both ears in 5 to 40% of patients. We have seen a num-

ber of patients in whom the second ear became involved 20 years after the first ear became affected.

8. In capsular otosclerosis, the disease process involves large areas of the periotic capsule instead of limiting itself to the oval window and adjacent bone. It is usually referred to as "cochlear otosclerosis," but the term "capsular," or "periotic," otosclerosis, is preferred because it emphasizes that the disease is a disorder of bone rather than of the cochlea itself. For reasons which are not yet clear, the disorder produces principally a sensorineural hearing loss with little if any conductive component. The diagnosis should be made only when there exists a history of a progressive hearing loss, usually bilateral, a clear family history of typical oval window otosclerosis, and positive radiologic findings of otosclerotic changes of bone on polygrams of the ears (Linthicum, 1972).

9. Acute and chronic noise exposure damages the organ of Corti, causing a loss of hair cells and secondary degeneration of auditory nerve fibers. It is a fairly common cause of sensorineural hearing loss in all age groups (Ward, 1973).

10. Occlusion of the vascular supply to the ear should result in the death of the ear, since the blood supply comes from one vessel, with no collateral supply. However, otologic methods have not yet been developed which allow us to diagnose with any degree of confidence cases of hearing loss due to vascular occlusion. Therefore, the actual incidence of deafness due to vascular obstruction is unknown at the present time.

11. "Presbycusis" refers to the hearing loss which occurs with advancing age. Before the conclusion is reached that a case of deafness is due simply to aging, a very careful history must be elicited to rule out all the other additive and known causes of gradual, progressive bilateral deafness.

12. The so-called "collagen diseases" attack the ears, along with numerous other organs of the body. Many of these diseases are now known to be autoimmune disorders. Sensorineural deafness has been seen in patients with lupus erythematosus, Wegener's granulomatosis, chronic relapsing polychondritis, cranial (temporal) arteritis, and periarteritis nodosa, and in Cogan's syndrome. In these patients, the vestibular system is likely to be involved along with the cochlea; the damage to both systems is caused by an inflammatory obliteration of the blood vessels.

13. Trauma is a relatively frequent cause of deafness, though it fortunately involves only one ear in most instances. The trauma can be due to external blows to the head or to sudden pressure changes in the spinal fluid system. External trauma can result in fractures through to the inner ear or auditory nerve, in hemorrhage into the labyrinth, or in an actual concussion of the cochlea and vestibular end-organs. Pressure changes in the cerebrospinal fluid, if they are sufficiently sudden and intense, can

cause the middle-ear windows to rupture. Since this mechanism was described by Goodhill in 1971, it has been observed with increasing frequency in patients who become deaf while performing strenuous physical activity. It is important to diagnose this condition, because prompt middle-ear surgery to seal the round or oval window leak may sometimes reverse the sensorineural hearing loss.

D. Acoustic Nerve

Nerve degeneration occurs in many disorders of the end-organs, as described in the preceding listing of common inner-ear disorders. There are several unusual disease processes which may primarily involve the acoustic nerve (arachnoidal cysts and vascular malformation), but they are encountered rarely. At this point, only two fairly common conditions of the audio-vestibular nerve will be described.

1. The otologist depends greatly on the audiologist to aid in the diagnosis of acoustic neuroma. It is only in the last 10 years that it has been demonstrated clearly that the first symptoms of this benign tumor are auditory, i.e., progressive deafness and constant tinnitus. Prior to that time, these tumors were diagnosed only after they were large enough to cause serious neurological symptoms, such as blindness, cerebellar ataxia, facial paralysis, and swallowing difficulty. By careful otologic evaluation, radiological studies, and audiological tests, it is now often possible to diagnose these tumors when they are quite small and causing little in the way of symptoms other than hearing loss and tinnitus. Small acoustic neuromas can be removed surgically with little morbidity, whereas the large growths sometimes cannot be removed completely and without serious complications, including death. Current otologic and audiological thinking suggests that any patient with a unilateral sensorineural hearing loss that is not due to an easily identifiable cause should be very carefully evaluated for a possible small acoustic neuroma.

2. Approximately 50% of patients with multiple sclerosis have involvements of the audio-vestibular system (Noffsinger et al., 1972). The symptoms and audiological findings can be similar to those seen in acoustic neuroma, i.e., those of a neural lesion. The diagnosis is made by careful neurological and otoneurological evaluation.

VIII. SUMMARY OF THE OTOLOGIC ASSESSMENT

The aims of the complete otologic assessment (including the audiological evaluation) are to arrive at a diagnosis of the cause of hearing loss, and to plan for the management of the patient. In the case of deafness, the final diagnosis most often concludes that the problem lies only within the ear. Occasionally, a more serious systemic disease, e.g., diabetes, multiple sclerosis, syphilis, or a more widespread anomaly, e.g., Alport's disease or Jervell's disease, is discovered while the otologic team is evaluating the patient's deafness. The patient with deafness must be considered in totality, so that associated disorders will not be overlooked. In the case of a problem with dysequilibrium, the diagnosis lies outside the ear more often than is the case with deafness (Drachman and Hart, 1972).

Having arrived at a diagnosis, the final charge to the otologic team is the management of the patient with a hearing or a vestibular disorder, more than it is the treatment of the deafness or vestibular problem as an isolated problem. The responsibilities of managing a child with a severe congenital or hereditary deafness are awesome, and include not only amplification of environmental sounds by means of a hearing aid, but the total psychosocial habilitation of the patient and psychological–educational counseling of the parents. Other forms of deafness, such as those caused by otosclerosis or chronic otitis media, are less complicated to manage, because the patient is usually in an otherwise healthy condition and requires only surgical correction and/or amplification.

REFERENCES

Black, F. O., Bergstrom, L., Downs, M., and Hemenway, W. (1971). "Congenital Deafness." Colorado Associated Univ. Press, Boulder, Colorado.

Bluestone, C. D., Paradise, J. L., and Berry, Q. C. (1972). *Laryngoscope* 82, 1654.

Busis, S. (1965). *Acta Oto-Laryngol. Suppl.* 209, 1.

Chusid, J. G., and McDonald, J. J. (1970). "Correlative Neuroanatomy and Functional Neurology," 15th ed. Lange Med. Publ., Los Altos, California.

Compere, W. E., Jr. (1958). *Trans. Amer. Acad. Ophthalmol. Otolaryngol.* 62, 444.

Drachman, D., and Hart, C. (1972). *Neurology* 22, 323.

Goodhill, V. (1971). *Laryngoscope* 81, 1462.

Hawkins, J. E., Jr. (1967). *In* "Deafness in Childhood" (F. McConnell and P. H. Ward, eds.), pp. 156–168. Vanderbilt Univ. Press, Nashville, Tennessee.

Hughes, J. (1971). "Synopsis of Pediatrics." Mosby, St. Louis, Missouri.

Jorgensen, M. B., and Schmidt, M. R. (1962). *Acta Oto-Laryngol.* 55, 537.

Konigsmark, B. W. (1969). *New England J. Med.* 281, 713, 774, 827.

Larsen, A. (1960). *Acta Oto-Laryngol. Suppl.* 154, 1.

Lindsay, J. (1973). *In* "Otolaryngology" (M. Paparella and D. A. Shumrick, eds.), Vol. 2, pp. 205–230. Saunders, Philadelphia, Pennsylvania.

Linthicum, F. H. (1972). *Arch. Otolaryngol.* 95, 564.

Mathog, R. H. (1970). *Arch. Otolaryngol.* 92, 7.

McGee, T. M. (1962). *Arch. Otolaryngol.* 75, 295.

Meyers, R. M. (1970). *Arch. Otolaryngol.* 92, 160.

Miller, G. F. (1965). *Arch. Otolaryngol.* 81, 41.

Nager, G. T. (1973). *In* "Otolaryngology" (M. Paparella and D. A. Shumrick, eds.), Vol. 2, pp. 3–23. Saunders, Philadelphia, Pennsylvania.

Noffsinger, D., Olsen, W. D., Carhart, R., Hart, C. W., and Sahgal, V. (1972). *Acta Oto-Laryngol. Suppl.* 303.

Proctor, C. A., and Proctor, B. (1967). *Arch. Otolaryngol.* **85**, 23.

Ward, W. D. (1973). *In* "Otolaryngology" (M. Paparella and D. A. Shumrick, eds.), Vol. 2, pp. 377–390. Saunders, Philadelphia, Pennsylvania.

Chapter Three
Electronystagmography[1]

Alfred C. Coats[2]

I. INTRODUCTION

Electronystagmography (ENG) refers to the application of an old technique of eye-movement recording, electro-oculography (EOG), to the recording of nystagmus. The ENG examination is essentially a series of tests taken from the clinical neuro-otologic examination. The tests done in the ENG laboratory do not differ in any substantive way from those done in the office or at the bedside except that nystagmus is recorded, rather than visually observed.

During the past decade, the clinical use of ENG has grown very rapidly, but dissemination of practical clinical knowledge about the examination has not kept pace with this growth. In this chapter, I shall attempt to provide a cohesive discussion of ENG technique and interpretation in a clinical setting.

Since an exhaustive presentation of all alternative tests and procedures is incompatible with my goal of cohesiveness, I shall limit my discussion to the following tests performed in my own routine clinical ENG examination: (1) ocular-dysmetria test ("calibration overshoot"), (2) gaze test, (3) sinusoidal tracking test, (4) optokinetic test, (5) paroxysmal

[1] Partial support for this work was provided by grant no. NS 10940 from the National Institute of Neurological Diseases and Stroke, and by grant no. HL 05435 from the National Heart and Lung Institute, National Institutes of Health, USPHS.

[2] Departments of Physiology and Otorhinolaryngology and Communicative Sciences, Baylor College of Medicine, Texas Medical Center, and the Audio-Vestibular Laboratory and Neurophysiology Services, The Methodist Hospital, Houston, Texas.

nystagmus test, (6) position test, and (7) bithermal caloric test. For more extensive outlines of the various vestibular-function tests, the reader may find Fields and Alford (1964), Henriksson *et al.* (1972), and Wolfson (1968) useful.

II. RECORDING PRINCIPLES

A. Electro-oculography (EOG)

1. Principle. Electrodes placed anywhere in the vicinity of the eyes record a voltage change when the eyes rotate. Early investigators assumed that this phenomenon (termed the "electro-oculogram" by Marg, 1951) was due to pickup of the extraocular muscle electromyogram. However, Mowrer *et al.* (1935) demonstrated that this voltage change is entirely independent of the extraocular muscles. It is now known that the EOG is due to a constant voltage generated within the retina (probably in the pigment epithelium) which is often called the "corneoretinal potential" (CRP).

Figure 1 illustrates the principle of EOG. The CRP and the sclera's insulating properties (Kris, 1960; Marg, 1951) cause the eyeball to behave like an electrical dipole. Rotation of the dipole creates a voltage change which, since the head is an electrical conductor, can be detected by electrodes placed on the surface of the head. This voltage change is amplified and made to drive a pen-writing recorder to produce the EOG. The EOG is usually recorded as a voltage difference between a pair of electrodes, and the EOG electrodes will record only eye movements in the plane of the electrode pair.

2. Electrode Placement. Figure 2 shows the EOG electrodes placed to record horizontal eye movements on one recorder channel (electrodes lateral to the outer canthi) and vertical eye movements on a second channel (electrodes above and below the eye). A ground electrode is placed in the center of the forehead to minimize 60-Hz hum interference. For a single-channel ENG, only the horizontal electrode pair is used.

3. Amplitude Calibration. Figure 3 illustrates the procedure for relating the angle through which the eye rotates to the amount of pen deflection (the "amplitude calibration"). The patient focuses alternately on two fixation points (small, examiner-controlled lights are convenient), which subtend a known angle of ocular rotation. A calibration angle of either 10° or 20° is acceptable. The measurement of calibration amplitude is shown at the bottom left of Figure 3.

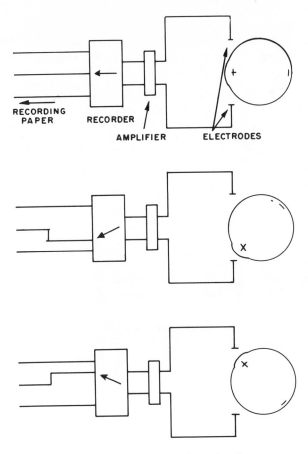

Figure 1 The principle of electro-oculography (EOG). The corneoretinal potential (CRP) is illustrated as a "+" (positive voltage) at the front of the eye and a "−" (negative voltage) at the back. Eye movement displaces this potential. This displacement is "seen" by electrodes placed in the plane of the eye movement because the head is an electrical conductor.

4. Potential Errors. (*a*) *Linearity.* Crucial to the application of EOG to clinical eye-movement recording is the question of linearity; e.g., does a 40° eye rotation produce a pen deflection twice that produced by a 20° eye movement? Geometric considerations suggest a sinusoidal relationship between pen deflection and eye rotation (Geddes *et al.*, 1973). However, several investigators have demonstrated that in actual practice, for eye rotation within ±45°, the deviation from a linear relationship is inconsequential (Geddes *et al.*, 1973; Hoffman *et al.*, 1939; Kris,

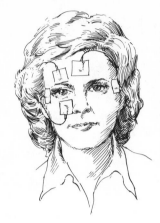

Figure 2 Electrode locations for recording vertical movements of the right eye (placed above and below the eye) and horizontal movements of both eyes (placed lateral to the outer borders of the eyes). The electrodes are placed in the plane of the pupils when the patient's gaze is straight ahead. The electrode in the center of the forehead connects the patient to ground to minimize 60-Hz hum interference. The electrodes are attached to the patient with squares of adhesive tape.

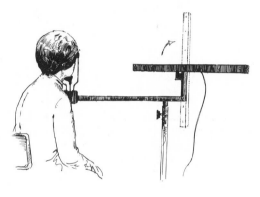

20° CALIBRATION

R

L

$\mathbf{I}$ 100 μV

Figure 3 Eye-movement calibrator and gaze tester (top). A hand-held control box (not shown) operates seven calibrating lights on the crossbar. The center light is in the midline. The two inner lights subtend an angle of 20° with the bridge of the subject's nose, i.e., each light is 10° from midline. The two middle lights are 20° from midline, and the outer two lights are 30° from midline. The 20° and 30° lights are used in the test for gaze nystagmus. The crossbar can be rotated either into the horizontal position for horizontal calibration and gaze testing or into the vertical position (dotted lines) for vertical calibration and gaze testing. Below the calibrator is shown a typical record of a 20° calibration (eyes moving back and forth between the two inner lights) obtained with an AC-coupled recorder. The method of measuring the calibration is shown at the left.

40

1960; Leksell, 1939; Shackel, 1960). Thus, for purposes of ENG, where recordings are generally less than ±30°, a linear EOG–pen deflection relationship can be assumed.

(b) *Sensitivity.* It has been reported that the EOG can record eye rotations as small as 0.5–1.0° (Fodor, 1968). However, in my experience, electrical "noise" produced by muscle potentials and the electroencephalogram (EEG) usually limits the sensitivity to 1–2°. We occasionally encounter patients with such a high noise level (particularly large-amplitude EEG in older patients, or small-amplitude corneoretinal potential, or both) that the sensitivity of the EOG is 5° or less.

The sensitivity of the EOG is much less than the sensitivity of direct visual observation (approximately 0.1°). Thus, in situations where one desires to detect small-amplitude eye movements with the patient's eyes open, e.g., during the gaze test, looking at the patient's eyes is superior to recording their movement with EOG.

(c) *Variability.* The CRP, on which EOG is based, is extremely labile, as might be expected, since it is a metabolically generated retinal event intimately related to visual function. Light adaptation has the most profound effect on EOG amplitude (Aantaa, 1970; Aserinsky, 1955; Homer, 1967; Munthe Fog, 1964). Figure 4 shows the striking effect of

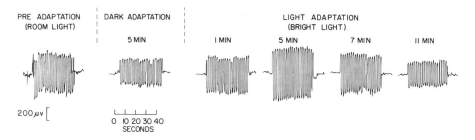

Figure 4 The effect of dark and light adaptation on EOG calibration amplitude. Paper speed was 50 mm per min. Records were obtained in the ENG laboratory under normal recording conditions. The time notations above the records show elapsed time from the beginning of adaptation.

light adaptation on CRP and, hence, on EOG calibration amplitude. In normal subjects, the maximum light-adapted EOG calibration is at least one and three-fourths (usually more than twice) as large as the minimum dark-adapted EOG (Aantaa, 1970).

The following precautions minimize the potentially serious effect of EOG amplitude fluctuations: (1) Do the ENG examination in a dimly lit room to minimize the amount of visual adaptation caused by opening and closing the eyes; (2) Repeat the calibration before each caloric irrigation (Hart, 1969; North, 1965).

B. The Electronystagmograph

An electronystagmograph is simply a standard biological pen-writing recorder, similar to the electrocardiograph and electroencephalograph. Table I lists the specifications that tailor the recorder to record nystagmus. Three of the more critical of these specifications will be discussed in detail.

TABLE I

SPECIFICATIONS OF AN ENG SUITABLE
FOR ROUTINE CLINICAL USE

I. Gain (sensitivity)
    25–500 μV/cm per deflection continuously variable with calibrated setting
II. Frequency response (3 dB down points)
    High   15 Hz
    Low   0.1 Hz (Time constant = 3 sec)
III. Common-mode rejection ratio
    Greater than 80 dB at 60 Hz
IV. Input impedance
    Greater than 1 megohm with differential input
V. Paper speed
    10 mm/sec
VI. Number of recording channels
    One or two (discussed in text)

1. Frequency Response. Bioelectric signals never occur as isolated phenomena. The particular event one wishes to record is always immersed in a milieu of competing electrical events of diverse origins. One important way of selectively recording the desired event is to tailor the frequency response of the recorder to reject unwanted signals. Care must be taken, however, not to restrict the recorder's frequency response to the point that the desired event is not recorded with fidelity.

In electronystagmography, 60-Hz hum and muscle potentials are probably the most serious of the rapidly changing interfering signals. These signals can be minimized, however, by restricting the high side of the frequency-response curve. Also, such slowly changing electrical signals as the electrodermal response (due to sweating) and electrolytic potentials at the electrode–skin interface can be eliminated by restricting the low side of the electronystagmograph's frequency response.

Figure 5 shows the effect of progressively restricting an electronystag-

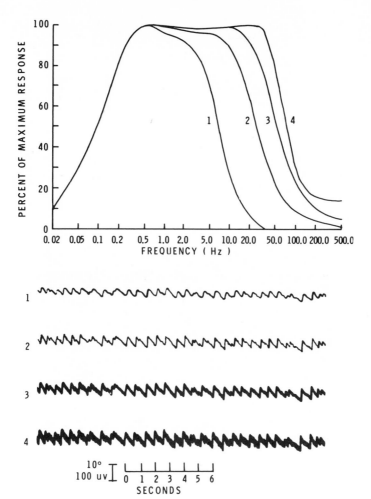

Figure 5 Effect of changing the high side of an electronystagmograph's frequency response. The recordings were made with four channels of a Beckman "Dynograph" recorder. Frequency-response curves are shown at the top, and recordings of the same nystagmus signal obtained by each channel are shown at the bottom. Channel 1 demonstrates degradation of the nystagmus signal when frequency response is restricted too far. Channel 4 demonstrates interference by high-frequency (60-Hz hum) electrical signals.

mograph's high-frequency response. With the highest cutoff (frequency-response curve 4), rapidly changing signals (60-Hz hum in this illustration) interfere with the nystagmus record. As the recorder's ability to respond to high frequencies is progressively restricted (curves 3 and 2), the rapidly changing signals are increasingly attenuated. However, re-

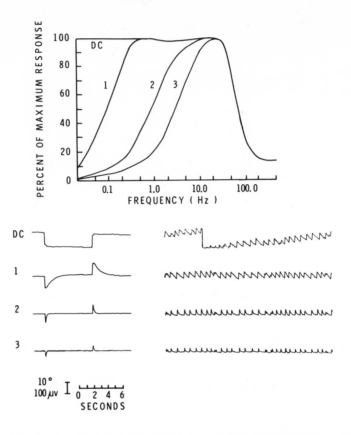

Figure 6 Effect of restricting the low side of an electronystagmograph's frequency response. The recordings were made with four channels of a Beckman "Dynograph" recorder. Frequency-response curves are shown at the top. Responses of the four channels to a "step function" are shown at bottom left, and responses to a nystagmus signal are shown at bottom right. The DC channel demonstrates interference by low-frequency electrical signals. When the recorder's ability to respond to low frequencies is restricted too severely, distortion of the nystagmus slow phase occurs (channels 2 and 3).

stricting the high side of the frequency-response curve too far (curve 1) distorts the most rapidly changing part of the nystagmus wave form, i.e., the transition between slow and fast phases.

Figure 6 illustrates the effect of progressively restricting the low side of an electronystagmograph's frequency-response curve. At bottom left of this figure is shown the recorder's response to a suddenly applied voltage change, such as closing a switch between the two poles of a battery might generate. The "DC" (which may be taken to mean either "direct coupled" or "direct current") recorder's pen remains deflected for as long as the voltage is applied. It thus reflects a voltage which is not changing at all and, hence, has a low-frequency response of zero.

With the lowest frequency cutoff ("DC"), slowly changing electrical events cause "baseline drift," requiring repeated pen recentering. As shown by record 1, the low side of the frequency-response curve can be restricted to filter out the slowly changing electrical events while still reproducing the nystagmus with fidelity. Records 2 and 3 demonstrate that restricting the low side of the recorder's frequency response too severely distorts the most slowly changing part of the nystagmus wave form, i.e., the slow phase.

Records 1, 2, and 3 in Figure 6 were obtained with an "AC"-coupled recorder. "AC" means "alternating current," so-called because the recorder will reproduce only changing electrical events. As shown at lower left, when a voltage-level change is applied to an AC-coupled recorder, the pen deflects when the change is applied but then returns to baseline. The "time constant" of an AC-coupled recorder is defined as the time required for the pen to return 63% of the way to baseline.

As Figure 6 demonstrates, the time constant and low-frequency response are related. The shorter the time constant, the higher the low side of the frequency-response curve.[3]

2. *Common-mode Rejection Ratio.* Biomedical recorders almost always use "differential amplifiers" to amplify the recorded signal. The main advantage of the differential amplifier is that it tends to reject interfering electrical "noise" radiated from nearby sources, e.g., 60-Hz power lines. In essence, a differential amplifier is two amplifiers connected so that their outputs subtract. Thus, signals that are the same at both inputs (common-mode signal) cancel out, whereas signals that differ at the two inputs pass through and are amplified.

Slight differences in the electronic components of the two sides of the differential amplifier will create slight differences in common-mode signals. Since electronic components are not perfectly uniform, real-life differential amplifiers never completely reject common-mode signals. However, some are better than others. The ability of the differential amplifier to reject common-mode signals is thus an important indication of its quality. This ability is measured by applying a signal, e.g., a 60-Hz sine wave, so that it is first in phase at the two inputs and then 180° out of phase. The ratio of in-phase to out-of-phase voltages required to produce the same output is termed the "common-mode rejection ratio."

---

[3] $T = \dfrac{1}{2\pi F_l}$ where: T = time constant
F_l = low-frequency cutoff (3 dB down points)

Thus, the 90-dB common-mode rejection ratio specified above means that an in-phase signal must be about 13,000 times as strong as an out-of-phase signal to produce the same output.

3. *Single- versus Dual-Channel Recorder.* In establishing a clinical ENG laboratory, one must decide whether to install a single- or dual-channel unit. Unfortunately, there is no clear answer. The *advantages* of a two-channel recorder over a one-channel recorder are:

1. Vertical eye movements can be recorded. As will be discussed, a vertical eye-movement channel occasionally reveals paroxysmal nystagmus that otherwise would be missed, and also, vertical ocular abnormalities may be important signs of central nervous system (CNS) pathology.
2. The vertical channel helps to detect eye blinks in the horizontal channel.
3. The second channel provides a backup channel so that the ENG lab need not shut down if one channel develops difficulties.
4. If the recorder has modular preamplifiers, the second channel can be used as a "velocity" channel which, in theory, provides a semi-automatic computation of nystagmus intensity.

The major *disadvantage* of the dual-channel recorder is that it costs about twice as much as a single-channel recorder. An additional minor disadvantage is that the dual-channel recorder is somewhat larger than the single-channel recorder (approximately 17 inches wide versus 10 inches wide).

III.   TEST PROCEDURE AND SIGNIFICANCE OF ABNORMAL FINDINGS

A.   General Clinical Significance

The ENG examination may help differentiate between pathology involving the peripheral vestibular system and that involving the central nervous system. We define the division between "peripheral" and "central" as the point at which the VIIIth nerve enters the brainstem (Reger, 1972). Electronystagmography is thus analogous to audiometry. The basic significance of both tests is their ability to localize pathology anatomically. Audiometry, however, provides more refined localization because it can separate nerve from end-organ lesions, whereas the ENG examination described herein cannot. Several ENG findings indicate pathology but do not distinguish between a peripheral and central location. I refer to this category of ENG abnormalities as "nonlocalizing."

In the remainder of this section, I shall discuss, in turn, each of the tests comprising the ENG examination. The discussion will include a description of each test's abnormal findings and the diagnostic significance of these findings.

B. Ocular-dysmetria Test

Ocular dysmetria is an over- or undershoot of the ocular rotation that occurs when visual fixation is transferred from one place to another (a "refixation movement" or "saccade"). Ocular dysmetria is thought to originate in the cerebellum (Cogan, 1954; Higgins and Daroff, 1966; Orzechowski, 1927), but in practical clinical application it should probably be considered indicative of either cerebellar or brainstem pathology.[4]

Because of the fleeting nature and small amplitude of the dysmetric ocular movement, obtaining a graphic record of it has obvious advantages. Noorden and Preziosi (1966), Ellenberger *et al.* (1972), and Haring and Simmons (1973) have published records of ocular dysmetria. Haring and Simmons point out that ocular dysmetria may be recorded in the course of the routine ENG calibration ("calibration overshoot"). Thus, a valuable central sign may be detected during the ENG examination with virtually no investment of additional examination time.

Most normal subjects demonstrate an occasional overshoot during the ENG calibration. Therefore, when inspecting the record for ocular dysmetria, one must have in mind some criterion for "limit of normal." Haring and Simmons (1973) require that 50% of the calibrations be overshot before ocular dysmetria is diagnosed. However, this criterion is based on an intuitive clinical impression. A systematic normative study would greatly enhance the clinical usefulness of the ocular-dysmetria test.

When inspecting the calibration record for ocular dysmetria, one must also keep in mind that eye-blink artifacts, which are often synchronized with the refixation movement, may produce a very good imitation of an overshoot. Since the vertical channel will register the eye blink but not the overshoot, it helps to distinguish between true and artifactual overshoots. If a vertical channel is not available, the examiner must observe

---

[4] Lesions involving the cerebellum (whether vascular or neoplastic) so frequently involve brainstem structures as well, that, when localizing central lesions, several authors (Coats, 1970; Daroff and Hoyt, 1971) group the cerebellum and brainstem together.

the patient's eyes during the calibration and record the occurrence of
eye blinks.

C. Gaze Test

Nystagmus may not be present with the eyes centered, but it may appear when they are deviated from center. The gaze test examines for
such a "gaze nystagmus"; it also examines for paresis of ocular deviation.

When present, gaze nystagmus almost always demonstrates the following characteristics: (1) It is divided into slow and fast phases, with the
fast phase in the direction of eye deviation; (2) its intensity (amplitude
and possibly slow-phase speed) increases with increasing eye deviation.
Congenital nystagmus (discussed later) presents the most notable exception to these characteristics.

1. *Technique.* Compared to the routine physical examination, the
gaze test done in the ENG laboratory usually incorporates the following
refinements: (1) The amount of eye rotation is quantitatively controlled;
and (2) the eye movements are recorded. The gaze test is done immediately after the calibration, while the patient is still in front of the fixation
points (Figure 3). The patient gazes steadily at the 20° and 30° fixation
points to right and left and above and below center. Gaze is maintained
for 30 sec in each of the eight eye positions.

Gaze nystagmus may be present but not recorded, either because its
amplitude is too low or because it is rotary. Also, paretic eye movements
may be easier to observe visually than to record. Therefore, during the
gaze test, it is very important to observe the patient's eyes visually as well
as to record their movements.

2. *Diagnostic Significance of Gaze Abnormalities.* With certain exceptions (discussed later), gaze nystagmus and gaze paresis indicate the
presence of CNS pathology. Particularly if persistent for a month or more,
these findings further suggest brainstem involvement (Daroff and Hoyt,
1971; Dow and Manni, 1964). (See footnote 4, p. 47.)

I have found the slightly modified Kestenbaum (1961) classification,
shown in Table II, to be useful in sorting out the localizing and etiologic
significance of gaze nystagmus. Figures 7 and 8 illustrate the different
types of abnormal gaze nystagmus. The significance of each type of gaze
nystagmus will be discussed.

(a) *End-point nystagmus* (Aschan *et al.*, 1957a; Kestenbaum, 1961;
Walsh and Hoyt, 1969). To my knowledge, there has been no systematic, quantitative study of end-point nystagmus. According to Aschan *et
al.* (1957a), "Gaze nystagmus [at] 20°–30° or less . . . should probably
be regarded as pathological." In Bloomberg's (1955) series of 100 normal

TABLE II

CLASSIFICATION OF GAZE NYSTAGMUS

I. Normal
   "End-point" or "end-position" nystagmus: a nystagmus which appears on
      extreme gaze (40° or more, rarely at 30°) in a large percentage of normals
II. Abnormal
   A. Vertical: present on up and/or down gaze (Figure 10)
   B. Horizontal (Figure 8)
      1. Bilateral, equal: nystagmus of approximately equal amplitude and
         frequency in both directions
      2. Bilateral, unequal: nystagmus of clearly unequal amplitudes in the
         two directions
      3. Unilateral: nystagmus present only in one direction of gaze

---

subjects, nystagmus was never present at "about 45°" from center. Our
experience supports these opinions; hence, we set gaze deviations at 20°
and 30° from center.

(*b*) *Vertical gaze nystagmus* (Figure 7). Vertical gaze nystagmus
indicates CNS pathology, probably involving the brainstem. Upward
vertical gaze nystagmus is much more common than downward vertical
gaze nystagmus. When vertical gaze nystagmus appears without associ-

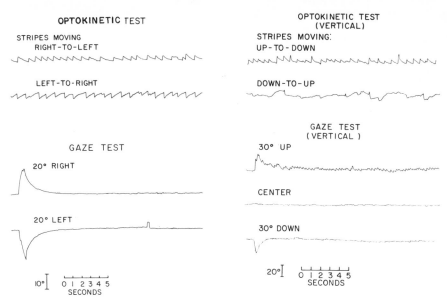

Figure 7 Gaze and OKN tests, demonstrating large vertical and minimal horizontal
abnormalities. The patient was a 55-year-old man with a large intrinsic glioma involving pons and possibly midbrain.

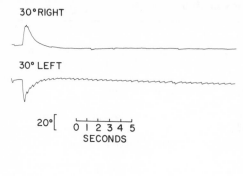

Figure 8 Examples of unilateral (top) and bilateral, unequal (bottom) horizontal gaze nystagmus. The patient with unilateral left horizontal gaze nystagmus had an acoustic neuroma on the left, approximately 2.5–3.0 cm in diameter. The patient with bilateral, unequal gaze nystagmus had an intrinsic pontine glioma.

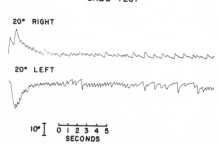

ated horizontal gaze nystagmus, it suggests either a midline or bilateral lesion in the upper pons or midbrain (Daroff and Hoyt, 1971; Kestenbaum, 1961).

(*c*) *Bilateral, equal horizontal gaze nystagmus.* As with other forms of gaze nystagmus, bilateral, equal horizontal gaze nystagmus indicates CNS pathology, probably involving the brainstem. However, when this form of gaze nystagmus appears as an isolated sign, one must rule out drug effects, particularly barbiturates (Bergman *et al.*, 1951), diphenylhydantoin (Dilantin) (Kutt *et al.*, 1964), and alcohol (Aschan, 1958).

(*d*) *Bilateral, unequal horizontal gaze nystagmus* (Figure 8, top). Since drug effects rarely produce asymmetrical abnormalities, bilateral, unequal gaze nystagmus argues against drug toxicity. Hence, this type of gaze nystagmus strongly suggests organic CNS pathology.

(*e*) *Unilateral horizontal gaze nystagmus* (Figure 8, bottom). A unilateral horizontal gaze nystagmus cannot be considered a central sign until one has ruled out the possibility that it is a manifestation of an intense vestibular spontaneous nystagmus. Visual fixation may suppress a spontaneous nystagmus so that it is not present with the eyes centered. However, deviating the eyes toward the fast phase may sufficiently enhance the nystagmus that it "breaks through" the visual fixation suppression and becomes visible.

The most straightforward way to determine if a unilateral horizontal gaze nystagmus is due to a vestibular spontaneous nystagmus is to have the patient close his eyes. If, on eye closure, there appears a spontaneous nystagmus in the same direction as the gaze nystagmus, with slow-phase speed greater than 8° per sec, then the gaze nystagmus is not a central sign (Coats, 1970).

D. Sinusoidal Tracking Test

1. Technique. The sinusoidal tracking test is done by having the patient fixate on a spot which is moving in a sinusoidal pattern (Benitez, 1970; Jung and Kornhuber, 1964; Ohm, 1940). We test with frequencies of 0.3 and 0.6 Hz, and the pattern subtends an angle of ±20° from center gaze. We obtain tracking movements in both the vertical and horizontal directions.

2. Clinical Significance. A normal individual should be able to track the pattern smoothly, although brief fixations on other objects may occasionally interrupt the smooth sinusoidal pattern. In the generally recognized abnormal sinusoidal tracking pattern, saccadic eye jerks in the direction of spot movement repeatedly "break up" the smooth sinusoidal pattern. Figure 9 illustrates these normal and abnormal patterns.

I have encountered an additional helpful abnormal sinusoidal tracking pattern—a tendency for gaze nystagmus to appear in an enhanced form at the extremes of the sinusoidal pattern. Figure 10 shows this pattern in a patient with an up-beating vertical gaze nystagmus. Often, the sinusoidal tracking abnormality combines the enhanced gaze nystagmus and "breakup" patterns.

The sinusoidal tracking test has been part of our routine ENG examination for only about 6 months. Our experience thus far supports the findings of Benitez (1970) and Jung and Kornhuber (1964) that (*1*) abnormal sinusoidal tracking occurs in central oculomotor lesions, usually involving the brainstem, (*2*) it is usually associated with gaze nystagmus and bilateral optokinetic diminution (see below), and (*3*) barbiturate sedation may cause it.

E. Spontaneous Nystagmus

1. Definition and Test Procedure. Spontaneous nystagmus is a nystagmus that is present in the absence of any known nystagmogenic stimulus. Assumption of a nonneutral position (positional nystagmus)

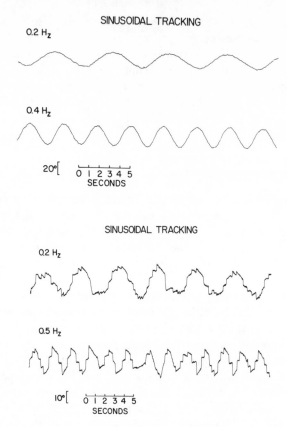

Figure 9 Sinusoidal tracking test, demonstrating normal smooth-pursuit movements (top) and abnormal "breakup" of smooth-pursuit movements in a patient with amyotrophic lateral sclerosis (bottom).

and deviating the eyes from center (gaze nystagmus) may be considered nystagmogenic stimuli. Therefore, I somewhat arbitrarily define spontaneous nystagmus as a nystagmus present in the head upright position (the best approximation of the "neutral" head position in the human) and with eyes centered.

We record spontaneous nystagmus while doing the gaze test. In addition to the eyes-deviated positions just listed, we record vertical and horizontal eye movements with the eyes centered for 30 sec to 1 min, first open and then closed. Since the patient's head is upright during the gaze test, this eyes-centered recording fulfills both criteria of spontaneous nystagmus.

2. *Clinical Significance.* I have found it useful to classify pathological spontaneous nystagmus according to its probable system of origin,

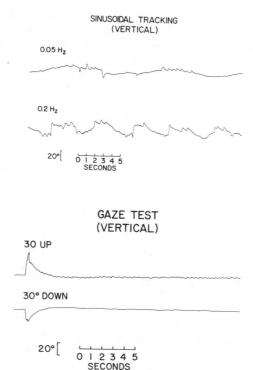

Figure 10 Vertical gaze and sinusoidal tracking tests, demonstrating "enhancement" of a vertical gaze nystagmus at the upward extreme of the sinusoidal tracking pattern.

i.e., *vestibular, ocular,* or *central*. This classification is analogous to Cogan's (1956) "otologic," "ocular," and "neurologic" divisions. Others have proposed similar classifications (Toglia and Moreno, 1971). My classification includes a fourth *normal* category not included in other classifications of spontaneous nystagmus. Table III summarizes my classifications. Each type of spontaneous nystagmus is discussed below in detail.

(*a*) *Normal spontaneous nystagmus with eyes closed.* (*1*) *Vertical.* Behind closed eyelids, a vertical, jerk-type nystagmus, usually up-beating, is present in about 80% of normal subjects (Fluur and Eriksson, 1961) and may be rather intense, i.e., slow-phase speed greater than 10° per sec.

(*2*) *Horizontal.* Although it is generally agreed that vertical spontaneous nystagmus behind closed eyelids occurs in normal persons, similar agreement about the presence of normal horizontal spontaneous nystagmus has not been reached. Although there were dissenters, most early investigators of clinical ENG reported (or implicitly assumed) that horizontal nystagmus present without visual fixation has the same clinical significance as spontaneous nystagmus present with visual fixation; i.e., it is always abnormal (see, for example, Aschan *et al.,* 1956a). However,

TABLE III

I. Normal
    Vertical, behind closed eyelids
    Horizontal, behind closed eyelids   7–8°/sec
    Voluntary
II. Vestibular (otologic)
    Fast and slow phases
    Horizontal
    Conjugate
    Suppressed by visual fixation
III. Ocular (ophthalmologic)
    Congenital
    Occupational
IV. Central (neurologic)
    Diagnosis made by excluding other types

considerable evidence has accumulated recently which supports the existence of a low-intensity horizontal spontaneous (or positional) nystagmus in 15–30% of otologically normal subjects (Barber and Wright, 1973; Bos *et al.*, 1963; Coats, 1969; Collins *et al.*, 1973; Fluur and Eriksson, 1961; Lansberg, 1962; Spector, 1971; Visser, 1962). The slow-component speed of this nystagmus is usually less than 7° per sec (Coats, 1969).

(*b*) *Normal spontaneous nystagmus with eyes open.* "Voluntary nystagmus" is the only known normal "spontaneous" nystagmus present with eyes open and fixed. Figure 11 (top) shows an example of voluntary nystagmus. It is a pendular (no division into fast and slow phases), conjugate, extremely rapid (3–15 oscillations per sec), small-amplitude nystagmus which is initiated and maintained by voluntary effort (Blair *et al.*, 1967; Lipman, 1972; Rosenblum and Shafer, 1966). Several reports indicate that voluntary nystagmus is rare (Rosenblum and Shafer, 1966; Walsh and Hoyt, 1969). However, my experience agrees with that of Blair *et al.* (1967), that voluntary nystagmus is relatively common.

The main clinical importance of voluntary nystagmus is that it could be mistaken for convergence nystagmus, which is a pathological nystagmus of dorsal midbrain origin. However, convergence nystagmus is a coarse, jerk-type, dysconjugate nystagmus (Figure 11, bottom). Once familiar with both types of nystagmus, one cannot possibly confuse them.

(*c*) *Vestibular (otologic) spontaneous nystagmus.* To be considered vestibular, a spontaneous nystagmus must have the following characteristics (Jung and Kornhuber, 1964):

1. divided into fast and slow phases ("jerk type");
2. horizontal or primarily horizontal (rotary component);
3. conjugate (both eyes move together);[5]
4. suppressed by visual fixation.

Figure 12 contrasts a vestibular spontaneous nystagmus with a central spontaneous nystagmus.

Vestibular spontaneous nystagmus, particularly if it is intense, is usually caused by a peripheral vestibular lesion (Coats, 1970). However, occasionally it may be caused by a central lesion which is localized to the vicinity of the vestibular nuclear complex on one side (Jung and Korn-

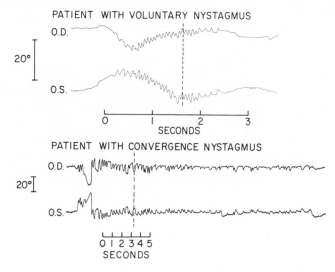

Figure 11 Voluntary nystagmus contrasted with convergence nystagmus. Movements of each eye were recorded individually with electrodes placed lateral to the outer canthus and on the bridge of the nose. Record from right eye (OD) and left eye (OS). The voluntary nystagmus was recorded with higher gain and faster paper speed than usual in standard clinical ENG (gain was 50μV per cm pen deflection; paper speed was 50 mm per sec). The dashed lines on each record connect equal points in time, demonstrating that the voluntary nystagmus is conjugate and the convergence nystagmus is dysconjugate. The patient with convergence nystagmus had a midbrain tumor which narrowed the sylvian aqueduct and displaced it posteriorly. The patient with voluntary nystagmus was referred by a neurologist, with a provisional diagnosis of midbrain tumor, but proved to be completely normal neurologically.

---

[5] This criterion of course does not apply if there is peripheral ocular paresis or paralysis.

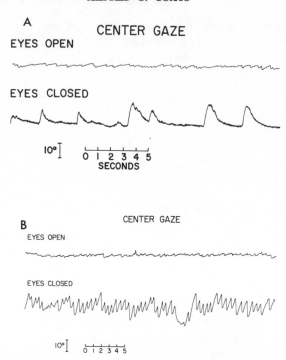

Figure 12 A. Vestibular spontaneous nystagmus in a patient with an acute right peripheral vestibular lesion. B. Central spontaneous nystagmus in a patient with a large right cerebellopontine meningioma. The vestibular and central types of spontaneous nystagmus are distinguishable only by the differing effects of closing the eyes.

huber, 1964; Scala and Spiegel, 1938). Because vestibular spontaneous nystagmus can be due to either peripheral vestibular or CNS pathology, it is a nonlocalizing abnormality.

(*d*) *Ocular (ophthalmologic) spontaneous nystagmus.* A synonymous term for this type of spontaneous nystagmus is "fixation nystagmus" (Jung and Kornhuber, 1964). Congenital nystagmus is by far the commonest type of ocular spontaneous nystagmus. Congenital nystagmus is present from birth or early infancy. It may have a pendular (Figure 13) or "spike-like" (Figure 14) wave form (Aschan and Bergstedt, 1955; Jung and Kornhuber, 1964). The wave form is extremely variable from patient to patient and often changes when fixation distance or direction of gaze is changed (Figures 13 and 14). Eye closure usually either abolishes or changes the direction of congenital nystagmus. It rarely enhances congenital nystagmus as it does vestibular nystagmus.

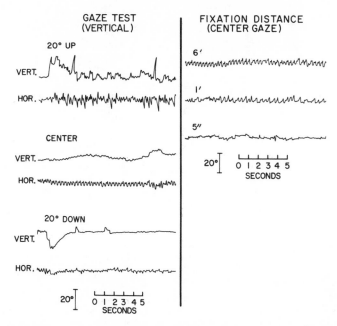

GAZE TEST
(VERTICAL)

FIXATION DISTANCE
(CENTER GAZE)

20° UP

VERT.

HOR.

CENTER

VERT.

HOR.

20° DOWN

VERT.

HOR.

6'

1'

5"

20°⌐ 0 1 2 3 4 5
      SECONDS

20°⌐ 0 1 2 3 4 5
      SECONDS

Figure 13 Effect of vertical gaze and of convergence on congenital nystagmus. On upward gaze, a large-amplitude horizontal pendular nystagmus develops (records at left). The nystagmus is suppressed when the eyes converge (records at right).

A visual abnormality may or may not accompany congenital nystagmus. Many neuro-ophthalmologists separate congenital nystagmus into different clinical types, depending on the presence or absence of a visual abnormality, as, for example, Cogan's (1967) "sensory defect" and "motor defect" types.

Congenital nystagmus may be mistaken for central spontaneous nystagmus, particularly in the patient with normal vision who does not discover his nystagmus until relatively late in life (Cogan, 1967). However, if the following distinctive characteristics of congenital nystagmus (Walsh and Hoyt, 1969) are recognized, it will rarely be mistaken for central nystagmus. (*1*) There is no oscillopsia, in spite of what is often a very large amplitude nystagmus. (*2*) Congenital nystagmus is almost always horizontal (Figures 13 and 14). (*3*) On vertical gaze, a vertical component rarely develops, and a horizontal pendular component may frequently appear (Figure 13). (*4*) Convergence usually suppresses congenital nystagmus (Figure 13).

In the presence of congenital nystagmus, both optokinetic and vestibu-

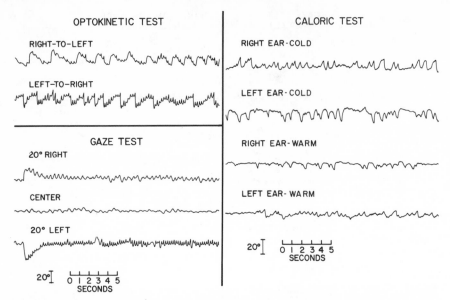

Figure 14 Gaze, OKN, and caloric tests of a patient with congenital nystagmus and essentially normal near vision. Records demonstrate severe disruption of the caloric and optokinetic responses, and change of nystagmus form with change in gaze direction ("pendular" form on right-lateral gaze and "spike-like" form on left-lateral gaze).

lar nystagmus are notoriously difficult to elicit, and even when elicited, they may be so grossly distorted as to preclude quantitation (Figure 14). The distortion of caloric responses makes quantitative vestibular-function assessment impossible in many congenital-nystagmus patients.

Noncongenital forms of ocular nystagmus are always associated with some sort of chronic abuse of the visual system. An example is "miner's nystagmus," which appears late in life in mine workers who have spent much of their lives in a dimly lit environment.

(*e*) *Central (neurologic) spontaneous nystagmus.* One concludes that a spontaneous nystagmus is of central origin by a process of exclusion. If the spontaneous nystagmus fails to meet one or more of the criteria of a vestibular type, and an ocular nystagmus has been ruled out as outlined above, then the nystagmus must be central. A central spontaneous nystagmus usually indicates a brainstem or cerebellar lesion (Jung and Kornhuber, 1964). Figure 12 illustrates a central spontaneous nystagmus which could be distinguished from vestibular spontaneous nystagmus only by observing the effect of eye closure on the nystagmus.

F. Optokinetic Test

Optokinetic nystagmus (OKN) occurs when one looks at a moving repetitive pattern (black stripes on a white background are usually used clinically) which fills most or all of the visual field. OKN has slow (following) phases in the direction of pattern movement and fast (refixation) phases opposite to the direction of pattern movement. Optokinetic nystagmus is probably involuntary if fixation on the moving pattern is maintained (Cogan, 1956; Smith, 1963). The larger the stimulus pattern, the less the variability in OKN due to voluntary visual-fixation changes.

An abnormal OKN test may be manifested as an *asymmetry* (difference in oppositely directed OKN in spite of equal stimulus speeds) or as a *bilateral diminution*. The OKN test is one of the more sensitive tests for central oculomotor pathology (Coats, 1970; Jung and Kornhuber, 1964).

1. Instrumentation and Test Technique. The OKN test is usually done with a hand-operated drum (Figure 15A). In order to fill the patient's visual field, some laboratories use a large, internally lighted cylinder which is lowered over the patient's head (Figure 15B). In our laboratory, a film-loop projector is used to evoke OKN (Figure 15C). This instrument is small and lightweight, yet its stimulus pattern fills most of the patient's visual field. Unlike the large cylinder, it can be used to evoke vertical OKN and allows rapid exchange of various stimulus patterns (including "sinusoidal tracking").

Basically, the clinical OKN test consists of eliciting nystagmus in opposite directions at the same stimulus speed. In the normal routine neurological examination, OKN is elicited only by two brief, oppositely directed horizontal stimuli. However, many ENG laboratories add the following to this basic test.

(a) Vertical OKN. Although early OKN studies involved only the horizontal response, the importance of vertical OKN testing has been emphasized recently (Coats, 1970; Jung and Kornhuber, 1964; Rosborg *et al.*, 1972; Smith, 1962). One reason for this emphasis is that if vertical OKN is excluded, a significant number of abnormalities will be missed. For example, in a recently reported large series of OKN tests (without ENG), one-fourth of the asymmetries were only in the vertical direction (Rosborg *et al.*, 1972; Tos *et al.*, 1972). In my experience, even in cases where both horizontal and vertical OKN asymmetries are present, the vertical asymmetry often is severe, whereas the horizontal asymmetry is minimal. (Figure 7 shows an example of this.) In addition, an isolated or predominant vertical OKN abnormality has localizing value, since

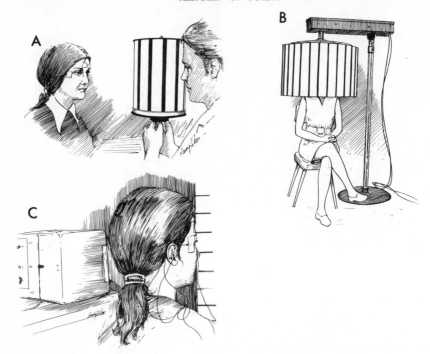

Figure 15 Alternative means of eliciting OKN in the clinical laboratory. A. Hand-held drum. B. Large, internally lighted cylinder, designed to provide a full-field stimulus. C. Film-loop projector (shown turned to provide a vertical OKN stimulus).

it is usually due to a high midbrain lesion (Jung and Kornhuber, 1964; Rosborg *et al.*, 1972; Smith, 1962).

(*b*) *Eliciting OKN at more than one stimulus speed.* OKN asymmetries are usually enhanced when stimulus speed is increased (Jung and Kornhuber, 1964; Susuki and Komatsuaki, 1962). Therefore, eliciting OKN at more than one stimulus speed often clarifies the presence of an asymmetry. Our stimuli are delivered at 15° per sec and 40° per sec "equivalent speeds," the speeds at which the eyes would rotate if they followed the stimulus exactly.

2. *Recognizing OKN Abnormalities.* (*a*) *Bilateral diminution.* Although OKN is involuntary if fixation is maintained, in practice it is under considerable voluntary control because of the patient's ability to influence it by varying fixation (Jung and Kornhuber, 1964; Smith, 1963). Hence, lack of cooperation must always be suspected when bilateral OKN diminution or absence is present.

(*b*) *Asymmetry.* There are two recognizable patterns of OKN asymmetry: (*1*) poorly formed, and (*2*) slow-phase speed. Figure 16

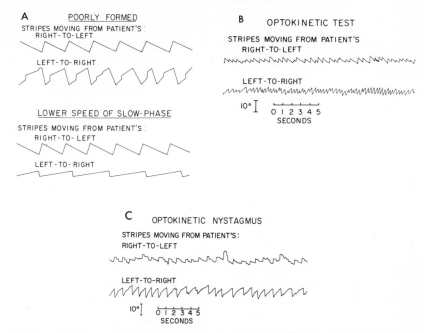

Figure 16 Patterns of OKN asymmetry. A. Diagrammatic representation of the two basic patterns. B. Actual example of slow-phase-speed pattern (left-beating response predominant). C. Actual example of a poorly formed pattern (left-beating response predominant). The patient with poorly formed asymmetry had a very large left acoustic neurinoma which displaced the brainstem and cerebellum medially. "Pure" asymmetries such as these are unusual. Usually, OKN asymmetry is a mixture of both the poorly formed and the slow-phase-speed patterns.

illustrates these two asymmetrical patterns. Both patterns involve the slow phase. In a poorly formed asymmetry, the slow phase is repeatedly broken up by rapid jerks in the same direction as the slow phase. This pattern is reminiscent of the breakup of smooth pursuit demonstrated by the sinusoidal tracking test, and may be due to the same pathophysiological mechanism (Jung and Kornhuber, 1964). Usually, an OKN asymmetry presents as a combination of the two patterns, and a slow-phase-speed asymmetry can often be converted into a poorly formed asymmetry by increasing stimulus speed.

(c) *Importance of conservatism in interpreting OKN abnormalities.* It is very important that OKN abnormalities be clearly present before being considered significant (Coats, 1970; Smith, 1963). We require abnormalities to be present at both stimulus speeds. If there is any doubt about an abnormality, we repeat the stimulus to confirm its presence.

3. *The Clinical Significance of OKN Abnormalities.* (a) *Detection*

of central pathology. If the patient has been cooperative, OKN asymmetry and bilateral diminution usually indicate the presence of CNS pathology. However, intense (greater than 8° per sec) vestibular spontaneous nystagmus can produce an OKN asymmetry with the predominant OKN response in the same direction as the spontaneous nystagmus (Coats, 1968; Jung and Kornhuber, 1964). Therefore, as with unilateral horizontal gaze nystagmus, intense spontaneous nystagmus (observed in darkness or behind closed eyelids) must be ruled out as a potential cause of OKN asymmetry. Peripheral ocular pathology, e.g., strabismus, severe extraocular muscle paresis, and long-standing unilateral blindness, must also be ruled out as a cause of OKN asymmetry (Coats, 1970).

(b) *Localization of central pathology.* (1) *Association with gaze abnormalities (paresis or nystagmus).* OKN abnormalities due to cerebral and brainstem lesions can be distinguished on the basis of associated gaze-test findings. An OKN abnormality due to brainstem or cerebellar pathology is always accompanied by either a gaze nystagmus or a gaze paresis (Coats, 1970; Jung and Kornhuber, 1964). In contrast, an OKN abnormality with a normal gaze test is usually due to a cerebral-hemisphere lesion (Coats, 1970; Cogan and Loeb, 1949; Davidoff *et al.*, 1966; Jung and Kornhuber, 1964).

(2) *Vertical OKN asymmetry.* In contrast to horizontal OKN asymmetry, vertical OKN asymmetry is rarely caused by cerebral-hemisphere pathology, and then only if the pathology is diffuse and severe (Jung and Kornhuber, 1964; Rosborg *et al.*, 1972; Smith, 1962). Therefore, a vertical OKN asymmetry suggests pathology involving the brainstem. An isolated vertical OKN asymmetry further suggests bilateral or midline lesions in the midbrain or upper pons (Jung and Kornhuber, 1964; Rosborg *et al.*, 1972; Smith, 1962).

Precautions must be observed in interpreting the vertical OKN test: (1) A slight vertical OKN asymmetry (down-beating response usually predominant) may be present in some normal subjects (Jung and Kornhuber, 1964). Therefore, if a vertical OKN asymmetry is present as an isolated finding, it must be very large before it can be considered significant. (2) Vertical electrodes record eyelid movements with extreme sensitivity. Therefore, the possibility that an apparent abnormally formed vertical OKN is due to superimposed eye blinks or other eyelid movements must be ruled out.

(3) *Bilaterally absent or deficient OKN.* Provided that failure to fixate on the stimulus has been ruled out, bilaterally absent or deficient OKN (either horizontal or vertical or both) has essentially the same localizing significance as vertical OKN asymmetry; i.e., it suggests a high bilateral or midline brainstem lesion.

(4) *Lateralizing significance of horizontal OKN asymmetry in brain-stem–cerebellar lesions.* In animal experiments, lateral lesions of the pons and midbrain below the level of the oculomotor nucleus cause a predominance of the OKN beating away from the side of the lesion (Teng *et al.*, 1958). A similar OKN asymmetry has been reported in humans with well-localized upper brainstem lesions (Tos *et al.*, 1972). However, in my experience and the experience of most others (Cogan and Loeb, 1949; Daroff and Hoyt, 1971), the lateralizing value of OKN asymmetry in brainstem lesions is poor in the routine clinical situation, probably because the lesion usually is large relative to the size of the structures responsible for the OKN asymmetry.

(5) *Lateralizing significance of horizontal OKN asymmetry in cerebral-hemisphere lesions.* In contrast to brainstem–cerebellar lesions, the lateralizing significance of OKN asymmetry in cerebral-hemisphere lesions is quite good. All reports agree that when a hemisphere lesion produces an OKN asymmetry, the predominant OKN beats toward the side of the lesion, and the lesion probably involves the temporal, parietal, or occipital lobe (Cogan and Loeb, 1949; Smith and Cogan, 1960; Tos *et al.*, 1972).

G. Paroxysmal Nystagmus Test

1. Nomenclature. In 1952, Dix and Hallpike described a maneuver (Figure 17) for eliciting what they termed "positional nystagmus of the benign paroxysmal type." In normal subjects, the Dix–Hallpike maneuver elicits no nystagmus, or possibly only a brief, weak nystagmus behind closed eyelids. However, in patients with certain types of vestibular-

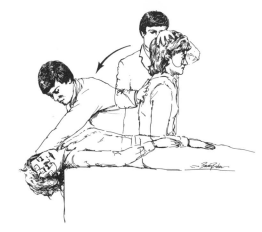

Figure 17 The Dix–Hallpike maneuver for eliciting paroxysmal nystagmus.

system disorders, the maneuver elicits a usually rather intense, transient nystagmic response (Figures 18 and 19).

An important point of nomenclature is whether "positional" should be used when referring to the abnormal nystagmus elicited by the Dix–Hall-pike maneuver. Barany first observed that some patients exhibited dizzi-ness and nystagmus only when they assumed a particular "critical posi-tion" (Barany, 1921; Jongkees, 1961). Later, Nylen devoted many years to systematic clinical study of this phenomenon, which is now termed "positional nystagmus." Nylen (1953) emphasized that positional nys-tagmus is caused only by a particular head position. He therefore stressed

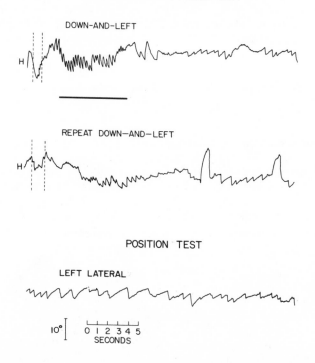

Figure 18 "Classical" paroxysmal nystagmus with oppositely directed positional nystagmus. When the patient was brought rapidly from the sitting to the head-hanging-and-left position, a burst of intense right-beating nystagmus appeared. However, when the patient was moved slowly into the left-lateral position, a per-sistent, moderate, left-beating nystagmus was present (below). After the transient paroxysmal nystagmus disappears, the patient's left-beating positional nystagmus can be seen in the records of the paroxysmal nystagmus test. The solid black bar below the top record indicates approximate duration of dizziness. The dashed lines show the period during which the patient was being moved.

PAROXYSMAL NYSTAGMUS TEST

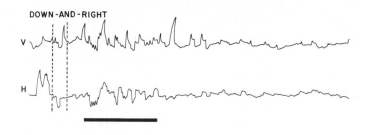

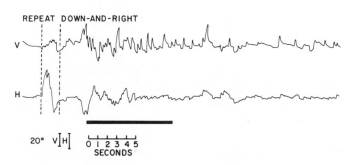

20° V⌊H⌋   0 1 2 3 4 5
            SECONDS

Figure 19 Example of "nonclassical" type of paroxysmal nystagmus. V = vertical eye movements; H = horizontal eye movements. Most of the recordable response is in the vertical direction.

that possible effects of head movement must be excluded by moving the patient as slowly as possible into the test position. However, several other writers advocated moving the patient rapidly into the various test positions, under the assumption that the rapid movement might "provoke" a positional nystagmus which would otherwise be missed (Lindsay, 1951; Williams, 1947). The Dix-Hallpike test evolved from this "rapid-movement" school of position testing.

Several independent observers have demonstrated that, if the Dix–Hallpike maneuver and the standard position test both elicit a nystagmus, the responses are often oppositely directed (Aschan *et al.*, 1957b; Stenger, 1955). Figure 18 shows an example of this. It therefore seems evident that "positional nystagmus of the benign paroxysmal type" is not dependent on the final head position but on the violent maneuver preceding it. Hence, I prefer not to use the word "positional" in describing a positive response to the Dix–Hallpike maneuver.

2. *Test Procedure.* The patient is first seated on the examining table with head straight ahead. He is then rapidly brought backward into the

head-hanging-and-turned position (Figure 17). He is left in this position for 30 sec or, if a nystagmic response appears, for as long as the response persists. If the response persists for more than 1½ min, the test position is terminated and the response considered "persistent." After this maneuver, the patient is brought back to the sitting, eyes-front position, and left there for about 30 sec, and then the maneuver is repeated with the neck twisted in the opposite direction.

If either maneuver produces a nystagmic response, the maneuver is repeated to see if the response is fatigable. If the response does not decrease significantly by the third elicitation, it is declared "nonfatigable."

In the ENG-recorded paroxysmal nystagmus test, the eyes are closed, and the nystagmic response is recorded rather than visually observed. Although paroxysmal nystagmus is usually primarily rotatory, it almost always has sufficient vertical or horizontal components, or both, to be recordable (Preber and Silfverskiöld, 1957; Stahle and Terins, 1965). However, since the vertical component is often predominant (Cawthorne, 1954; Preber and Silfverskiöld, 1957), paroxysmal nystagmus frequently will be missed if vertical eye movements are not recorded. Figure 19 demonstrates a paroxysmal nystagmus which is almost entirely vertical.

3. *Diagnostic Significance.* (a) *"Classical" paroxysmal nystagmus.* Following are the salient features of "positional nystagmus of the benign paroxysmal type" as it was originally described by Dix and Hallpike (1952). Figure 18 shows a typical example.

1. *Latent period.* The nystagmic response does not begin for 0.5–8.0 sec after the patient arrives at the test position.
2. *Transient "paroxysmal" response.* The nystagmus "increases in a rapid crescendo in a period which may be as short as 2–3 seconds, or as long as 10 seconds. Thereafter it rapidly declines." [6]
3. *Dizziness (usually severe).* The paroxysmal nystagmic response is accompanied by dizziness which is often so severe that "the patients may close their eyes, cry out in alarm, and make active efforts to sit up again."
4. *Fatigability.* When the maneuver is repeated, the response either does not reappear or reappears with significantly reduced intensity.

I regard all of the above criteria except latency as essential for designating a paroxysmal nystagmus as "classical." Dix and Hallpike (1952)

---

[6] Dix and Hallpike (1952) did not fix the total duration of the response, but other authors (Aschan *et al.*, 1956a; Lindsay, 1951) mention durations of 20–60 seconds.

originally described the latent period as "nearly always" present, implying that sometimes it was not present. Not infrequently, I encounter paroxysmal nystagmus that clearly fits all criteria of the "classical" type, except that it has no well-defined latent period. Recording the response behind closed eyelids may well reduce or abolish a latent period which would be observed if the nystagmus were suppressed by visual fixation.

The following additional characteristics of classical paroxysmal nystagmus are not essential criteria but are often helpful in classifying doubtful responses: (1) The response is usually unilateral; (2) the nystagmus usually is directed toward the downward ear, which is also the pathological ear; and (3) the caloric and audiometric tests are usually normal.

(b) *Pathophysiological types of "classical" paroxysmal nystagmus.* My experience parallels Schuknecht's (1969), that patients with classical paroxysmal nystagmus tend to cluster into the following rather well-defined clinical types.

1. *Elderly patients* (Lindsay, 1967). A large percentage of patients with classical, positive Dix–Hallpike tests are older than 55 years. Although not life-threatening, paroxysmal nystagmus tends to persist in the elderly.

2. *Posttraumatic dizziness.* Many authors (Barber, 1964; Cawthorne, 1954; Cope and Ryan, 1959; Dix and Hallpike, 1952; Gordon, 1954; Harrison, 1956; Preber and Silfverskiöld, 1957; Schuknecht, 1969) have noted that paroxysmal nystagmus occurs in a large percentage (about 15%, in my experience) of patients complaining of posttraumatic dizziness following head trauma, and is often the only objective abnormal finding. The prognostic implication of paroxysmal nystagmus after head trauma is relatively good, since most of the patients can expect to be symptom-free within 2–6 months.

3. *Middle-ear pathology.* A significant proportion of patients with chronic middle-ear infection who complain of episodic dizziness have classical paroxysmal nystagmus (Barber, 1964; Dix and Hallpike, 1952; Schuknecht, 1969). As Jongkees (1961) has pointed out, when such a patient is encountered, the possibility of a labyrinthine fistula must be ruled out.

4. *Middle-ear surgery.* Classical paroxysmal nystagmus is occasionally encountered after stapes surgery (Barber, 1964; Schuknecht, 1969; Spector, 1961; Terins, 1963). It is probably related to mechanical manipulation of structures in the vestibule. Paroxysmal nystagmus is uncommon following other types of temporal-bone surgery such as mastoidectomy, labyrinthectomy, and tympanoplasty (Schuknecht, 1969).

5. *Rare types.*   An idiopathic "paroxysmal positional vertigo of child-hood" has been described (Chutorian, 1972). Also, Mahmud *et al.* (1970) reported a case of classical paroxysmal nystagmus in pernicious anemia.

(*c*) *Localizing value of paroxysmal nystagmus.*   (*1*) *Classical par-oxysmal nystagmus.*   The pathophysiological mechanism of classical paroxysmal nystagmus has not yet been established (Stahle and Terins, 1965). Although some animal experiments suggest that cerebellar lesions may produce a syndrome resembling paroxysmal nystagmus (Fernandez and Lindsay, 1960), the available clinical evidence argues overwhelm-ingly for a peripheral origin. Therefore, I regard a classical positive Dix–Hallpike test as a peripheral sign.

(*2*) *Nonclassical paroxysmal nystagmus.*   Figure 19 shows an ex-ample of nonclassical paroxysmal nystagmus. Cawthorne (1954) and Harrison (1968) suggested that nonclassical paroxysmal nystagmus indicates CNS pathology. However, in my experience, this finding, al-though more likely to be due to central pathology than is a classical re-sponse, nevertheless is frequently of peripheral origin. I therefore regard a nonclassical positive Dix–Hallpike test as a nonlocalizing sign.

H.   Position Test

1. *Nomenclature.*   The position test explores a series of standard head positions to determine if the patient has positional nystagmus. Unlike the paroxysmal nystagmus test, movement into each position is as slow as possible, to exclude effects of movement.

To permit reasonably concise communication of position-test results, a positional-nystagmus terminology has developed. Although alternate terminologies are used, the following is currently probably the most prevalent (Henriksson *et al.,* 1972).

(*a*) *"Spontaneous" versus "positional" nystagmus.*   (*1*) *Spontaneous nystagmus.*   Any nystagmus present in the head-upright position with eyes centered. (*2*) *Positional nystagmus.*   A nystagmus that is not present with head upright, but is present in one or more other positions. (*3*) *Spontaneous and positional nystagmus.*   A nystagmus present in the head-upright position, but modified either in intensity or direction by assumption of one or more other positions.

(*b*) *Classification of positional nystagmus.*   Most authorities (Barber, 1964; Fernandez and Lindsay, 1960; Jongkees, 1961; Lindsay, 1967) use the Aschan *et al.* (1957a) modification of Nylen's classification, as out-lined in Table IV. Figures 20 and 21 show examples of the persistent

TABLE IV
CLASSIFICATION OF POSITIONAL NYSTAGMUS

I. Persistent—continues for at least 1 min after assuming the test position.
  A. Type I (direction changing)—beats in one direction in one (or more) position(s) and in the opposite direction in other position(s). Figure 20 shows an example.
  B. Type II (direction fixed)—beats in the same direction whenever present. Figure 21 shows an example.
II. Transitory—goes away within 1 min after the test position is assumed. Called "type III positional nystagmus"; also called "positioning" nystagmus.

forms of positional nystagmus (types I and II). Type III includes all varieties of pathological transitory positional nystagmus. A transitory positional nystagmus is usually a partially elicited paroxysmal nystagmus, and some authors (Aschan, 1961) regard type III positional nystagmus and paroxysmal nystagmus as synonymous. However, a small minority of the transient positional responses do not have a typical "paroxysmal" time course; I therefore prefer to replace the term "type III positional nystagmus" with "positioning nystagmus" (Henriksson *et al.*, 1972; Stenger, 1955).

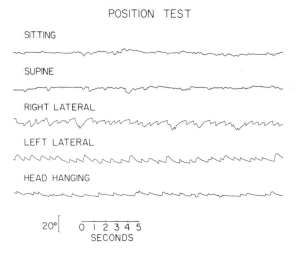

Figure 20 Example of a moderate-to-intense, direction-changing positional nystagmus (left-beating in right-lateral and right-beating in left-lateral and head-hanging positions). The patient was a 65-year-old man with "senility" and presumptive diagnosis of "abnormal cerebral blood flow."

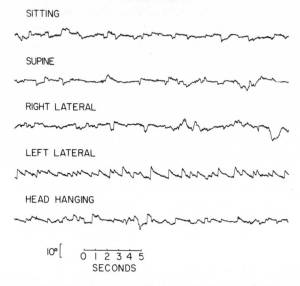

Figure 21 Example of a moderate, direction-fixed positional nystagmus (right-beating in left-lateral position). The patient was a 21-year-old man with sudden left hearing loss 3 weeks before testing. Caloric test showed borderline left unilateral weakness.

2. Position Test Technique. We obtain eyes-closed records of at least 30 sec with the patient in each of the following positions:[7]

1. sitting (patient seated comfortably, facing straight ahead);
2. supine (patient lying on his back, head level with chest);
3. right lateral (patient lying on right side with a pillow under his head so his neck is straight);
4. head right (patient lying on his back with his head turned as far right as possible);
5. left lateral (as with right lateral except lying on left side);
6. head left (as with head right except head turned to the left);
7. head hanging (patient lying on his back with his head as far below the horizontal as possible).

---

[7] Positions (4) and (6) were included to test for possible nystagmogenic neck-twisting effects, e.g., proprioceptive, vascular. However, in some 5000 consecutive patients, I have not found a significant difference between nystagmus in the lateral neck-twisted and neck-straight positions. Possibly a more dynamic testing procedure, such as Jongkees and Philipszoon (1964) describe, is needed to demonstrate pathological "neck-torsion nystagmus."

The patient is moved into each position as slowly as is practicable. Since spontaneous and positional nystagmus are subject to central suppression (discussed with the caloric test), it may be desirable to have the patient perform a concentration task while in each test position. However, this may reduce record quality by introducing voluntary eye movements, muscle potentials, and eye blinks. Therefore, one must use judgment in applying the concentration task to the position test.

3. *Diagnostic Significance of Position Test Results.* (*a*) *"Idiopathic" positional nystagmus.* Idiopathic nystagmus (see previous section) is often seen when the patient is in positions other than sitting, and hence, in such instances, must be called "positional" rather than "spontaneous." As with spontaneous nystagmus, I consider a positional nystagmus with slow-phase speed less than 7° per sec to be idiopathic.

(*b*) *Drugs causing positional nystagmus.* Alcohol, sedatives (particularly barbiturates), and salicylates (quinine and aspirin) may cause direction-changing positional nystagmus (Nylen, 1950). Therefore, when a direction-changing positional nystagmus is encountered as an isolated finding, the possibility of drug ingestion must be ruled out.

The positional nystagmus produced by alcohol (positional alcohol nystagmus, or PAN) is the only drug-induced nystagmus that has been studied extensively with ENG (Aschan *et al.*, 1956b; Hill *et al.*, 1973). Behind closed eyelids, PAN may persist for many hours after all other drug effects have worn off. If other types of drug-induced positional nystagmus demonstrate a similar persistence, then residual drug effects might explain most or even all instances of direction-changing idiopathic positional nystagmus.

(*c*) *Pathologic positional nystagmus (slow-phase speed greater than 7° per sec).* Although some authors report a statistical tendency for direction-changing positional nystagmus to occur in central lesions, and direction-fixed positional nystagmus to occur in peripheral lesions (Henriksson *et al.*, 1972; Nylen, 1950), it is generally agreed that this tendency is not sufficiently strong to be useful clinically (Aschan *et al.*, 1956a; Jongkees, 1961; Jongkees and Philipszoon, 1964; Schiller and Hedberg, 1960). Therefore, positional nystagmus with slow-phase speed over 7° per sec, whether type I or type II, is a nonlocalizing abnormality.

I. Bithermal Caloric Test

Brown–Sequard first described the human caloric response in the latter part of the nineteenth century. However, it was not until Barany's early twentieth-century work that the caloric test found widespread clinical application (Jongkees, 1949). In the 1920–1940 period, variations of

Barany's original technique proliferated (Arslan, 1955; Jongkees, 1949), but the caloric test achieved acceptance among clinical practitioners only as a rather unreliable qualitative procedure.

The hindsight with which we are now able to view this early period suggests that the Barany caloric test was subject to three fundamental weaknesses.

1. A difference between the cold caloric responses could be due to a difference between left- and right-beating nystagmus (which could be the result of either a brain lesion or a peripheral vestibular deficit) or to a difference in the responsiveness of the peripheral labyrinths. The inability of the cold-water caloric test to distinguish between these two possibilities limited its localizing value.
2. Caloric nystagmus could be observed only while suppressed by visual fixation. As a consequence, uncomfortable degrees of caloric stimulation were required to break through this suppression, and even then only a fine, comparatively difficult-to-observe nystagmus was available for analysis.
3. The measurement parameters available with naked-eye observation (latency, duration, and a subjective assessment of nystagmus "vigor") were not optimal.

The ENG-recorded bithermal caloric test overcomes all of the these weaknesses. The use of warm as well as cold caloric stimuli allows nystagmus-direction differences to be distinguished from vestibular-responsiveness differences (Fitzgerald and Hallpike, 1942; Kobrak, 1943; Thornval, 1932). The use of ENG to record the nystagmus allows removal of visual fixation, thus providing a much larger and more easily measured caloric nystagmus (Figure 27, top). Recording the nystagmus also allows measurement of slow-phase speed, which is generally acknowledged to provide a more accurate assessment of nystagmus intensity than any parameter measurable by direct visual observation (see discussion, following).

1. *Test Technique.* The bithermal caloric test consists essentially of obtaining cold and warm caloric responses from each ear, with the temperatures equally above and below body temperature (Fitzgerald and Hallpike, 1942). Figure 22 illustrates a caloric irrigation. The patient is supine, with head inclined 30°, to bring the horizontal canal into the vertical position. In our laboratory, each ear is irrigated for 40 sec at temperatures of 31°C and 43°C.[8] A rest period of at least 5 min is al-

---

[8] The technique as originally described (Fitzgerald and Hallpike, 1942) used temperatures of 30°C and 44°C and was intended for use with eyes open and fixed.

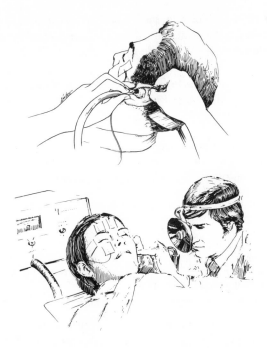

Figure 22 Performing the caloric irrigation. Dual constant-temperature reservoirs can be seen behind the patient. The outlet is controlled by a footswitch-operated timer. The tubing leading to the subject's ear is insulated with foam rubber. Note the use of a head lamp to visualize the position of the irrigating tube in the ear canal. The top drawing shows technician's view of inserted tube. A catch basin, normally placed under the patient's ear, is not shown.

lowed between the disappearance of one caloric response and the beginning of the next irrigation.

In order to minimize central suppression of the caloric responses (Barber and Wright, 1967; Coats, 1966), the patient is instructed to perform aloud a "concentration task," e.g., subtracting serial sevens, during each

---

With eyes open and fixed, 40-sec irrigations at temperatures of 30°C and 44°C were thought to be "minimal" stimuli. However, when later investigations of the test were done with eyes closed, it quickly became apparent that the stimulus was, in fact, rather intense. Aschan (1955) recognized the necessity of reducing stimulus intensity and chose to reduce duration rather than the difference between body and irrigation temperatures. Our preliminary studies suggest that reducing duration increases the response variability, whereas reducing temperature difference (within certain limits) does not. Therefore, we prefer to reduce temperature difference rather than duration.

response. The difficulty of the task is adjusted to match the patient's ability. Because of the possibility of large fluctuations in corneoretinal-potential amplitude (Figure 4), we repeat the amplitude calibration before each irrigation.

2. *Quantifying the Caloric Test.* (a) *Which is the "best" measurement of caloric-response magnitude?* Table V lists the various caloric-

TABLE V

ALTERNATIVE MEASUREMENTS OF CALORIC-RESPONSE MAGNITUDE

  I. Response duration—time elapsed from first beat to last beat
 II. Total response magnitude
    A. Total number of beats during response
    B. Total amplitude (sum of the amplitudes of all beats occurring during the response)
III. Maximum response magnitude
    A. Maximum amplitude
    B. Maximum frequency
    C. Maximum slow-component speed

---

response measurements proposed by different writers. It is generally agreed that maximum speed of slow component (SSC) is a better measure of caloric-response magnitude than duration because:

1. Maximum SSC correlates better with stimulus intensity (Aschan, 1955; Henriksson, 1956), probably because the temperature-change time course, rather than the end-organ response, is the primary determinant of caloric-response duration (Cawthorne and Cobb, 1954; Ishiyama and Keels, 1970).

2. In patients with unilateral sensorineural hearing loss, maximum SSC demonstrates vestibular pathology much more often than does caloric-response duration (Fodor, 1968; Henriksson, 1956; Jongkees and Philipszoon, 1964; Koch *et al.*, 1959; Stahle and Bergman, 1967).

The other caloric-response measurements are not as unequivocally inferior to SSC (Gulick and Pfaltz, 1964; Stahle, 1958; Torok, 1969) as is duration. However, the other measurements have not been studied as extensively as the SSC has been.

Convenience is the main argument for the various alternatives to maximum SSC. However, this argument's force is reduced by the availability of "shortcut" hand measurements (see the following), differentiator or "velocity" channels (Henriksson, 1956), and a recently developed instrument which automatically calculates and digitally displays maximum caloric SSC (Coats and Black, 1973).

(*b*) *Determining maximum caloric-response SSC.* The most direct way of determining SSC is to measure its amplitude and duration, and divide duration into amplitude. In terms of the record's appearance, this determines slow-phase *steepness* or *slope*.[9] Figure 23 illustrates "exact" and approximate (shortcut) methods of determining SSC. The effect of random slow-phase-speed fluctuations is minimized by averaging SSCs across several beats (at least ten, in our laboratory). The approximate measurements may occasionally yield false–negative results (Henriksson, 1956). Therefore, a borderline-significant difference in caloric responses obtained by an approximate measurement may prove significant if the responses are remeasured the "exact" way.

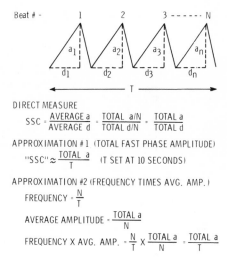

Figure 23 Exact and approximate methods of determining slow-phase speed. *N* beats occur during the period over which the average is obtained. The two approximate methods yield essentially the same result.

DIRECT MEASURE

$$SSC = \frac{AVERAGE\ a}{AVERAGE\ d} = \frac{TOTAL\ a/N}{TOTAL\ d/N} = \frac{TOTAL\ a}{TOTAL\ d}$$

APPROXIMATION # 1 (TOTAL FAST PHASE AMPLITUDE)

$$"SSC" \approx \frac{TOTAL\ a}{T} \quad (T\ SET\ AT\ 10\ SECONDS)$$

APPROXIMATION #2 (FREQUENCY TIMES AVG. AMP.)

$$FREQUENCY = \frac{N}{T}$$

$$AVERAGE\ AMPLITUDE = \frac{TOTAL\ a}{N}$$

$$FREQUENCY\ X\ AVG.\ AMP. = \frac{N}{T} \ X \ \frac{TOTAL\ a}{N} = \frac{TOTAL\ a}{T}$$

(*c*) *Measuring caloric unilateral weakness and directional preponderance.* Caloric-nystagmus SSCs cannot be used directly to evaluate the vestibular system, because absolute values in normals vary widely (Aschan *et al.*, 1956a; Jongkees, 1948; Jung and Kornhuber, 1964; Stahle, 1958). Therefore, comparative measurements are used (Jongkees, 1948). Two comparisons are made: (*1*) a comparison of the responses from the right versus the left ear (unilateral weakness or canal paresis), and (*2*) a comparison of right- versus left-beating nystagmus (directional preponderance). Figure 24 shows a left unilateral weakness, and Figure 25 shows a directional preponderance to the left.

---

[9] Protractor-like instruments have been proposed to directly measure slow-phase slopes but in my experience such instruments save less time than might be supposed, and yield relatively inaccurate results.

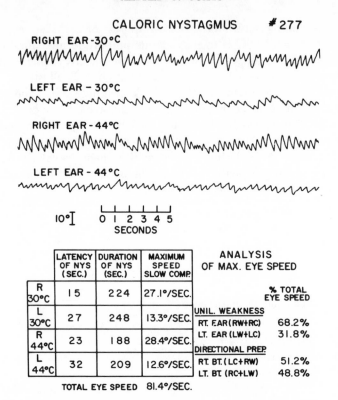

Figure 24 Caloric test, showing a unilateral weakness on the left. The large difference between ears shown by the maximum slow-phase speeds (right-hand column in box at bottom) was not demonstrated by caloric-response duration (time from first to last beat). The patient was a 59-year-old man with intermittent dizziness and severe sensorineural hearing loss on the left.

Absolute differences between ears and between right- and left-beating responses become more variable as the responses become more intense (Jongkees and Philipszoon, 1964). Therefore, we express unilateral weakness and directional preponderance in *relative* terms, i.e., as a percentage of the total of all four response intensities. Thus, caloric unilateral weakness (UW) and directional preponderance (DP) are calculated by equations (1) and (2), respectively (Coats, 1965; Jongkees and Philipszoon, 1964):

$$(1) \quad UW = \frac{\text{Response from right ear} - \text{Response from left ear}}{\text{Total of all four responses}} \times 100$$

$$= \frac{(RC + RW) - (LC + LW)}{RC + LC + RW + LW} \times 100$$

$$(2) \quad DP = \frac{\text{Right-beating response} - \text{Left-beating response}}{\text{Total of all four responses}} \times 100$$

$$= \frac{(LC + RW) - (RC + LW)}{RC + LC + RW + LW} \times 100$$

Where

RC = Maximum SSC of right–cold response
LC = Maximum SSC of left–cold response
RW = Maximum SSC of right–warm response
LW = Maximum SSC of left–warm response

3. *Normal Limits of Caloric-Test Results.* (*a*) *Unilateral weakness* (*UW*) *and directional preponderance* (*DP*). Table VI summarizes the

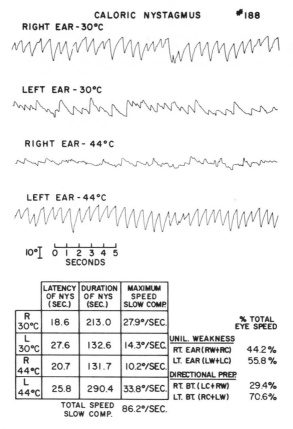

Figure 25 Caloric test showing a relatively large directional preponderance to the left. The patient was a 75-year-old woman with moderate left sensorineural hearing loss, tinnitus, and occasional episodes of dizziness.

TABLE VI
STANDARD DEVIATIONS OF NORMAL CALORIC UW AND DP
(MEASURED BY MAXIMUM SLOW-COMPONENT SPEEDS)

Reference and methods	Unilateral weakness	Directional preponderance
Aschan *et al.* (1956a). 30-sec irrigations at 30°C and 44°C, eyes closed. 25 subjects, 25–50 years old.	8.6%	8.8%
Henriksson (1956). 40-sec irrigations at 30°C and 43.6°C, in dark. 25 subjects, 19–45 years old.	9.5%	8.5%
Jongkees *et al.* (1962). 30-sec irrigations at 30°C and 44°C, eyes closed. 47 subjects.	7.5%	8.7%
Preber (1958). 40-sec irrigations at 30°C and 44°C, eyes closed. 50 subjects.	5.3%	5.8%
Coats (1965). 40-sec irrigations at 30°C and 44°C, eyes closed. 30 subjects.	9.5%	13.2%
Brookler and Pulec (1970). 30-sec irrigations at 30°C and 44°C, eyes closed. 839 "patients without neuro-otologic disease."	11.5%[a]	13.5%[a]

[a] Measured by the author from frequency-distribution curves.

results of six independent normal bithermal caloric-test series. In each series, UW and DP were calculated according to equations (1) and (2).

UW standard deviations vary from 5.3% to 11.5%. It is standard practice to set the normal limit of a quantitative clinical test at twice the standard deviation. In our laboratory, the normal limit of UW is set at 20%, thus assuming a "true" standard deviation of 10%.

In all but one of the normal series (Henriksson, 1956), DP was more variable than UW. DP's greater variability makes its normal limit less well-defined than that of UW. Further complicating the determination of DP's normal limit is the possible existence of a "physiologic" DP in some normals (Coats, 1966, 1969; Hallpike *et al.*, 1951; Jongkees *et al.*, 1962). In our laboratory, a DP of 20–30% is regarded as "questionably" pathologic; a DP greater than 30% is considered pathological.

(*b*) *Bilateral weakness (BW)*. Although absolute maximum SSCs vary widely in normals, it is a general clinical impression that a very weak (or absent) caloric response from both labyrinths is abnormal. Some difficulty arises, however, when one attempts to define "very weak," because normative data on absolute values of maximum caloric SSC are scanty. Preber (1958) found a mean normal maximum SSC of about 22° per sec and a standard deviation (S) of about 6° per sec. Subtracting 2S from the mean SSC would give a lower limit of 10° per sec. Henriksson

(1956) found comparable values of 29° per sec and 11° per sec, giving a lower limit of 7° per sec. My present criterion for BW is a caloric test with average responses from each ear of less than 7.5° per sec. Figure 26 shows a caloric test demonstrating BW.

(*c*) *Failure of fixation suppression (FFS)*. In normal individuals, visual fixation either suppresses or abolishes caloric nystagmus. Several

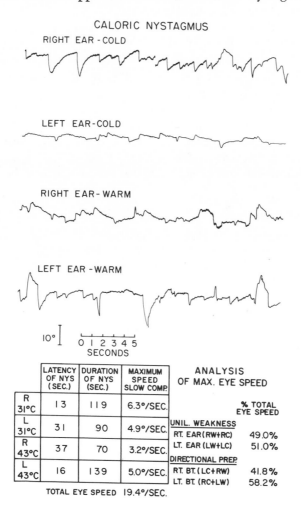

	LATENCY OF NYS (SEC.)	DURATION OF NYS (SEC.)	MAXIMUM SPEED SLOW COMP.	ANALYSIS OF MAX. EYE SPEED	
R 31°C	13	119	6.3°/SEC.		% TOTAL EYE SPEED
L 31°C	31	90	4.9°/SEC.	UNIL. WEAKNESS RT. EAR(RW+RC)	49.0%
R 43°C	37	70	3.2°/SEC.	LT. EAR (LW+LC)	51.0%
L 43°C	16	139	5.0°/SEC.	DIRECTIONAL PREP. RT. BT. (LC+RW)	41.8%
				LT. BT. (RC+LW)	58.2%

TOTAL EYE SPEED 19.4°/SEC.

Figure 26 Caloric test, showing bilateral weakness in a patient with possible streptomycin toxicity. The average response from each ear is less than 7.5° per sec. For example, the average response from the right ear is:

$$\frac{RC+RW}{2} = \frac{6.3+3.2}{2} = 4.8° \text{ per sec.}$$

reports suggest that failure to suppress caloric nystagmus with visual fixation is a pathological sign, indicating CNS pathology (Hart, 1967; Maccario *et al.*, 1972; Naito *et al.*, 1963; Preber and Silfverskiöld, 1960). I termed this sign "failure of fixation suppression" (FFS) and defined it as "SSC with eyes open and fixed as great or greater than with eyes closed" (Coats, 1970). Figure 27 contrasts FFS with the normal effect of visual suppression on caloric nystagmus.

Quantifying the amount of fixation suppression may provide a more sensitive test (Demanez and Ledoux, 1970). Our own investigation suggests that (1) slow-phase speed is the best nystagmus parameter to quantify FFS, and (2) suppression of SSC by 20% or less is abnormal (Alpert and Coats, in preparation).

4. *Diagnostic Significance of Caloric-Test Results.* (a) *Unilateral weakness.* A caloric UW can only be caused by a lesion of the vestibular end-organ or the primary vestibular nerve fibers. It is therefore a *peripheral* finding (Aschan, 1955; Aschan *et al.*, 1957b; Jongkees, 1948; Jung and Kornhuber, 1964; Stahle, 1958). We should note here that the

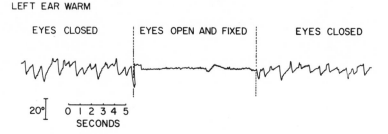

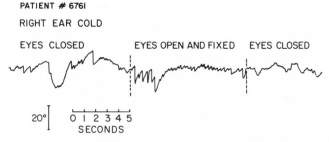

Figure 27 Demonstration of "failure of fixation suppression" (FFS) of caloric nystagmus. The top record demonstrates normal suppression of caloric nystagmus by visual fixation. It was obtained from a patient with a small right acoustic neurinoma. The bottom record demonstrates FFS. It was obtained from a patient with multiple sclerosis.

TABLE VII

DIAGNOSTIC SIGNIFICANCE OF ENG ABNORMALITIES[a]

Test	Normal or of questionable pathological significance	Nonlocalizing	Peripheral	Central (R/O ocular for all signs)
Calibration				Ocular dysmetria ("calibration overshoot") (R/O eye blinks)
Gaze test				Gaze nystagmus: Vertical; Unilateral (R/O intense spontaneous NYS); Bilateral, equal (R/O sedation); Bilateral, unequal
Optokinetic test				Asymmetry (R/O intense spontaneous NYS); Bilateral diminution (R/O lack of voluntary visual fixation and sedatives); "Breakup" of smooth pursuit (R/O sedation); Central spontaneous NYS
Sinusoidal tracking test				
Position test	Horizontal and vestibular spontaneous NYS and positional NYS less than 7.0°/sec; Vertical spontaneous NYS behind closed eyelids	Vestibular spontaneous NYS and positional NYS greater than 7.0°/sec		
Paroxysmal nystagmus test		Nonclassical	Classical	
Bithermal caloric test	DP between 20 and 30%	DP greater than 30%	UW; BW (R/O central interruption of V-O reflex)	FFS (R/O sedation)

[a] R/O = Rule out; NYS = Nystagmus; V-O = Vestibulo-ocular

81

division between "central" and "peripheral" is to some extent arbitrary, since a vestibular-nucleus lesion could involve primary vestibular nerve fibers and thereby produce a UW. In my experience, however, such a lesion nearly always produces central findings along with the UW (Coats, 1970).

(b) *Directional preponderance.* A caloric DP can be due to either peripheral or central pathology (Brookler, 1970; Cawthorne *et al.*, 1942; Fitzgerald and Hallpike, 1942; Koch *et al.*, 1959). It is therefore a non-localizing abnormality.

(c) *Bilateral weakness.* Caloric BW may be due to either bilateral peripheral vestibular pathology, e.g., as streptomycin toxicity might produce, or central pathology which interferes with the vestibulo-ocular reflex arc. However, most BWs seen in our laboratory are due to bilateral peripheral pathology. Furthermore, the occasional patient with BW due to central pathology almost always has associated central oculomotor signs. In particular, the OKN test is usually abnormal.

Thus, I consider BW a peripheral sign, with the proviso, however, that brainstem oculomotor pathology be ruled out.

(d) *Failure of fixation suppression.* FFS is a central sign. However, two benign causes of FFS have been demonstrated and must be ruled out: (1) sedation, particularly by barbiturates (Coats, 1970; Rashbass and Russell, 1961), and (2) contact lenses, particularly if they are new or uncomfortable. In addition, as with all other central ENG abnormalities, peripheral ocular pathology must be ruled out in the patient demonstrating FFS.

IV. SUMMARY

Table VII summarizes the diagnostic significance of the ENG tests discussed in this chapter.

REFERENCES

Aantaa, E. (1970). *Acta Oto-Laryngol. Suppl.* **267**, 1.
Alpert, J. N. (1974). *Neurology* **24**, 891.
Arslan, M. (1955). *Acta Oto-Laryngol. Suppl.* **122**, 1.
Aschan, G. (1955). *Acta Soc. Med. Upsal.* **60**, 99.
Aschan, G. (1958). *Acta Oto-Laryngol. Suppl.* **140**, 69.
Aschan, G. (1961). *Acta Oto-Laryngol. Suppl.* **159**, 90.
Aschan, G., and Bergstedt, M. (1955). *Acta Soc. Med. Upsal.* **60**, 1.

Aschan, G., Bergstedt, M., and Stahle, J. (1956a). *Acta Oto-Laryngol. Suppl.* **129**, 1.
Aschan, G., Bergstedt, M., Goldberg, L., and Laurell, L. (1956b). *Quart. J. Stud. Alcohol* **17**, 381.
Aschan, G., Bergstedt, M., Drettner, B., Nylen, C. O., and Stahle, J. (1957a). *Laryngoscope* **67**, 884.
Aschan, G., Bergstedt, M., and Stahle, J. (1957b). *Acta Oto-Laryngol. Suppl.* **129**, 5.
Aserinsky, E. (1955). *Amer. Med. Ass. Arch. Ophthalmol.* **53**, 542.
Barany, R. (1921). *J. Laryngol. Otol.* **36**, 229.
Barber, H. O. (1964). *Ann. Otol. Rhinol. Laryngol.* **73**, 838.
Barber, H. O., and Wright, G. (1967). *Laryngoscope* **77**, 1016.
Barber, H. O., and Wright, G. (1973). *Advan. Otorhinolaryngol.* **19**, 276.
Benitez, J. T. (1970). *Laryngoscope* **80**, 834.
Bergman, P. S., Nathanson, M., and Bender, M. B. (1951). *Trans. Amer. Neurol. Ass.* **76**, 232.
Blair, C. J., Goldberg, M. F., and von Noorden, G. K. (1967). *Arch. Ophthalmol.* **77**, 349.
Bloomberg, L. (1955). *Acta Psychiat. Scand. Suppl.* **96**, 1.
Bos, J. H., Oosterveld, W. J., Philipszoon, A. J., Wozza, J., and Zelig, S. (1963). *Pract. Oto-Rhino-Laryngol.* **25**, 282.
Brookler, K. H. (1970). *Laryngoscope* **80**, 747.
Brookler, K. H., and Pulec, J. L. (1970). *Trans. Amer. Acad. Ophthalmol. Oto-Laryngol.* **74**, 563.
Cawthorne, T. E. (1954). *Trans. Amer. Otol. Soc.* **42**, 265.
Cawthorne, T. E., and Cobb, W. A. (1954). *Acta Oto-Laryngol.* **44**, 580.
Cawthorne, T. E., Fitzgerald, G., and Hallpike, C. S. (1942). *Brain* **65**, 161.
Chutorian, A. M. (1972). *Develop. Med. Child Neurol.* **14**, 513.
Coats, A. C. (1965). *Med. Rec. Ann.* (Houston) **58**, 48.
Coats, A. C. (1966). *Ann. Otol. Rhinol. Laryngol.* **75**, 1135.
Coats, A. C. (1968). *Ann. Otol. Rhinol. Laryngol.* **77**, 938.
Coats, A. C. (1969). *Acta Otolaryngol.* **67**, 33.
Coats, A. C. (1970). *Arch. Otolaryngol.* **92**, 43.
Coats, A. C., and Black, K. H. (1973). *Trans. Amer. Acad. Ophthalmol. Otolaryngol.* **77**, 106.
Cogan, D. G. (1954). *Acta Ophthalmol.* **51**, 318.
Cogan, D. G. (1956). "Neurology of the Ocular Muscles," 2nd ed. Thomas, Springfield, Illinois.
Cogan, D. G. (1967). *Can. J. Ophthalmol.* **2**, 4.
Cogan, D. G., and Loeb, D. R. (1949). *Arch. Neurol. Psychiat.* **61**, 183.
Collins, W. E., Schroeder, D. J., and Hill, R. J. (1973). *Advan. Oto-Rhino-Laryngol.* **19**, 295.
Cope, S., and Ryan, G. M. S. (1959). *J. Laryngol. Otol.* **73**, 113.
Daroff, R. B., and Hoyt, W. F. (1971). *In* "The Control of Eye Movements" (P. Bach-y-Rita, C. C. Collins, and J. E. Hyde, eds.), pp. 175–235. Academic Press, New York.
Davidoff, R. A., Atkin, A., Anderson, P. J., and Bender, M. B. (1966). *Arch. Neurol.* **14**, 73.
Demanez, J. P., and Ledoux, A. (1970). *Advan. Otolaryngol.* **17**, 90.
Dix, M. R., and Hallpike, C. S. (1952). *Proc. Roy. Soc. Med.* **45**, 341.
Dow, R. S., and Manni, E. (1964). *In* "The Oculomotor System" (M. B. Bender, ed.), pp. 280–292. Harper, New York.

Ellenberger, C., Keltner, J. L., and Stroud, M. H. (1972). *Brain* **95**, 685.

Fernandez, C., and Lindsay, J. R. (1960). *J. Nerv. Ment. Dis.* **130**, 488.

Fields, W. S., and Alford, B. R. (eds.) (1964). "Neurological Aspects of Auditory and Vestibular Disorders." Thomas, Springfield, Illinois.

Fitzgerald, G., and Hallpike, C. S. (1942). *Brain* **65**, 115.

Fluur, E., and Eriksson, L. (1961). *Acta Oto-Laryngol.* **53**, 486.

Fodor, F. (1968). *In* "The Vestibular System and Its Diseases" (R. J. Wolfson, ed.), pp. 309–321. Univ. of Pennsylvania Press, Philadelphia, Pennsylvania.

Geddes, L. A., Bourland, J. D., Steinberg, R., and Wise, G. (1973). *Med. Biol. Eng.* **11**, 73.

Gordon, N. (1954). *Lancet* **1**, 1216.

Gulick, R. D., and Pfaltz, C. R. (1964). *Ann. Otol. Rhinol. Laryngol.* **73**, 893.

Hallpike, C. S., Harrison, S., and Slater, E. (1951). *Acta Oto-Laryngol.* **39**, 151.

Haring, R. D., and Simmons, F. B. (1973). *Arch. Otolaryngol.* **98**, 14.

Harrison, M. S. (1956). *Brain* **79**, 474.

Harrison, M. S. (1968). *In* "The Vestibular System and Its Diseases" (R. J. Wolfson, ed.), pp. 404–427. Univ. of Pennsylvania Press, Philadelphia, Pennsylvania.

Hart, C. W. (1967). *Laryngoscope* **77**, 2103.

Hart, C. W. (1969). *Ann. Otol. Rhinol. Laryngol.* **78**, 181.

Henriksson, N. G. (1956). *Acta Oto-Laryngol. Suppl.* **125**, 1.

Henriksson, N. G., Pfaltz, C. R., Torok, N., and Rubin, W. (1972). "A Synopsis of the Vestibular System." Gasser and Cie AG, Basel.

Higgins, D. C., and Daroff, R. B. (1966). *Arch. Ophthalmol.* **75**, 742.

Hill, R. J., Collins, W. E., and Schroeder, D. J. (1973). *Ann. Otol. Rhinol. Laryngol.* **82**, 103.

Hoffman, A. C., Wellman, B., and Carmichael, L. (1939). *J. Exp. Psychol.* **24**, 40.

Homer, L. D. (1967). *Pflugers Arch.* **296**, 133.

Ishiyama, E., and Keels, E. W. (1970). *Pract. Oto.-Rhino.-Laryngol.* **32**, 231.

Jongkees, L. B. W. (1948). Value of the caloric test of the labyrinth. *Arch. Otolaryngol.* **48**, 402.

Jongkees, L. B. W. (1949). *Arch. Otolaryngol.* **49**, 594.

Jongkees, L. B. W. (1961). *Acta Oto-Laryngol. Suppl.* **159**, 78.

Jongkees, L. B. W., Maas, J. P. M., and Philipszoon, A. J. (1962). *Pract. Oto.-Rhino.-Laryngol.* (Basel) **24**, 65.

Jongkees, L. B. W., and Philipszoon, A. J. (1964). *Acta Oto-Laryngol. Suppl.* **189**, 1.

Jung, R., and Kornhuber, H. H. (1964). *In* "The Oculomotor System" (M. B. Bender, ed.), pp. 428–482. Harper, New York.

Kestenbaum, A. (1961). "Clinical Methods of Neuro-Ophthalmologic Examination," 2nd ed. Grune and Stratton, New York.

Kobrak, F. (1943). *J. Laryngol. Otol.* **58**, 167.

Koch, H., Henriksson, N. G., Lundgren, A., and Andren, G. (1959). *Acta Oto-Laryngol.* **50**, 517.

Kris, C. (1960). *In* "Medical Physics" (O. Glasser, ed.), Vol. 3, pp. 692–700. Year Book Publ., Chicago, Illinois.

Kutt, H., Winters, W., Kokenge, R., and McDowell, F. (1964). *Arch. Neurol.* **11**, 642.

Lansberg, M. P. (1962). *Ned. Tijdschr. Geneesk.* **106**, 398.

Leksell, L. (1939). *Acta Chir. Scand.* **82**, 262.

Lindsay, J. R. (1951). *Ann. Otol. Rhinol. Laryngol.* **60**, 1134.

Lindsay, J. R. (1967). *Arch. Otolaryngol.* **85**, 544.

Lipman, I. J. (1972). *Dis. Nerv. Syst.* **33**, 200.

Maccario, M., Backman, J. R., and Korein, J. (1972). *Neurology* 22, 781.

Mahmud, K., Ripley, D., and Doscherholmen, A. (1970). *Arch. Otolaryngol.* 92, 278.

Marg, E. (1951). *Amer. Med. Ass. Arch. Ophthalmol.* 45, 169.

Mowrer, O. H., Ruch, T. C., and Miller, N. E. (1935). *Amer. J. Physiol.* 114, 423.

Munthe Fog, C. V. (1964). *Acta Oto-Laryngol. Suppl.* 188, 414.

Naito, T., Tatsumi, T., Matsunaga, T., and Matsunaga, T. (1963). *Acta Oto-Laryngol. Suppl.* 179, 72.

Noorden, C. K. von, and Preziosi, T. J. (1966). *Arch. Ophthalmol.* 76, 162.

North, A. W. (1965). *Invest. Ophthalmol.* 4, 343.

Nylen, C. O. (1950). *J. Laryngol. Otol.* 64, 295.

Nylen, C. O. (1953). *Acta Oto-Laryngol. Suppl.* 109, 125.

Ohm, J. (1940). *Graefes. Arch. Ophthalmol.* 142, 482.

Orzechowski, C. (1927). *J. Psychol. Neurol.* 35, 1.

Preber, L. (1958). *Acta Oto-Laryngol. Suppl.* 144, 1.

Preber, L., and Silfverskiöld, B. P. (1957). *Acta Oto-Laryngol.* 48, 255.

Preber, L., and Silfverskiöld, B. P. (1960). *Acta Oto-Laryngol.* 51, 153.

Rashbass, C., and Russell, G. F. M. (1961). *Brain* 84, 329.

Reger, S. N. (1972). *In* "Guidelines for Clinical Auditory Evaluation" (W. H. Williams, ed.), pp. 90–96. Amer. Acad. Ophthalmol. and Otolaryngol., Rochester, Minnesota.

Rosborg, J., Tos, M., and Adser, J. (1972). *Acta Neurol. Scand.* 48, 621.

Rosenblum, J. A., and Shafer, N. (1966). *Arch. Neurol.* 15, 560.

Scala, N. P., and Spiegel, E. A. (1938). *Trans. Amer. Acad. Ophthalmol. Otolaryngol.* 43, 277.

Schiller, F., and Hedberg, W. C. (1960). *Amer. Med. Ass. Arch. Neurol.* 2, 309.

Schuknecht, H. F. (1969). *Arch. Otolaryngol.* 90, 113.

Shackel, B. (1960). *Brit. J. Ophthalmol.* 44, 89.

Smith, J. L. (1962). *Neurology* 12, 48.

Smith, J. L. (1963). "Optokinetic Nystagmus." Thomas, Springfield, Illinois.

Smith, J. L., and Cogan, D. G. (1960). *Neurology* 10, 127.

Spector, M. (1961). *Ann. Otol. Rhino. Laryngol.* 70, 251.

Spector, M. (1971). *J. Laryngol. Otol.* 85, 1039.

Stahle, J. (1958). *Acta Oto-Laryngol. Suppl.* 137, 1.

Stahle, J., and Bergman, B. (1967). *Laryngoscope* 77, 1629.

Stahle, J., and Terins, J. (1965). *Ann. Otol.* 74, 69.

Stenger, H. H. (1955). *Arch. Ohren. Nasen. Kehlkopfheilk.* 168, 220.

Susuki, J. I., and Komatsuaki, A. (1962). *Acta Otolaryngol.* 54, 49.

Teng, P., Shanzer, S., and Bender, M. B. (1958). *Neurology* 8, 22.

Terins, J. (1963). *Nord. Med.* 70, 1329.

Thornval, A. (1932). *Acta Oto-Laryngol.* 17, 163.

Toglia, J. U., and Moreno, S. (1971). *Dis. Nerv. Syst.* 32, 623.

Torok, N. (1969). *Arch. Otolaryngol.* 90, 78.

Tos, M., Adser, J., and Rosborg, J. (1972). *Acta Neurol. Scand.* 48, 607.

Visser, S. L. (1962). *Ned. Tijdschr. Geneesk.* 106, 2139.

Walsh, F. B., and Hoyt, W. F. (1969). "Clinical Neuro-Ophthalmology," 3rd ed. Williams and Wilkins, Baltimore, Maryland.

Williams, H. L. (1947). *Ann. Otol. Rhinol. Laryngol.* 56, 614.

Wolfson, R. J. (ed.) (1968). "The Vestibular System and Its Diseases." Univ. of Pennsylvania Press, Philadelphia, Pennsylvania.

Chapter Four

Acoustic Impedance–Admittance Measurements

Alan S. Feldman[1]

I. INTRODUCTION

Acoustic measurements provide a direct, objective means of evaluating the status of the transformer function of the middle ear. The major function of the middle ear is to overcome the impedance mismatch generated by signals in our environment traveling from an air medium to the fluid medium of the cochlea. A prerequisite of maximum power transfer is a good impedance match between the two media. The middle-ear system functions as an impedance matching transformer in accomplishing this task, by matching the low impedance of air in the ear canal to the high impedance of the fluid in the inner ear. Pathology of the middle ear modifies the efficiency of this system.

Analysis of the function of the middle ear is accomplished by various measurements of the flow of acoustic energy through the middle ear. One may measure the *static* acoustic impedance or the *dynamic* acoustic impedance (Dallos, 1964; Jerger, 1972; Lilly, 1964, 1973; Lilly and Shepherd, 1964; Metz, 1946; Møller, 1960, 1961, 1962, 1963; Pinto and Dallos, 1968; Zwislocki, 1957a,b, 1961, 1963a). The former is a measurement of one or several parameters of steady state acoustic impedance, usually at ambient atmospheric pressure, while the latter is a measurement of some changing acoustic impedance characteristics measured at the eardrum.

[1] Department of Otolaryngology. State University of New York College of Medicine, Upstate Medical Center, Syracuse, New York.

These may be either a measurement of the changing transmission characteristics as air pressure is varied across the plane of the tympanic membrane (tympanometry), or a measurement of change in a steady state of impedance that occurs as a consequence of the contraction of one or both intraaural muscles (intraaural muscle reflex).

The clinical measurement of acoustic impedance was first described by Metz in 1946, but only recently has it been widely adopted. In the decade from 1960 to 1970, there was a rapid advancement in clinical instrumentation and techniques (Brooks, 1968, 1971; Feldman, 1963; Klockhoff, 1961; Liden *et al.*, 1970a,b; Newman and Fanger, 1973; Terkildsen and Scott Nielsen, 1960; Zwislocki, 1963b). Instrumentation and clinical techniques available to us today permit the examiner not only to establish the presence or absence of pathology in the middle-ear system, but also to provide information, in many instances, about the specific pathology which may be present.

The battery of acoustic impedance measurements is most effectively used as the first measurement in the clinical setting. When this battery of tests establishes the normality of function of the middle ear, it eliminates the need for the measurement of bone conduction as performed in traditional audiometry. The only reason to measure bone-conduction thresholds is to obtain an inferential measurement of the middle ear as revealed by the presence or absence of an air–bone gap. In the presence of normal acoustic impedance findings, such a measurement would be unnecessarily redundant. Only in those cases when a measure of the magnitude of a conductive pathology is desired is bone-conduction audiometry necessary.

II. PRINCIPLES OF ACOUSTIC IMPEDANCE

The measurement of acoustic impedance at the eardrum is quite separate from audiometry. In traditional audiometry, the concern is with some aspect of hearing, either threshold, discrimination, jnd's (just noticeable difference), or the like. These measurements involve the totality of the auditory system, including the hearing centers in the brain. In opposition to this, most of the battery of measurements of acoustic impedance have nothing to do with hearing per se. No correlation yet has been demonstrated between hearing loss magnitude and acoustic impedance. The measurement of acoustic impedance is fundamentally a measure of the efficiency of the mechanical middle-ear system and, thus, is a measure of transmission function, not hearing. For this reason, the battery of acoustic impedance tests *should not* be referred to as "impedance audiometry."

Impedance measurements are an expression of the difficulty encountered in the transfer of acoustic energy from one point to another, and acoustic impedance measurements describe either the difficulty attributed to individual factors impeding the flow of acoustic energy or to a combination of those factors expressed as the complex acoustic impedance.

A. Mechanics of the Middle-Ear System

The middle-ear mechanical system possesses a certain amount of stiffness, mass, and resistance (Onchi, 1949), and the impedance, which is a combination of these variables, may be understood as the opposition this system offers to the flow of energy through it. In the ear, for example, a force exerted on the eardrum is not completely transmitted through the mechanical system of membranes, ossicles, ligaments, and air space to the cochlea. Instead, depending on the stiffness, mass, and resistance of the system, a portion of the energy is reflected back toward its source. For example, a very stiff, noncompliant system will reflect more energy than a loose, compliant system.

The stiffness of a system may be understood as a spring which, when compressed, stores energy that is not transmitted or lost, but, to the contrary, is returned to the source. At the same time, the mass of a system offers another form of resistivity to motion. This is the inertial component of the mechanical middle-ear system. The two, stiffness and mass, store energy and return it to the source, but in a time relationship in which they are 180° out of phase with each other. In both stiffness and mass systems, energy is stored during the portions of the pressure cycle in which the pressure is moving from zero to either its maximum positive or negative value. Then the stored energy is released 90° out of phase as the pressure move returns from maximum toward zero values (Figure 1).

In the normal human ear, the relative contribution of the mass or in-

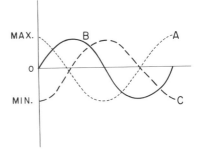

Figure 1 Phase relationships between pressure (B) and flow for stiffness (A) and mass (C) dominated systems. (A) and (C) are each 90° out of phase with pressure and 180° out of phase with each other.

ertial component is minimal in the lower frequencies but increases as frequency increases. The predominant factor affecting the flow of energy in the ear is related to the stiffness of the system in the lower frequencies. As the effect of the two are 180° out of phase with each other, their combined effect is algebraically additive. When they are equal, they cancel each other out, and the systrem at that point is said to be in resonance. Thus, as the frequency increases, the relative contribution to the total impedance of stiffness and mass shifts, so that at about 800 Hz the two components are about equal in the normal ear, and then the first resonant point of the ear is reached. The effect of pathology is such that stiffening pathologies, such as otosclerosis, increase the resonant point while loosening pathologies, such as ossicular discontinuity, lower the point of resonance. The stiffness and mass components are called *reactive* components of the total acoustic impedance. The unit of measurement of acoustic reactance is the acoustic ohm, and the identifying symbol is X_A or $-X_A$ for mass and stiffness components, respectively.

The flow of energy is also affected by a third factor, which is relatively stable across frequencies. This is the *resistance,* or friction. It constitutes the so-called "real" component of the acoustic impedance, which results in a real loss of energy as a consequence of the friction in the system, including the cochlea. In this case, the flow through the system is in phase with the pressure introduced. The resistive component, R_A, is also expressed in acoustic ohms.

B. Complex Acoustic Impedance–Admittance

Impedance is referred to as a complex quantity because the three mechanical factors (stiffness, mass, and resistance) cannot be simply added to derive the total effective value. As shown in Table I, these three mechanical factors have both electrical and acoustic counterparts. The resultant value of acoustic impedance (Z_A) is generated through

TABLE I

MECHANICAL, ELECTRICAL AND ACOUSTIC FACTORS RELATED
TO THE FLOW OF ENERGY

Mechanical (impedance Z_M)	Electrical (impedance Z)	Acoustic (impedance Z_A)
Stiffness (springiness)	Capacitance	Negative reactance ($-X_A$)
Mass (inertia)	Inductance	Positive reactance (X_A)
Resistance (friction)	Resistance	Resistance (R_A)

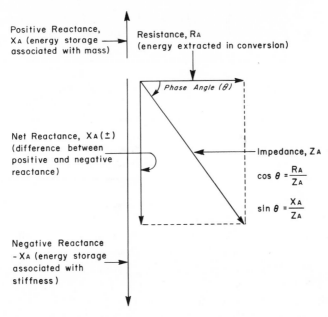

Figure 2   Vector diagram representing complex acoustic impedance (Z_A) and its components.

the use of vector plots (Lilly, 1972, 1973), whereby the magnitude and direction of the reactive and resistive components are summed according to the relationship between the legs of a right-angle triangle, and the acoustic impedance is represented by the hypotenuse of the triangle. The phase angle of Z_A is an essential component which describes the direction of that vector. Figure 2 displays this relationship between the component acoustic impedance vectors and the resultant acoustic impedance vector and angle.

C.   Impedance–Admittance Relationships

In current practice, the measurement of acoustic impedance is often inferential (Newman and Fanger, 1973). This is because electroacoustic instrumentation generally measures flow. Impedance is equal to the pressure divided by the flow, and when pressure is held constant, the measurement of flow is a measurement of the reciprocal of acoustic impedance. This is called *acoustic admittance* (Y_A), which is expressed in acoustic millimhos. If the acoustic impedance is understood as a *measure of the difficulty with which energy flows*, then acoustic admittance is simply a *measure of the ease with which energy flows* into or through

TABLE II

RELATIONSHIPS BETWEEN ACOUSTIC IMPEDANCE
AND ACOUSTIC ADMITTANCE PARAMETERS

Acoustic impedance (Z_A) (in acoustic ohms)	Acoustic admittance (Y_A) (in acoustic millimhos)
Negative reactance ($-X_A$)	Positive susceptance (B_A)
Positive reactance (X_A)	Negative susceptance ($-B_A$)
Resistance (R_A)	Conductance (G_A)

a system. Table II compares the components of impedance with the reciprocal components of admittance. Note that *acoustic conductance* (G_A) is the resistive component of acoustic admittance and is an expression of how much of the energy is being consumed by the resistance in the system. *Acoustic susceptance* (B_A) is an expression of how much of the energy is flowing into a medium of storage. Positive susceptance is directly related to the compliance of the system: The larger the susceptance, the greater the compliance. The less stiff a body is the more compliant it is and, as we shall see later, the measurement of acoustic impedance has often been expressed in terms of the compliance of an equivalent volume of air. The difficulty with expression in this form is that a volume of air has a different compliance at different altitudes and temperatures, and Lilly (1972, 1973) has accurately pointed out that the storage component of the acoustic impedance is more accurately described in either acoustic ohms (acoustic reactance) or acoustic millimhos (acoustic susceptance).

When a signal is introduced through a probe sealed in the ear canal, the sound wave travels along the canal until it strikes the tympanic membrane. The physical properties of the tympanic membrane and its attachments determine how much of this incident wave is transmitted through the middle ear and on to the cochlea, and how much will be reflected back toward the source. The measurement of acoustic impedance–admittance involves a measurement of the acoustic parameters of the reflected wave and a comparison of that wave with the incident wave.

Because of the minimal size of the ear canal relative to the wave length within the measurable frequency range, the ear canal contains only a small portion of the incident and reflected waves. At any point in space, a resultant wave develops that is a consequence of the frequency, phase, and amplitude characteristics of the two sound waves. Insofar as the parameters of the incident wave can be specified, it then becomes possible to determine the contributing properties of the reflected wave. Depending on the measuring tool used, with today's clinical instruments, one may obtain information about either acoustic impedance–admittance components or estimates of the complex acoustic impedance itself. These measurements provide information about the static impedance properties of the ear and also are used to describe the tympanometric function (Liden *et al.*, 1970a,b; Terkildsen, 1962; Terkildsen and Thomsen, 1959; Thomsen, 1958). In addition, descriptive information about the properties of the intraaural muscle reflex also become available (Djupesland, 1962, 1965, 1967, 1969b; Hung and Dallos, 1972; Jepson, 1953, 1955, 1963; Klockhoff, 1961; Yonovitz and Harris, 1972). The equipment also permits assessment of the patency and function of the Eustachian tube (Holmquist, 1969, 1972a,b).

III. INSTRUMENTATION

Regardless of the specific instrument used, there are fundamental similarities that are common to all impedance measuring devices. Most instruments used to measure acoustic impedance are referred to as "bridges." An acoustic bridge is a device that may be coupled to an unknown impedance, the ear, which possesses a variable system that is balanced against the unknown (Zwislocki, 1961). When a balance in the system is obtained, readings from the variable adjustments tell us something about some parameters of the acoustic impedance of the ear. Mechanical bridges (Metz, 1946; Zwislocki, 1961, 1963b) simulate an impedance that is analogous to the impedance at the eardrum. Electroacoustic bridges vary the parameters of the signal introduced into the ear canal, thereby providing information about some values of the signal reflected off the eardrum as compared to known values of the incident or probe signal.

As with the mechanical bridges, most electroacoustic instruments operate on a balancing principle. One, the Grason–Stadler Otoadmittance meter, is, as its name indicates, not a bridge. With this instrument, the operator does not balance or adjust either incident or resultant signals. This is accomplished within the instrument by an automatic volume control and electronic multipliers.

A. Mechanical Acoustic Bridges

The first clinical measurements of acoustic impedance were reported by Metz in 1946. The instrument he used was a modification of a Schuster

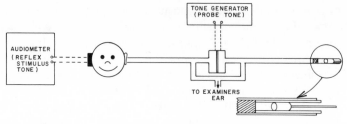

MECHANICAL ACOUSTIC BRIDGE (METZ)

Figure 3   Schematic diagram of the Metz mechanical acoustic bridge.

(1934) acoustic bridge, which is essentially a mechanical balancing null detector, as shown schematically in Figure 3.

Metz's bridge was a mechanical acoustic impedance bridge in which the impedance on the side of the bridge coupled to the ear could be matched by a variable resistance and volume, together serving as the resistance and stiffness components on the variable side of the acoustic bridge. However, problems of instability of the mechanical components as well as the failure of the instrument to accommodate for the very significant volume of the ear canal, which was interposed between the front of the bridge and the eardrum, mitigated against the effectiveness of this instrument as a valid means of obtaining precise measurements of static acoustic impedance. It was, however, quite effective in dynamic measurement of acoustic impedance changes associated with the stapedius reflex.

The control of these problems was accomplished with the introduction of the Zwislocki acoustic bridge (Zwislocki, 1963b; Zwislocki and Feldman, 1963). Two features provided this instrument with the capability for the precise measurement of static acoustic impedance. One was the addition of a variable volume of air on the balancing side of the bridge, which would compensate for the volume of air in the ear canal interposed between the tip of the bridge and the eardrum. The other was the extreme stability of the variable resistance and compliance elements.

1. Principle of Operation. The Zwislocki acoustic bridge is shown schematically in Figure 4. It consists essentially of two main tubes (A) and (B) of exactly equal internal diameter and length, with a miniature electroacoustic transducer (E) secured symmetrically between them. The transducer is connected to an external signal source that provides any desired probe tone. A variable acoustic impedance terminates the matching side of the bridge, and a tube (Y) connects the two main tubes. Tube (A) fits within a specially designed speculum that is fitted

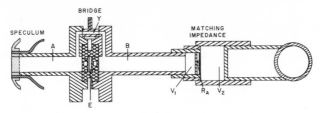

ZWISLOCKI ACOUSTIC BRIDGE

Figure 4 Schematic diagram of Zwislocki mechanical acoustic bridge showing symmetrical tubes (A) and (B), monitoring communicating (Y) tube, diaphragm (E) and variables (V_1), (R_A), and (V_2).

with different sized plastic tips. This permits an airtight coupling to the ear canal. Tube (B) terminates in the matching impedance. The transducer (E) radiates sound waves of equal amplitude, but in opposite phase, into the main tubes. These waves are partially reflected at the ends of the tubes, one at the eardrum, the other at the variable impedance. The resultant sound pressure in each tube is generated by both the original and the reflected waves. Since the phase and amplitude of the reflected waves depend on the acoustic impedance terminating the tubes, the sound pressure in tube (A) leading to the ear canal is equal to the sound pressure in tube (B) when both are terminated by an equal impedance. The sole difference between the waves is that they are 180° out of phase with each other. This results in a sound cancellation in the (Y) tube. Such a cancellation can be detected by listening through a stethoscope connected to the third branch of the (Y) tube. The balancing side of the Zwislocki bridge contains three variable elements. One, (V_1), is a predetermined volume of air that compensates for the volume of the ear canal between the eardrum and the tip of the speculum and the bridge. This volume is critical for precise static acoustic impedance measurements at the eardrum. The other two variables are a variable slit resistance element (R_a) and a compliance element (V_2), which is a variable air volume. The resistance may be calibrated in acoustic ohms. The compliance may be calibrated in an equivalent volume of air which has a compliance equivalent to that at the eardrum, or in acoustic ohms. This latter can be converted to acoustic reactance ($-X_A$).

In addition to obtaining static acoustic impedance measurements, the Zwislocki mechanical acoustic bridge also can be used as a measure of dynamic acoustic impedance change as a consequence of the acoustic reflex (Deutsch, 1968, 1972; Feldman, 1967b; Feldman and Zwislocki, 1965). Once a null has been obtained, a signal can be introduced to the contralateral ear that is loud enough to induce a contraction of the sta-

pedius muscle. Contraction of this muscle will modify the wave reflected off the eardrum as it changes the impedance characteristics of
the ear, and consequently, it will destroy the null that has been obtained.
The examiner hears a surge or return of the signal. With removal of the
contralateral signal, the null returns.

Measurements with this instrument are both reliable and valid, and
contribute readily to the differential diagnosis of middle-ear pathologies,
as well as just answering the question of whether or not there is middle-
ear pathology. Such a differential distinction is shown in Figure 5, which
compares diametrically opposed impedance in otosclerosis and discontinuity of the ossicles. The former represents a stiff, noncompliant, high-
impedance system, while the latter is a loose, compliant, low-impedance
system.

2. *Limitations of the Mechanical Bridge.* Despite its extreme precision and reliability, certain problems have limited the use of the Zwislocki bridge to a few sophisticated clinical settings. Consequently, it
has been used mostly in experimental studies of middle-ear function,
with comparatively little clinical usage. While there has appeared to be
a problem in mastering the technique for precision of measurement, of
even greater importance is the inability to perform tympanometric measurements with this instrument. In recent years, tympanometry has proven
to be a vital component of the impedance test battery (Brooks, 1968;
Liden *et al.*, 1970a,b; Terkildsen, 1962, 1964). Furthermore, the size of
the instrument as it is coupled to the ear generally excludes its use in the
young pediatric population, where considerable need for the measurement of middle-ear function exists. Finally, the measurement of the
acoustic reflex can only be performed at ambient atmospheric pressure
with this instrument. In those conditions where the middle-ear pressure
deviates from normal, the reflex must be performed at the deviant peak-
pressure values.

B. Electroacoustic Instruments

Problems associated with the Metz mechanical acoustic bridge, in terms
of both instrumentation and individual differences, tended to obscure
pathological effects and were the source of early major objections to the
use of static, or, as it was then called, "absolute" acoustic impedance,
as a diagnostic procedure. Furthermore, from a design standpoint, the
instrumentation necessary simply to detect an acoustic impedance change,
but not necessarily to quantify it, required a less technical engineering
sophistication. This provided the impetus for the development of probe
tube electroacoustic impedance bridges (Figure 6), such as the electro-

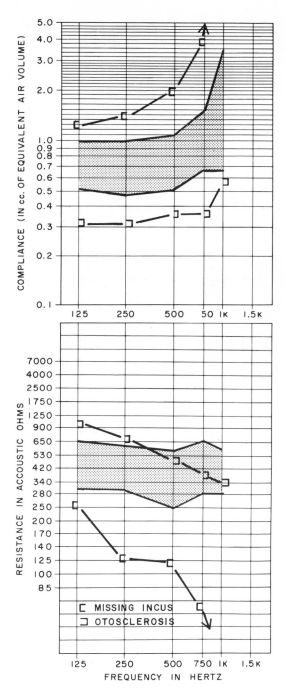

Figure 5 Plot of normal ranges (shaded) for compliance and resistance as measured with a Zwislocki acoustic bridge, and comparing values for a typical otosclerotic ear and an ear with a missing incus.

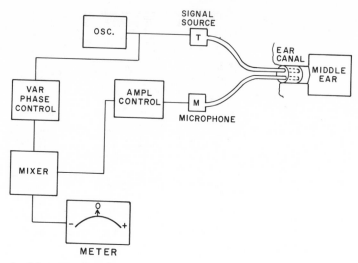

Figure 6 Schematic for electroacoustic impedance bridge (after Terkildsen and Scott Nielsen, 1960) with phase and amplitude balancing system.

acoustic bridge developed by Terkildsen and Scott Nielsen (1960), which resulted in the production, in 1961, of the first commercially available clinical electroacoustic bridge, the Madsen Z061. Although the Terkildsen and Scott Nielsen design included a phase control capable of potentially isolating the in-phase and out-of-phase acoustic impedance components of acoustic resistance and acoustic reactance, its measurement was not considered to be of clinical significance, and the clinical instrument did not provide for either component or complex acoustic impedance read-out. The instrument only balanced in terms of the absolute magnitude of the resultant wave, and was used essentially as a reflex and tympanometry indicator. As a result of this, the technique for clinical measurements continued to emphasize what was originally referred to as "relative" acoustic impedance but which was later, and more appropriately, labeled "dynamic" acoustic impedance (Pinto and Dallos, 1968).

The ease of clinical operation of electroacoustic instruments, plus their greater flexibility, suggests that clinical instrumentation will continue to be of this type rather than the mechanical acoustic type. The fundamental contribution of the Zwislocki acoustic bridge was the demonstration that, with precision instrumentation, static acoustic impedance measurements do have clinical usefulness and can effectively contribute to the differential diagnosis of middle-ear pathologies (Feldman, 1964; Preide, 1970; Zwislocki and Feldman, 1970). As a consequence of this, the newer electroacoustic instruments provide, in addition to dynamic measures, one or another form of measurement of some parameters of static acoustic impedance.

1. *Principle of Operation.* The principle of operation of the electro-acoustic instruments is schematically illustrated in Figures 7, 8, and 9. The fundamental principle is similar in all of the instruments. As shown in Figure 7, a signal is generated and propagated by a microphone through

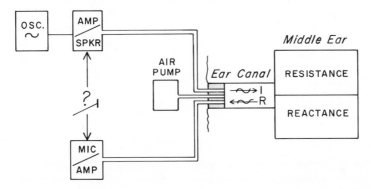

Figure 7 Schematic of a basic electroacoustic system for impedance measurement of a middle ear. Variable control (?) provides the means of balance of the system.

a capillary tube to the ear canal, which is sealed by an air-tight fitting from the environment. A second probe tube conveys the resultant sound wave in the ear canal to a microphone–amplifier system. Some means of either adjusting the amplitude of the probe tone to balance the system, or analyzing the resultant wave in relation to some parameters of the probe tone, provides the examiner with information about the acoustic impedance as measured at the entrance to the ear canal. The contribution of the ear-canal volume to the total measurement is minimized by a pressure system that places the eardrum under maximum positive and negative stress. The ability of the eardrum and ossicles to vibrate is restricted under stress. This effectively decouples the middle ear from the measurement. When this is compared to the measurement under ambient pressure, the difference between stress and ambient measurements is a consequence of the middle-ear acoustic impedance.

Current clinical instrumentation differs according to the principles demonstrated by Figures 8 and 9. In all instances, the returning signal is the same through the pickup receiver system.

Most electroacoustic bridges use a low-frequency probe tone (220 Hz), and measure amplitude differential that occurs between the incident and resultant signals. As shown in Figure 8, the resultant wave is rectified to a DC voltage, thereby discarding information about the phase param-

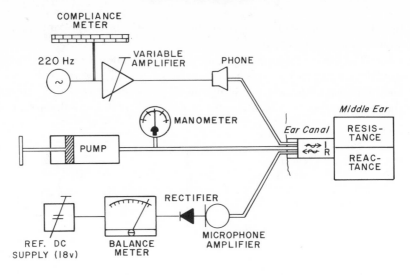

Figure 8 Schematic of a common electroacoustic impedance bridge which measures and balances amplitude differentials between incident (I) and resultant (R) waves in the ear canal.

eters of the signal. A constant voltage to a meter is offset when the returning voltage is applied to it. Rotation of the variable control or potentiometer of the instrument modifies the level of probe-tone output until the meter is in balance. In effect, this readjusts the level of the signal in the ear canal to a specified sound pressure level (SPL), usually 85 dB or 95 dB. The readout system may be calibrated in cubic centimeters of an equivalent volume of air or acoustic ohms, or both, depending on the instrument. This approach presumes that the impedance is reactive, with only a negligible resistive contribution.

When the air pressure in the ear canal is increased to 200 mm H_2O, the reflected signal will be at its maximum because, under such pressure, the middle ear is theoretically decoupled from the system, and the ear canal simulates a hard-walled cavity. The same is true for measurements under negative pressure of 200 mm H_2O. When the bridge is balanced at midmeter, values recorded at these points represent a measurement of the decoupled ear canal (Brooks, 1971). As the pressure across the plane of the tympanic membrane is returned to normal ambient atmospheric pressure, the flow of energy through the middle ear will normally reach its maximum. Values recorded at this point reflect a combination of ear-canal and middle-ear impedance ($Z_{A(amb)}$). The static acoustic impedance of the middle ear alone is the complex interaction between the average of the two stress measurements and the total measurement at ambient atmospheric pressure. In clinical practice, there is generally an insignificant difference between the two stress measurements for low-frequency probe tones, and static middle-ear values are usually computed from the values at only positive 200 mm of pressure and ambient atmospheric pressure. With an instrument such as that shown in Figure 8, computation of Z_A involves the conversion from separate measurements according to the formula in equation (1):

$$(1) \qquad Z_A = \frac{Z_{A \text{ (stress)}} \times Z_{A \text{ (amb)}}}{Z_{A \text{ (stress)}} - Z_{A \text{ (amb)}}}$$

This can also be derived from a nomogram provided in the instrument manuals. In fact, this formula represents an estimate of Z_A due to its failure to account for the phase angle (Lilly, 1972, 1973).

The essential distinction between the two popular types of commercially available electroacoustic instruments is their use of different approaches to analysis of the resultant wave in the ear canal for the measurement of static acoustic impedance. Electroacoustic bridges, such as the Madsen Z070, American Electromedics 81, and Peters AP61, rectify the signal, disregard the phase, and consequently, essentially ignore the resistive component. Because the primary contribution to the impedance at low frequencies is the negative reactance, enough information is usually available to contribute to differential diagnosis of the ear in many pathological conditions. What these instruments can tell us is something about the magnitude of the acoustic impedance vector, e.g., high, low, or normal impedance. However, one cannot, with this information, plot the angle of the vector or derive the resistance contribution to the complex acoustic impedance. This shortcoming may tend to increase the likelihood of overlap between normal and pathological ears.

The other type of electroacoustic instrument is one that measures the reciprocal of the parameters measured by the mechanical acoustic bridge. The Grason Stadler Model 1720 Otoadmittance meter differs from the previous bridges, as shown in Figure 9. As with the other instruments, this one contains a pressure-pump system which varies the air pressure gradient across the tympanic membrane, and a small probe tip with tubes for air pressure, transmission, and pickup of acoustic signals. However, instead of rectifying the resultant wave monitored in the ear canal, the signal is first split and compared, both in phase and 90° out of phase with the original probe tone. The resultant signal is also fed through an automatic volume control circuit which electronically modifies the level of the probe tone fed to the ear canal, maintaining it at 85-dB SPL. This is the reason for not referring to the instrument as a bridge. The examiner does not adjust a variable control. Instead, levels are internally

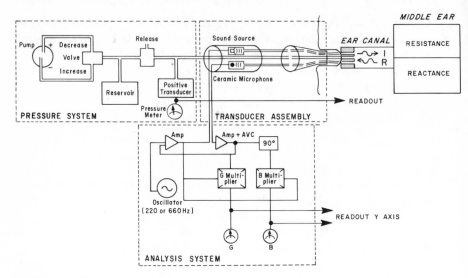

Figure 9 Schematic of monitoring electroacoustic otoadmittance meter which measures phase and amplitude differentials between incident (I) and resultant (R) waves in the ear canal.

monitored and displayed on meters in the form of acoustic millimhos of susceptance (B_A) and conductance (G_A), which are the acoustic admittance (Y_A) counterparts of the reactive and resistive components of acoustic impedance. The other distinction of this instrument is that it has a 660-Hz probe tone in addition to the 220-Hz probe tone common to most other instruments. This provides a measurement at a point closer to, but just below, the resonant point of the ear, thereby enabling the examiner to evaluate the possible effect of pathology on resonance in pathological ears. With this type of instrument, computation of Z_A involves conversion from its reciprocal Y_A. Because data is revealed in admittance components, it is possible to directly derive the vector angle as well as phasor amplitude. The formula for converting the data appears in equation (2).

(2)
$$\frac{1}{Z_A} = Y_A = \sqrt{B_A{}^2 + G_A{}^2}$$

where

$$B_A = B_{A\ (amb)} - B_{A\ (stress)}$$
$$G_A = G_{A\ (amb)} - B_{A\ (stress)}$$

These values of Z_A, Y_A, and phase angle can be derived from the tables provided in the instrument handbook.

In addition to providing information about static impedance at atmospheric pressure, the measurement with variable pressure across the eardrum also reveals those points, negative or positive, which represent optimal transmission pressures for certain pathological conditions. For example, ears with resolving serous otitis will display maximum flow at negative atmospheric pressures.

While the static acoustic impedance computation is determined in part from the value at ambient atmospheric pressure, the determination of the peak point of the tympanogram, which may deviate from ambient pressure, is an important consideration from at least two standpoints. First, it may give some indication of the potential transmission characteristics of the middle ear, and second, it is at this pressure value that measurement of the acoustic reflex is made.

IV. PRELIMINARY STEPS IN MEASUREMENT

Regardless of the instrument used, there are some fundamental principles essential to the successful measurement of acoustic impedance. No measurement of this type will be successful without an effective seal of the ear canal. The examiner must first make a careful visual inspection of the ear canal to (1) insure the absence of potentially obstructive cerumen, (2) establish the proper angle of insertion of the probe, and (3) determine the size and shape of the tip (plastic or other material) to be placed on the probe ending.

A. Problems of Obstructive Cerumen

The presence or absence of cerumen in the ear canal does not appear to be as critical a factor in electroacoustic measurements as it is in measurements made with a mechanical acoustic bridge. With the latter instrument, absorption of the signal by a plug of cerumen affects the total measurement because a similar absorption is not present on the balancing side of the bridge. However, in electroacoustic measurements, cerumen is a constant factor in both stress and nonstress measurements and, consequently, is effectively eliminated in the final computational process to determine static values. However, cerumen that obliterates or obstructs the tympanic membrane, or that adheres to it, obviously will interfere with a middle-ear measurement. Of perhaps even greater significance is what appears to be innocuous or insignificant amount of cerumen in the orifice. In this instance, two potential problems exist. One is the flake of cerumen that sits in front of a probe and which will act as a valve as pressure is varied from normal to positive and back to negative states. The other problem is the danger of plugging one of the capillary probe tubes. This results in either an inability to obtain a measurement, or, with small amounts of cerumen in the tube, an alteration of the calibration for static measurements.

B. Determination of Angle and Depth of Probe Insertion

Ear canals vary in a number of critical dimensions, and the angle of insertion of the probe tip is important. While not required to be directly facing the tympanic membrane, the probe must not be against the canal wall. Consequently, visual inspection of the external meatus is a critical first step in the measurement. By pulling the pinna upward and backward, with the examiner sitting so as to permit visibility into the patient's ear canal, a deep penetration into the lumen of the canal and not against the canal wall will be facilitated. Soft tips will usually be more comfortable than hard ones, but comfort must not be considered a prerequisite of the measurement.

C. Achieving an Airtight Seal

The major reason for failure to obtain valid measurements in clinical settings can be attributed to an inability to achieve or maintain an airtight seal of the ear canal. This problem was difficult to overcome in mechanical acoustic bridge measurements because the only feedback to the examiner about the effectiveness of the seal was in the quality of the signal monitored. In electroacoustic measurements, validation of a seal is achieved simply by monitoring the air pressure manometer. If a seal is not obtained, the positive and negative pressures will not be maintained. Inspection of the lumen of the ear canal reveals the size and shape of the canal, and the innovative examiner should have as wide a selection of tips as possible. Once a tip has been selected, insertion of the probe should be deep and firm. Light lubrication of the selected tip will sometimes facilitate a seal but has the disadvantage of creating a greater potential for extrusion of the tip when positive pressure is introduced into the canal.

The varied sizes and shapes of ear canals has tended to preclude a single type of ear tip as being universally effective in achieving an hermetic seal. The use of air-filled inflatable cuffs dates back to the Madson Z061. These were replaced by molded hard plastic, hard rubber, or soft silicon and foam tips of varying sizes and shapes. The inflatable cuff was reintroduced with the Grason Stadler 1720. The cuff, however, was fluid-filled in order to eliminate the problem of an added variable introduced by a compliant air-filled cuff. The fluid-filled inflatable cuff has the unique advantage of complete adaptability to an infinite variety of ear canal shapes and sizes. However, it has the disadvantage of being relatively expensive, sensitive to rupture, and more time-consuming than is desirable for clinical applications. As a consequence, all manufacturers provide a variety of sizes of molded and other tips, and the adept and innovative clinician will add to these a variety of commercially available stock earmold and other tips that may be adapted as probe tips. Individually molded tips have also been used (Lilly, 1970; Pinto and Dallos, 1968). With only one exception, one may expect little difference in the measurement results with the different tips (Richards and Kartye, 1973). However, the foam tips supplied with some instruments can affect static acoustic impedance values. Unlike the other tips, the surface of some foam rubber is such that it will introduce a surface that offers both resistance and compliance.

V. CLINICAL ACOUSTIC IMPEDANCE EVALUATION

The clinical evaluation of middle-ear function with an electroacoustic measuring device actually consists of a battery of measurements (Table III). As with other differential diagnostic tests, one looks for intertest consistency to obtain a meaningful interpretation of the results. Inconsistencies must be interpreted in light of possible pathological entities or, as is sometimes the case, present limitations of our expertise, or test

TABLE III

THE EVALUATION OF ACOUSTIC IMPEDANCE:
BATTERY OF MEASUREMENTS

A. Static acoustic impedance
   1. Resistive component
   2. Reactive component
   3. Phase angle between (1) and (2)
   4. Complex acoustic impedance–admittance
B. Dynamic acoustic impedance
   1. Tympanometry
      (a) Pressure point
      (b) Amplitude
      (c) Shape
   2. Intraaural muscle reflex
      (a) Acoustic
      (b) Nonacoustic
C. Tests of Eustachian-tube patency and function

limitations. For example, while stiffening pathology should result in high static acoustic impedance, complications due to eardrum pathology may result in misleading low static impedance measurements. Such findings should not be disconcerting, because the other tests in the battery—tympanogram pressure points and shape, and interaural reflexes —will usually provide validating data to help establish a diagnosis. Furthermore, the results of the battery of impedance measurements must be viewed in relation to the history, otologic findings, and audiological tests. The acoustic impedance evaluation of middle-ear function should be expected to reinforce other established diagnostic procedures, not to completely replace them.

A. Static Acoustic Impedance

Because static acoustic impedance is either increased or decreased by middle-ear pathology, its measurement can help differentiate between normal and pathological middle ears (Bicknell and Morgan, 1968; Feldman, 1963, 1964, 1967a, 1969, 1971; Jerger, 1970; Nilges et al., 1969; Preide, 1970; Wilber, 1972; Wilber et al., 1970; Zwislocki, 1957a,b, 1961, 1963a,b, 1968; Zwislocki and Feldman, 1970). In the latter category are such clinical entities as stapedial otosclerosis, malleolar fixation from otosclerosis or tympanosclerosis, adhesions of the ossicular chain, serous otitis media, acute otitis media, inadequate pressure equalization, and middle-ear tumors. Many of these conditions provide uniquely different results in the individual tests within the battery of impedance tests and can frequently be distinguished from one another as well as from an interruption of the ossicular chain, a condition which results in diametrically opposed lower impedance. The absolute parameters of the transmission characteristics of the middle ear in normal and pathological ears at ambient atmospheric pressure have been extensively described in both laboratory studies (Møller, 1961, 1963; Onchi, 1949, 1961; Zwislocki, 1957a,b, 1962, 1963b) and clinical studies (Brooks, 1971; Burke et al., 1970a,b; Feldman, 1963, 1964, 1967a, 1969; Jerger, 1970; Lilly, 1972, 1973; Wilber, 1972; Wilber et al., 1970; Zwislocki and Feldman, 1970). The measurements in these studies were made with either mechanical or electroacoustic systems or, in some instances, with both. Table IV is a comparison, from several different sources, of static acoustic impedance ranges of normal ears, obtained with a Madsen Z070 electroacoustic bridge, a Grason Stadler Model 1720 Otoadmittance meter, and a Zwislocki acoustic bridge.

   1. Relationship between Static Acoustic Impedance Measurements Obtained with Mechanical and Electroacoustic Bridges. Correlations

TABLE IV

NORMAL RANGES FOR ACOUSTIC IMPEDANCE (Z_A) OBTAINED WITH MADSEN Z070,[a] GRASON STADLER 1720,[b] AND ZWISLOCKI ACOUSTIC BRIDGE,[c] EXPRESSED IN 90TH, 50TH, AND 10TH CENTILE

		Source							
		Madsen Z070 (Jerger)		Madsen Z070 (Wilber et al.)		Grason Stadler 1720 (Feldman)		Zwislocki (Lilly)	
Probe frequency	Range (in centiles)	Z_A in Ac. Ohms	Phase angle	Z_A in Ac. Ohms	Phase angle	Z_A in Ac. Ohms	Phase angle	Z_A in Ac. Ohms	Phase angle
220/250 Hz	90th	2750	—[d]	1890	—	3048	/−70°	2060	/−72.2°
	50th	2050	—	1395	—	1856	/−69.5°	1530	/−74.1°
	10th	1750	—	880	—	1124	/−75°	1075	/−74.8°
660/750 Hz	90th	—	—	—	—	715	/−44°	798	/−37.9°
	50th	—	—	—	—	409	/−31°	521	/−41.6°
	10th	—	—	—	—	215	/−39°	329	/−45.6°

[a] Jerger, 1970; Wilber et al., 1969. Data with the Madsen Z070 are approximated from figures in original references.
[b] Feldman, 1973, 1974.
[c] Lilly, 1972.
[d] Second frequency and phase angle cannot be measured with Madsen Z070.

107

between mechanical and electroacoustic bridges have been found to be high in normal ears (Burke *et al.*, 1970b; Feldman *et al.*, 1971; Stone and Feldman, 1971; Wilber, 1971). However, some discrepancies have been observed between static measurements in pathological ears with the same instruments (Wilber *et al.*, 1970; Stone and Feldman, 1971). In part, some of these discrepancies are a consequence of the failure to equate measurement points with the two instruments. The measurements with a mechanical acoustic bridge are confined to ambient atmospheric pressure. When static measurements are performed with the electroacoustic bridge, there must be a distinction made between maximum transmission at ambient atmospheric pressure and some other pressure point if the maximum point deviates from normal (Jerger, 1972). For example, an ear with middle-ear effusion has a very high acoustic impedance, but under negative pressure in the canal, a point of greater compliance may be achieved. If the static acoustic impedance is computed from values measured at this point rather than at ambient atmospheric pressure, it is conceivable that the acoustic impedance would appear normal. However, when the comparison is made as it should be, between stress and 0-mm (ambient) pressure, the ear will be found to have a very high acoustic impedance. The former measurement is informative and of some value in the total diagnostic battery. The negative pressure peak may indicate something about potential maximum compliance and the appropriate point for testing the acoustic reflex, but it is not an indication of the patient's static acoustic impedance.

Another reason exists for discrepancies between mechanical and some electroacoustic bridges. When the latter perform their function by rectifying the resultant wave in the analysis of a signal, there is a loss of the phase relationships involved, and the instrument cannot isolate the separate impedance components. In normal ears, resistance is a relatively constant factor across frequencies and exerts a minimal contribution to the total impedance in the lower frequencies (Burke *et al.*, 1970a; Zwislocki, 1961). Thus, correlations will not be adversely affected in measurements of normal ears made with the two instruments. However, in an ear with otosclerosis, the resistance is not stable across frequencies (Feldman and Zwislocki, 1965; Lilly, 1970; Metz, 1946; Zwislocki, 1957b, 1962, 1963b). It is higher than normal in the lower frequencies and would thus contribute substantially to the amplitude and direction of the acoustic impedance phasor for a 220-Hz probe tone (Lilly, 1970, 1972, 1973). This probably contributes to some discrepancies that have been observed in absolute values obtained with the Zwislocki and Madsen bridges. In two studies of otosclerotics (Wilber *et al.*, 1969; Zwislocki and Feldman, 1970), using the Zwislocki acoustic bridge, median reactance values of approximately 3500 acoustic ohms were obtained with a 250-Hz probe tone, whereas for the Madsen Z070 in the study by Wilber *et al.* (1970), the median otosclerotic impedance was 2250 acoustic ohms at 220 Hz. On the other hand, using an electroacoustic system that does isolate impedance components, the Grason Stadler Model 1720 Otoadmittance meter, a median value of 3160 acoustic ohms at 220 Hz was obtained for a group of 15 otosclerotic patients (Feldman, 1973). This finding compares quite favorably with the mechanical acoustic bridge measurements.

When static measurements are derived with a continuously changing pressure across the plane of the tympanic membrane, results may differ from those obtained with a mechanical acoustic bridge. The static acoustic impedance is computed from the amplitude of the tympanogram in electroacoustic instruments, and the amplitude and configuration of the derived tympanograms do appear to be affected by the rate of change of pressure as well as the direction of changing pressure (Figure 10). Research has yet to be reported as to which rate of speed and direction of pressure change yields the most valid measurement of static acoustic impedance.

2. *Frequency of Probe Tone.* The major advantage of the mechanical acoustic bridge is the greater flexibility afforded by its lack of limitation to a single low-frequency probe tone. It has been noted that the

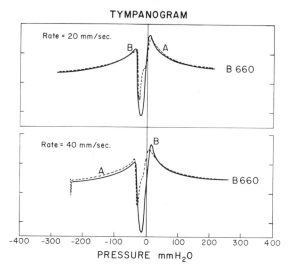

Figure 10 Tympanograms derived at two different rates of speed and from negative to positive (A) and positive to negative (B) pressure change. The notch is deeper for (B) than for (A), and the faster speed has a broader and deeper notch than the slower speed.

effect of pathology is most evident at middle frequencies approaching the first resonant point of the ear. Whereas the normal ear begins to spread out in distribution by 750 Hz, the stiffening pathologies tend to shift the resonant point upward in frequency and should be more clearly differentiated from normal at a higher frequency than at a lower frequency. This is demonstrated in Figure 11, which compares the acoustic impedance for normal and otosclerotic ears measured with an otoadmittance meter at 220 Hz and at 660 Hz; the latter is a frequency close to the first resonant point of the normal ear. The much reduced overlap at 660 Hz is probably a consequence of this upward shift in resonance caused by the stiffening pathology of otosclerosis.

A further advantage of the higher frequency probe tone is that it provides the examiner with a clue as to whether or not eardrum pathology is complicating the measurement (Alberti and Jerger, 1973; Feldman, 1974; Terkildsen, 1964; Terkildsen and Thomsen, 1959; Wilber et al., 1970). Scarring of the tympanic membrane lowers the static acoustic impedance measured with the electroacoustic bridge, and confirmation of this may only be available with a higher frequency probe tone. If one wishes to measure static acoustic impedance, the nature of the middle-ear system, as well as the effect of pathology on it, would suggest that the measurement not be confined to a low-frequency probe tone.

3.   *Standard Measurement Notation for Static Acoustic Impedance.* Unfortunately, no single standard notation has been established for the plotting or recording of static acoustic impedance. With the Zwislocki

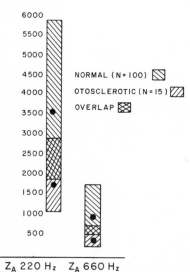

Figure 11   Bar graph ranges of Z_A and overlap for normal and otosclerotic ears.

acoustic bridge (Figure 5), results were commonly expressed in terms of a volume of air having a compliance equivalent to the compliance measured at the eardrum (reactive component) and in arbitrary degrees of rotation of the resistance element, which for each instrument could be converted to acoustic ohms. Lilly (1972, 1973) has very astutely demonstrated that the use of an equivalent volume of air has serious shortcomings, in that it is critically dependent on such variables as altitude and barometric pressure, as well as temperature and humidity. It also leads to a skewing of the distribution toward larger volumes. He converted the Feldman (1967a) and Zwislocki and Feldman (1970) equivalent-volume data to the more appropriate acoustic reactance ($-X_A$) expressed in acoustic ohms, and computed the acoustic impedance and phase angles from that data. The Grason Stadler Model 1720 Otoadmittance meter does not measure or read out an equivalent volume but, instead, measures the separate admittance components of susceptance (B_A) and conductance (G_A) in acoustic millimhos, which are quite appropriate for clinical use. If one desires, conversion to either acoustic admittance (Y_A) or acoustic impedance (Z_A) is accomplished simply by reference to conversion tables (Burke, 1972; Rose, 1973).

The earlier Madsen Model Z061 did not measure static acoustic impedance, but the Madsen Model Z070 and American Electromedics Model 81, while they do not separate or measure the resistive component, read out in equivalent volume on one scale and acoustic impedance on another. The Peters Model AP61 reads out only in equivalent volume. Thus, much of the static data reported from use of these instruments, as with the Zwislocki acoustic bridge, have been expressed in terms of equivalent volume.

Continued use of measurement in equivalent volume to express the magnitude of static acoustic impedance is inadvisable. It will be a considerable advantage to the clinician when some single universal notation is established, either the acoustic ohm or the reciprocal acoustic millimho, and when read-out systems, as well as reporting of results, are consistent (Burke et al., 1967; Lilly et al., 1968). Until that time, the clinician must adjust to the interrelationships between the notations and convert from one notation system to the other in order to compare data.

4. *Overlap between Normal and Pathological Ears.* Even with these problems and limitations, when the measurements are made properly, all electroacoustic instruments provide the examiner with good approximations of the absolute magnitude of the static acoustic impedance at the plane of the eardrum. For the most part, static acoustic impedance overlap between normal and pathological ears is small (Brooks, 1968; Jerger, 1970; Nilges et al., 1969; Wilber et al., 1970; Zwislocki and Feldman,

1970), and other tests in the battery often provide enough information about the overlapping group to minimize its significance even further. It is only about 10% of pathological middle ears that overlap on either side of the normal distribution. Some of this overlap comes from otherwise normal ears which have atypically high acoustic impedance, and some from pathological ears falling within the normal range. As has already been noted, the use of high frequency tympanometry has made it possible to explain why some patients with pathology that results in stiff middle-ear systems, but who also have healed perforations of the tympanic membrane, have acoustic impedance that overlaps into the normal range. While it has not yet been demonstrated, it is possible that some pathological thickening and scarring of an eardrum may also contribute to a higher acoustic impedance.

5. *The Use of Phase Angle in Interpretation of Clinical Data.* The inclusion of phase angles, as suggested by Lilly (1972, 1973), has not yet been applied on a broad enough clinical scale to evaluate its contribution to the differential diagnostic battery. In theory, differential pathological effects on the resistive component will be revealed by shifts in the phase angle. Table V is a tabulation of a sample of data from otosclerotic ears measured with the Grason Stadler Otoadmittance meter compared with previously reported data obtained with a Zwislocki acoustic bridge. All data is reported in acoustic ohms and phase angle. With both instruments, when compared to the normative data in Table IV, not only is there an approximate doubling of the acoustic ohm value in otosclerosis but also a shift in phase angle, which implies that the preponderant effect on the impedance is reactive. Phase angle derivation is possible with instruments that provide the resistive and reactive components. Given this information, the phase angle can be computed from a conversion chart (Newman and Fanger, 1973).

6. *Interpretation and Reporting of Static Acoustic Impedance.* As displayed in Table IV, normative data for static acoustic impedance has been developed (Feldman, 1973, 1974; Jerger *et al.*, 1972) for both the Madsen Z070 electroacoustic bridge and the Grason Stadler Model 1720 Otoadmittance meter. This can be displayed in either numerical or template form. However, no standard report form between instruments has been developed. In most clinical situations, it is sufficient to determine simply whether the static acoustic impedance falls within or outside the normal ranges. When it falls outside that range it may be described as high or low impedance, whichever may be the case, and the appropriate pathologies that fit these categories must be ruled out. An example of one way of plotting results is shown in Figure 12, which displays static acoustic impedance obtained on a normal ear and an abnormal ear (oto-

TABLE V

RANGES (10TH, 50TH, AND 90TH CENTILE) OF ACOUSTIC IMPEDANCE (z_A), ACOUSTIC ADMITTANCE (y_A), AND PHASE ANGLE FOR 15 OTOSCLEROTIC EARS MEASURED WITH THE GRASON STADLER 1720 OTOADMITTANCE METER, COMPARED WITH SIMILAR RANGES OF ACOUSTIC IMPEDANCE (z_A) AND PHASE ANGLE FOR 23 OTOSCLEROTIC EARS MEASURED WITH A ZWISLOCKI MECHANICAL ACOUSTIC BRIDGE

| Otoadmittance meter data, 15 otosclerotic ears | | | | | Zwislocki bridge data,[a] 23 otosclerotic ears | | |
Probe frequency	Z_A (in acoustic ohms)	Phase angle	Y_A (in acoustic mmho)	Range (in centiles)	Probe frequency	Z_A (in acoustic ohms)	Phase angle
220 Hz	6020	$\underline{/-77°}$	.14	90th	250 Hz	6002	$\underline{/-78.6°}$
220 Hz	3162	$\underline{/-79°}$	.31	50th	250 Hz	2568	$\underline{/-81.6°}$
220 Hz	1961	$\underline{/-79°}$	.50	10th	250 Hz	2354	$\underline{/-82.1°}$
660 Hz	2040	$\underline{/-72°}$	.53	90th	750 Hz	1607	$\underline{/-66.3°}$
660 Hz	1047	$\underline{/-44°}$	.95	50th	750 Hz	1023	$\underline{/-73.2°}$
660 Hz	642	$\underline{/-45°}$	1.55	10th	750 Hz	652	$\underline{/-70.4°}$

[a] From Lilly, 1972.

NOTE: Phase angle for admittance would be positive.

113

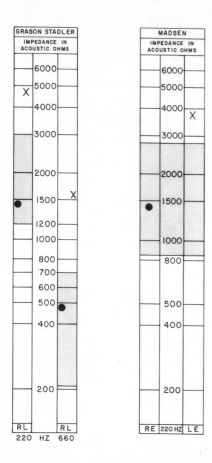

Figure 12 Normal right ear (filled circle) and otosclerotic left ear (X) of a patient measured with Grason Stadler 1720 Otoadmittance meter and Madsen Z070 electroacoustic bridge. Shaded area represents normal range for each instrument.

sclerosis), each measured with the two different instruments. This sort of display form quickly reveals the relationship to normal range of any individual ear.

B. Tympanometry

The changing transmission characteristics of the middle ear accompanying a change of air pressure in the sealed ear canal are displayed by a curve called a "tympanogram" (Terkildsen, 1962, 1964). Placing the tympanic membrane under stress with positive and negative pressure decreases the flow of energy through the middle ear by increasing its impedance (von Békésy, 1932). This results in the reflection of a major portion of a signal directed toward the eardrum. Although in theory, with the drum under stress, a probe hermetically sealed in the ear would be directing the signal into a rigid walled cavity, some transmission still occurs under this condition, and the reflection of the signal is not complete. However, a sufficient decoupling of the middle ear is achieved in this manner to allow for the electroacoustic analysis of the middle-ear function. The stress measurement is primarily a consequence of the ear-canal volume (Terkildsen and Thomsen, 1959). As the air pressure across the plane of the tympanic membrane is returned to normal, the impedance of the system becomes minimal and flow is maximized through the middle ear. This flow reaches its peak at ambient atmospheric pressure, and the measurement at this point is a combination of ear-canal volume and the static acoustic impedance of the middle ear (Figure 13). Deviations in amplitude, location, and shape of the derived tympanogram provide the examiner with considerable information about the possible pathological conditions that may exist to interfere with normal middle-ear function.

Thomsen (1958) first suggested pressure balance methods using the Metz mechanical acoustic bridge in a pressure chamber as a means of measuring middle-ear pressure and Eustachian-tube function. However, tympanometry as a clinical test of middle-ear function was developed with the advent of the electroacoustic impedance bridge, first described by Terkildsen and Scott Nielsen (1960) and initially reported as a test of various pathologies of the middle ear by Terkildsen and Thomsen (1959) and Terkildsen (1962, 1964). A number of authors have since described the application of this approach, which serves as the foundation of electroacoustic impedance measurements (Brooks, 1968, 1969; Fulton and Lamb, 1970; Lamb and Norris, 1969; Liden *et al.*, 1970a,b; Newman and Fanger, 1973; Peterson and Liden, 1970). Depending on the instrumen-

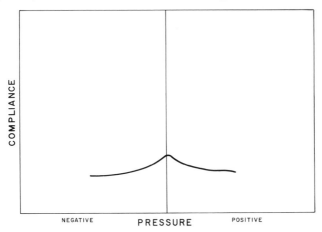

Figure 13 Changing compliance as a function of pressure in a normal ear.

tation, readout of tympanometric function may be plotted either manually or automatically, each yielding the same essential data, although very distinct differences in detail are present with different instruments or different plotting modes.

1. *Interpretation of Tympanogram.* There has been some tendency in the past to fit tympanograms into categories (Jerger, 1970, 1973). Such an approach may prove too restrictive. As more versatile instrumentation is developed, confusing subcategories and a proliferation of classifications is a likely natural consequence. Already, the once-simple three categories described by Jerger (1970) have grown to at least six basic curves (Rock, 1972). The clinician is often in the position of having to report the results of impedance evaluations to referring sources, many of whom know nothing about impedance, let alone how some subtests may be typed. As a result, reporting a "Type A_S" or "A_{dd}" would be meaningless. In the end, the results must be interpreted and communicated in terms of the possible clinical entities a particular tympanogram may represent. It would be far more appropriate for the clinician to think directly in these terms rather than including the unnecessary and often misinforming intermediate step of typing or classifying data into a noncommunicative category.

Each tympanogram can be interpreted with respect to (*1*) *its peak pressure point*, (*2*) *its peak amplitude*, and (*3*) *its shape.* These three factors provide the examiner with maximum information about the middle ear under test, which may be conveyed in a descriptive manner. One has a better chance of understanding the effect of pathology on impedance when thinking in these terms.

(*a*) *Pressure point of tympanograms.* (*1*) *Normal pressure tympanogram.* The origins of tympanometry stem from an attempt to find a simple clinical means of assessing the status of air pressure in the middle ear. Dishoeck's (1938) pneumophone method involved a subjective impression by the patient of maximum signal loudness when the state of pressure was varied in the ear canal, and Thomsen (1958) demonstrated that the impedance measurement could objectively evaluate the state of middle-ear pressure. Various estimates have been made as to the range of air pressure in the normal middle ear relative to the ear canal. Brooks (1969) found that, in 92% of a pediatric population, pressure ranged between 0 and −170 mm H_2O, and considered this range the limit for normality, while Jerger (1970) used a −100 mm criteria. Porter (1972) used a ±50 mm criteria in a study of normal children and adults. Rock (1972) considered a pressure deviation of −60 mm pathological although he reported only five of 153 normal ears to demonstrate more than −30 mm pressure. Holmquist (1972a) reported a range of ±25 mm to be the limits

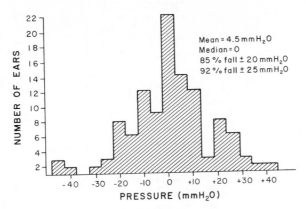

Figure 14 Histogram of distribution of middle-ear pressure of 100 patients with no middle-ear pathology.

of normal for a series of 160 ears. In a study of 100 children and adults with normal middle ears, Feldman (1973) found 92% of the subjects to fall within a range of ± 25 mm H_2O. As seen in Figure 14, which displays that distribution of middle-ear pressure, the mean pressure is 0 mm and the distribution is quite symmetrical, being equally distributed on the negative and positive side of ambient atmospheric pressure. Using a ± 30 mm H_2O as the anticipated range of normal would encompass 95% of this population and would appear to be a far more reasonable figure than even the popular ± 50 mm H_2O. Description of such a tympanogram would simply be that the middle ear functions best at ambient pressure. In these ears, pathology that may exist is unrelated to where the optimal pressure point is. In addition to normal ears, those with otosclerosis and interruption of the ossicular chain can be expected to have normal tympanometric pressure function. The distinction between these two pathologies is in the amplitude and shape, not the peak pressure point.

(2) *Negative pressure tympanogram.* Tympanograms that peak at some point negative to this recommended range will do so because of (1) poor Eustachian-tube function, either acute or chronic, (2) residual adhesive otitis, or (3) middle-ear effusion or serous otitis, usually in the resolving or developing stage, but occasionally in the acute stage. Most ears with serous otitis and so-called "glue" ears have essentially flat tympanograms, without a peak at any pressure point. This implies a rigidly fixed system that does not improve in transmission under any pressure state. Figure 15 shows tympanograms of the ears of three patients, each demonstrating one of these negative pressure conditions. It is important to note that, when a peak has not been attained by a -200 mm pressure, additional negative pressure may reveal the existence of a peak point.

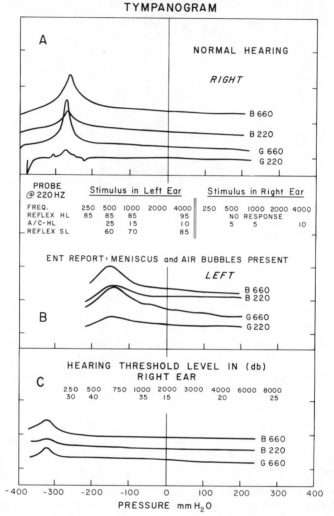

TYMPANOGRAM

A

NORMAL HEARING

RIGHT

B 660

B 220

G 660
G 220

PROBE @ 220HZ	Stimulus in Left Ear					Stimulus in Right Ear			
FREQ.	250	500	1000	2000	4000	250	500	1000 2000	4000
REFLEX HL	85	85	85		95			NO RESPONSE	
A/C-HL		25	15		10		5	5	10
REFLEX SL		60	70		85				

ENT REPORT: MENISCUS and AIR BUBBLES PRESENT

LEFT

B 660
B 220

G 660
G 220

B

HEARING THRESHOLD LEVEL IN (db)
RIGHT EAR

250	500	750	1000	2000	3000	4000	6000	8000
30	40		35	15		20		25

C

B 660

B 220

G 660

-400   -300   -200   -100   0   100   200   300   400

PRESSURE mm H$_2$O

Figure 15 Tympanogram of three patients with negative-pressure peaks illustrating: (A) probable adhesions and tympanosclerosis but normal hearing; (B) serous otitis media in a resolving stage; and (C) negative pressure but no apparent fluid or visible retraction.

Thus, had the pressure not been extended beyond −200 mm in the patient with adhesive otitis (Figure 15A), the tympanogram would have appeared flat. In none of these patients is it possible to say which of the conditions is acting to produce the derived tympanograms. All that is revealed by the tympanometry is that the middle ear transmits energy best at a negative pressure. They can all be described as *negative pressure tympanograms*. This does not necessarily mean that air pressure behind the eardrum is negative. In an ear with adhesions, the pressure in the middle ear may be completely normal, but the adhesions may affect the position of the eardrum and ossicles in such a way that transmission is best when the system is pulled into a different position by the negative canal pressure.

One of the difficulties in validating tympanometry is that the test itself is more sensitive than most other examining methods (Bluestone *et al.*, 1973). Pressure deviations of -100 to -200 mm H_2O do not always reveal themselves to otoscopic examinations. For example, the patient with poor Eustachian-tube ventilation shown in Figure 15C was repeatedly examined by the otologist, who continued to be unimpressed with the physical findings. However, an unexplained bilateral 30-dB mixed but primarily conductive hearing loss, along with the repeated negative pressure tympanograms, finally led to the decision to perform an exploratory myringotomy. The findings were negative in that no fluid was found, but pressure equalization tubes were placed in both eardrums. Following this, hearing improved 20-dB, and Eustachian-tube function tested with the pressure equalization tubes in place was normal. This conflict with otoscopic examination is quite common, and tympanometry is generally found to be the better judge of the middle-ear pressure status.

(3) *Positive pressure tympanogram.* Pathologically positive pressure peak tympanograms are less common than those with negative pressure peaks. Middle-ear diseases generally result in the latter pathology and rarely exhibit positive pressure peaks. It is conceivable that, if a patient were tested immediately following a forceful sneeze, the tympanogram would peak on the positive pressure axis. The same would be true following a Valsalva maneuver. However, evacuation through the Eustachian tube is more easily accomplished when pressure in the middle ear is positive than when it is negative, and pressure equalization will occur quickly as the patient swallows.

The one pathological condition that can result in a positive pressure peaked tympanogram is acute otitis media. An example of this transient condition is shown in Figure 16, which plots the tympanometric function measured over the course of acute otitis media accompanying an upper respiratory infection and following recovery. Antibiotic treatment was started just prior to the first measurement. It should be noted that, from the first to second day, the pressure shift was $+100$ mm in the right ear. By the third day, the shift was back to a $+40$ mm value but with a more shallow peak. Three days later, the pressure peak was measured at -120 mm. At this time, the acute otitis disease process had resolved, and the

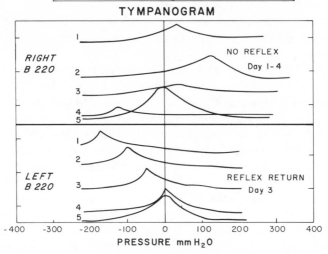

	Stimulus in Left Ear					Stimulus in Right Ear				
	250	500	1000	2000	4000	250	500	1000	2000	4000
12/14	10	15	5	5	0	10	5	5	10	-5
12/16	5	0	-10	0	0	0	0	5	5	15

TYMPANOGRAM

Figure 16 Serial tympanograms for right and left ears of patient with right acute otitis media and left Eustachian-tube blockage. Also shown is the pure-tone audiogram obtained on the first and third examinations. Curves 1 to 3 were recorded on successive days, curve 4, 3 days later, and curve 5, 3 months later.

pathology now was diagnosed as a serous otitis, which was treated by myringotomy. When tested 6 months later, the tympanogram appeared normal in all respects except for an increased amplitude of the tympanogram, probably because of the healed myringotomy. The opposite ear is also shown for comparison along with air-conduction thresholds for both ears. It is of interest that there was neither a complaint by the patient nor otoscopic evidence of an abnormality in the left ear, which over the course of the examinations moved from a −170 mm H_2O pressure to normal. The ear that simply showed evidence of poor ventilation may have been described as "blocked" by the patient, had not that feeling been overshadowed by the rather painful acute otitis in the right ear. Amplitude of this tympanogram did not change significantly at any time.

Another common index of middle-ear function is the audiogram. The hearing loss in both ears shown in Figure 16 never really exceeded the limits of normal by usual standards, although a symmetrical mild shift in air-conduction threshold was clearly evident in each ear. Brooks (1971) has advocated tympanometry as a more effective screening device in a pediatric population. Eagles *et al.* (1967) pointed out that screening audiometry fails to identify a significant number of children with middle-ear disease. Jerger *et al.* (1972) found 8% of a sample of 1133 normal patients to demonstrate abnormal tympanometry without audiometric evidence of a conductive loss. Subtle pathology of the middle-ear system is frequently first detected by the acoustic impedance measurement, which is a more sensitive index of the transmission characteristics of the middle ear than is audiometry. Presumed unilateral otosclerotic patients have been found to demonstrate increased acoustic impedance in the "uninvolved" ear (Feldman, 1969), implying that the otosclerotic process had already begun before the audiogram revealed it.

(b) *Amplitude of tympanograms.* The amplitude of the tympanogram is a function of the compliance of the system. A stiff, noncompliant middle ear is revealed by a shallow amplitude curve, while a loose, flaccid system yields a large amplitude tympanogram. Ears with high acoustic impedance fit the former category, and low acoustic impedance ears the latter. For systems that are self-balancing, such as the Grason Stadler Model 1720, one may compute the absolute magnitude of the acoustic impedance or admittance components by calculating the values of the eardrum under positive and negative stress, averaging them, and subtracting the derived value from the amplitude of the appropriate tympanogram (1) at ambient pressure and (2) at peak amplitude. For normal-pressure tympanograms, these will be the same points; but in negative and positive pressure tympanograms, the latter points deviate from ambient pressure. If desired, this value can be used as an estimate of a potential impedance. However, sufficient research has yet to be reported on the relationship between the optimal impedance in pathological ears and the impedance in those ears when they revert to normal. The probability that pathology such as serous otitis will reduce the amplitude (Bluestone *et al.*, 1973; Brooks, 1968, 1969) was noted in the ear with acute otitis, shown in Figure 16.

When the tympanogram is plotted, either automatically or manually, the use of a template provides a quick indication of whether or not the amplitude of the tympanogram deviates from anticipated normal ranges. The technique for this is not the same with all instruments. The Madsen Z070 and the American Electromedics 81, for example, plot in relative units with a preprinted template referred to a baseline on the tympanogram (Figure 17). The Grason Stadler 1720, because it is calibrated in absolute units which record both B_A and G_A for two frequencies, uses a template overlay (Figure 18). These templates cannot be preprinted on the tympanogram form with this instrument, not only because of the calibrated multiple readouts, but also because the position of the positive and negative stress points is a function of the ear-canal volume in front of the

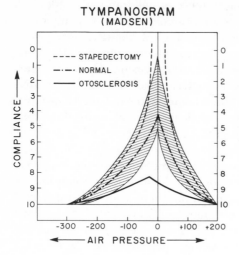

Figure 17 Tympanogram showing the range of normal compliance as a function of pressure (striated area) for Madsen Z070 electroacoustic bridge. Typical tympanograms for ears with high impedance (otosclerosis), low impedance (stapedectomy), and normal impedance are shown relative to the normal range.

probe, which will vary with both the ear-canal size and the depth of insertion of the probe. With any instrument, it is evident that the static acoustic impedance for negative and positive pressure tympanograms will always be identified as high because the amplitude at ambient pressure is negligible. When the peak amplitude is within the ambient-pressure range, however, high-impedance ears will peak below the template, and

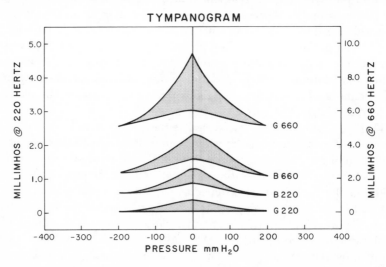

Figure 18 Templates of normal tympanometric ranges for conductance (G) and susceptance (B) at 220 and 660 Hz with the Grason Stadler 1720 Otoadmittance meter.

low-impedance ears will peak above it, as demonstrated by the two examples in Figure 17.

For noncalibrated readout systems, such as the Madsen, Peters, and American Electromedics, the tympanogram amplitude is a relative index of compliance and not an absolute reading of static impedance. In tympanometry with calibrated systems, the measurement of the amplitude of the derived curves is the method for deriving the static acoustic impedance values. The location of the peak of the curve on the pressure axis is the index of eardrum position and middle-ear pressure. This allows for differentiation of those pathologies that may be similar in static acoustic impedance but which differ on the pressure axis. Of course, the clinician must bear in mind that, just as some normal-hearing people may exhibit negative pressure tympanograms as residuals from old pathology, similarly, some otosclerotics will present the same complicating phenomenon. In these instances, the clinician must rely on other aspects of the test battery to attempt to clarify the nature of the basic problem.

Since the advent of tympanometry, it has been evident that healed perforations of the tympanic membrane have an effect on the amplitude of the tympanogram (Terkildsen and Thomsen, 1959). Although Liden *et al.* (1970a,b) emphasized the effect of healed perforations on the shape of a tympanogram for high frequency probe tones, as will be discussed later, Feldman (1974) and Alberti and Jerger (1974) also noted the effect of that condition on amplitude. This is demonstrated in Table VI,

TABLE VI

MEDIAN AND 80% RANGE OF B_A, G_A, Y_A, AND Z_A FOR POPULATION OF 17 PATIENTS WITH ONE NORMAL EARDRUM AND ONE EARDRUM WITH EVIDENCE OF HEALED PERFORATION[a]

	80% Range in mmho		Medians in mmho	
	TM Pathology	Normal	TM Pathology	Normal
B_A 220	.75 — 2.25	.45 — 1.25	1.40	.7
G_A 220	.1 — .9	.05 — .40	.45	.15
B_A 660	2.3 — 4.55	.8 — 3.65	2.70	1.65
G_A 660	4.25 — 10.75	1.45 — 5.3	6.80	2.50
Y_A 220	.8 — 2.4	.45 — 1.25	1.5	.75
Y_A 660	4.55 — 11.6	1.65 — 6.45	7.4	3.4
Z_A 220	412 — 1235	798 — 2223	656	1333
Z_A 660	86 — 220	155 — 602	135	295

[a] From Feldman, 1972.

which compares medians and ranges of B_A, G_A, Y_A, and Z_A for a group of patients with a normal tympanic membrane on one side and a healed perforation on the other. It is clearly evident that the effect of a healed perforation is to lower markedly the static acoustic impedance (increase the amplitude of the tympanogram), not only for higher frequency probe tones, but also at the commonly used 220-Hz probe frequency. This effect would cause otherwise stiff, pathological ears to appear as normal or loose pathological ears, and explains why the static acoustic impedance of some otosclerotics appears normal. It must be emphasized that interpretation of the static acoustic impedance, as revealed by the amplitude of the tympanogram, is of minimal validity unless the examiner is aware that the derived tympanogram is showing an effect of eardrum, not middle-ear, pathology. This is often impossible to achieve without the use of higher frequency probe tones whose tympanogram shape as well as amplitude provide this information. The implication, of course, is that when there is a healed perforation of the tympanic membrane, valid measurement of middle-ear static impedance is not feasible. The scarred eardrum functions as an uncontrollable variable which prevents accurate static acoustic impedance evaluation of the middle-ear system.

(c) *Shape of the tympanogram.* The third aspect of interpretation of tympanograms relates to the shape of the curve. Slope and smoothness are the essential features differentiating this variable.

(1) *Slope of the tympanogram.* The sharpness of the tympanogram at the point of maximum compliance has been suggested as an index of pathology (Brooks, 1969). By measuring the height of the curve from a perpendicular bisecting the tympanogram between two points ±50 mm of pressure around its peak, an amplitude gradient is derived (Figure 19). The normal gradient value is about 40% of the compliance. The gradi-

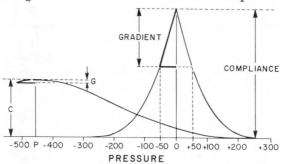

Figure 19 Computation of pressure gradient (G) based on variations of compliance (C) in response to pressure changes for a normal middle ear (right tympanogram) and an ear with fluid in the middle-ear space (left tympanogram). (From Brooks, 1969).

ent can drop to less than 10% in ears with fluid and can reach as much as 80% in cases of healed perforation. Thus, stiffening pathologies reduce the gradient as well as the amplitude to which it is related, and loosening pathologies increase it. This is an extension of a template application, in that it views amplitude in relation to the slope. One problem when using gradient values for diagnostic purposes is that the slope in normal ears is instrument-, not ear-, related, and slope-gradient norms would have to be developed for different instruments. Figure 20 compares basic curves

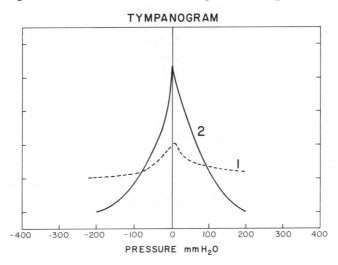

TYMPANOGRAM

PRESSURE mm H₂O

Figure 20   Comparison of tympanogram shape and amplitude on the same normal ear measured with a Grason–Stadler Otoadmittance meter (1) and a Madsen Electroacoustic bridge (2).

from the same ear obtained with two different instruments. It is evident that the slope gradient of each is different. This is a consequence of one instrument (Grason Stadler Model 1720) having an AVC circuit that internally adjusts the signal so that the SPL in the ear canal is maintained at a constant level. At each point on the curve, the value, in this instance susceptance, is an absolute measurement. The shape is directly related to the absolute change in impedance. With the Madsen-type instrument, the SPL is not constant because the control of SPL and air pressure are independently varied. Thus, this type of instrument does not generate a constant SPL of 95 dB, but, instead, the level in the canal changes as the impedance changes with modification of air pressure. This results in exaggerated and noncalibrated amplitude curves. With instruments of this sort, the tympanogram itself is strictly a relative indication of the actual acoustic impedance.

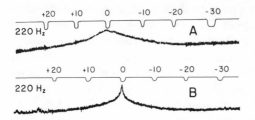

Figure 21 Comparison of tympanometric shape for a normal eardrum (A) and an eardrum with a healed perforation (B). (From Terkildsen and Thomsen, 1959.)

Changes in slope have been described since the advent of tympanometry. Terkildsen and Thomsen (1959) described a steepening of the tympanogram peak with atrophic healed tympanic membranes (Figure 21). Using the same kind of uncalibrated system, Liden *et al.* (1970a) studied notch depth and width for a 220-Hz, 625-Hz, and 800-Hz probe tone. They noted an increasing depth and width as well as the difference in SPL between the two stress points of the tympanogram. Each of these parameters increased with frequency. Thus, gradient values would be expected to change with higher probe-tone frequencies. A slight deviation from normal pressure was also noted for the higher frequencies. One additional aspect of slope is the configuration in instances of middle-ear effusion. When both low- and high-frequency probe tones are used, there is a tendency for the convergence of the susceptance tracings under negative pressure. This is demonstrated in Figure 22, which displays the sus-

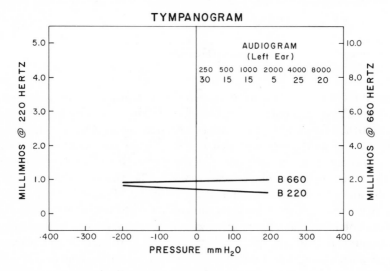

Figure 22 Flat tympanograms from an ear with serous fluid, showing the typical convergence of B 220 and B 660 tracings.

ceptance tympanograms of an ear with acute serous otitis but a very mild hearing loss.

(2) *Smoothness of the tympanogram.* The usual smooth, symmetrical tympanometric curve has been shown to be affected by pathology. The effect is greatest with high-frequency probe tones (Alberti and Jerger, 1974; Feldman, 1974; Liden et al., 1970a,b; Peterson and Liden, 1970). The four possible factors that have been identified as contributing to this effect include: (1) interruption of the ossicular chain; (2) healed perforations of the tympanic membrane; (3) hypermobility or flaccidity of the tympanic membrane; and (4) normal resonance of the system. In reality, the first three of these factors are special conditions that alter the normal resonance of the middle ear, shifting it lower in frequency. Most normal ears are stiffness-dominated in the probe tone range of current electro-acoustic bridges. As a consequence, the resonance of the normal ear is not generally revealed in tympanometry. As stiffness decreases and mass effects increase, notching of the tympanogram occurs. With the use of a probe-tone frequency as high as 800 Hz (Alberti and Jerger, 1974; Liden et al., 1970a,b; Peterson and Liden, 1970), it is predictable that a shifting of the stiffness–mass relationships would result in rather bizarre resonance effects and, consequently, a change in the smoothness of the tympanogram.

It has been demonstrated with a mechanical acoustic bridge that ossicular discontinuity lowers the resonant point of the ear (Feldman, 1964; Preide, 1970). This is revealed by a deep "W" patterning of the tympanogram, as shown by Liden et al. (1970a,b) and Peterson and Liden (1970). An example of the effect of such an interruption, i.e., broadening the notch and introducing a "W" pattern, is displayed by the tympanogram, in Figure 23, of a patient with crural interruption associated with van der Hoeve's syndrome. It also increases the amplitude of the low-frequency tympanogram beyond normal limits and may be revealed by a tympanogram that goes off scale with noncalibrated readouts, as was noted in Figure 17. In these low-impedance systems, when the pressure in the ear canal is higher or lower than the pressure in the middle ear, the stiffness of the system is exaggerated. This increases the negative reactance. However, as the air pressure in the canal relative to the middle ear approaches a state of equality, positive reactance becomes a more dominant factor, resulting in a sudden marked change in the stiffness–mass relationships. This is revealed by the "W" patterning of the tympanogram, and the reversal of direction is an indication of the phase shift.

In the case of small healed perforations, the "W" patterning tends to be smaller than for interruptions (Figure 24). In the former condition, the

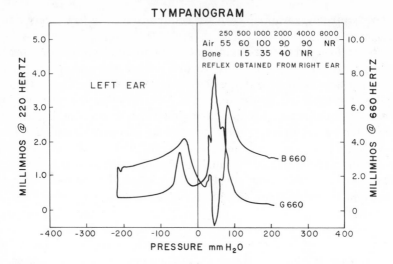

Figure 23 Tympanograms with marked multiple notching that is both broad and deep, observed in an ear with ossicular discontinuity. Notching occurs around peak pressure point and implies sudden shift from stiffness to mass control in the susceptance curve.

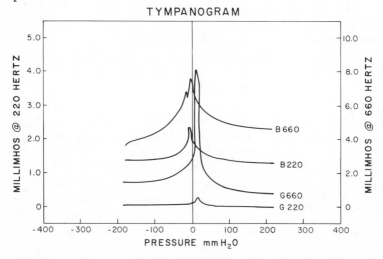

Figure 24 Notching of B 660 tympanogram and sharp peaking of the B 220, G 220, and G 660 tympanograms, all characteristic of a healed perforation pattern.

signal reflected from the eardrum is affected not only by the mechanical factors of the middle ear, the air pressure change across the eardrum, and the differences in vibration pattern of the eardrum as frequency increases, but also by the differences in reflected signals from the normal three-layer tympanic membrane and the thinner healed areas. This results in less marked "W" patterning or a peaking of the tympanogram for the higher frequency probe tones. The extent of the "W" pattern notching may depend on the size and location of the healed perforation.

The very flaccid eardrum may also behave in a manner similar to an ear with an interruption. This has been suggested by Alberti and Jerger (1974) and Liden et al. (1970a), who observed the "W" patterning in flaccid eardrums in otherwise normal ears. It may be that the 800-Hz probe tone used in those studies was too close to the natural first resonant point of the ear, and this effect may be noted as a consequence of resonance, not pathology. In the latter study, it was barely perceptible for a 625-Hz probe tone for a flaccid eardrum, but marked for one with a healed perforation.

The implication of these findings with higher frequency probe tones is that both eardrum and middle-ear pathology can affect the amplitude and shape of the tympanogram. The closer the probe tone is to the natural resonance of the ear, the more likely it is that the measurement will be contaminated by nonpathological factors. Consequently, it would appear that the upper probe tone frequency of choice should be set below the 800-Hz resonant point of the ear. This should probably be somewhere between 500 Hz and 700 Hz. At the same time, it is important to use a probe tone in this latter range because of the contrasting effects of pathologies on resonance. It is also a good means of validating amplitude as an index of static acoustic impedance. As noted earlier, when changes in shape associated with a healed perforation are observed with a higher frequency probe tone it also affects the lower frequency tympanogram amplitude, and thus would invalidate the static values of both low and high frequencies. In these instances, the condition of the tympanic membrane precludes the precise measurement of the middle ear itself. This is clearly demonstrated in Figure 25, which shows the tympanogram of a patient with confirmed otosclerosis. Tympanometric measurements at both low and high frequencies were suggestive of a loose, rather than a stiff, middle-ear system. Similar results were obtained with measurements made with a Zwislocki mechanical acoustic bridge. However, the ear had several large healed perforations; and it was the eardrum, more than the middle ear, that was affecting the measurement in this patient. Because of the healed perforations, it was not possible to measure accurately the stiffened middle-ear system secondary to the footplate fixation.

Figure 26 demonstrates an additional factor that alters the smoothness of the tympanogram. In the instance of vascular perturbations, there will be superimposed pulsations on the basic tympanograms. In this patient, the basic pattern is normal, and the pulsations are not indicative

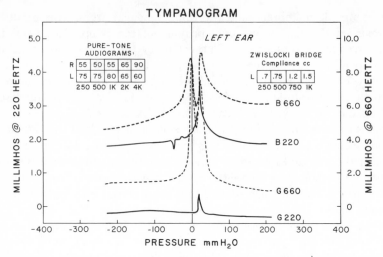

Figure 25 Marked notched "W" pattern and exaggerated conductance and susceptance values in one ear of a patient with otosclerosis and a large healed perforation of the tympanic membrane. Also shown are Zwislocki acoustic bridge compliance values and air-conduction thresholds.

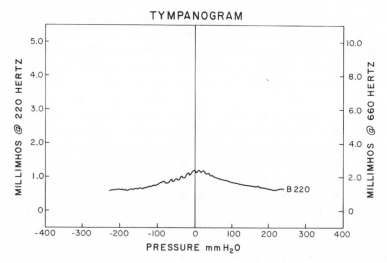

Figure 26 Tympanogram measured for B 220 Hz demonstrating superimposed vascular perturbations.

of pathology. However, similar perturbations on a flat tympanogram might be suggestive of a glomus jugulari tumor. Fluctuations occurring in synchrony with the respiration rate would imply abnormal patency of the Eustachian tube.

C. Intraaural Muscle Reflex

The early failures in the clinical use of static acoustic impedance measurements resulted in a reliance on the determination of relative impedance changes associated with the contraction of the intraaural muscles (Djupesland, 1962, 1964, 1967, 1969a,b; Jepsen, 1953, 1955, 1963; Klockhoff, 1961; Metz, 1946, 1952). The anatomical arrangement of the middle-ear muscles is such that the contraction of the tensor tympani pulls the manubrium of the malleus and the eardrum inward. The contraction of the stapedius muscle moves the stapes, stiffens the ossicular chain, and moves the eardrum outward or in a biphasic pattern (Yonovitz and Harris, 1972). The overall result of these ossicular displacements is a reduced mobility of the ossicular chain. This increased stiffness and possible modification of volume results in a simultaneous change in the impedance measured at the tympanic membrane (Feldman and Zwislocki, 1965; Hung and Dallos, 1972; Lilly and Shepherd, 1964; Møller, 1962). The result of this change can be determined in an absolute sense and is measured as an increase in impedance when the ear canal is sealed, or may simply be measured as a change in impedance when measured in dynamic terms. This dynamic change in impedance is what has been most broadly applied in many clinical settings. Because the reflex is bilateral to a unilateral stimulus, acoustic impedance changes in one ear may be studied with a stimulus presented to the contralateral ear. At the same time, the reflex-eliciting stimulus can provide some index of sensorineural function in the contralateral ear. The test ear in acoustic reflex measurements varies. If one is looking at the impedance change, then the ear in which the probe sits is the test ear. However, when measuring threshold for elicitation of the reflex, the test ear is the ear being stimulated with the eliciting signal.

Questions exist about the role of the tensor tympani in response to acoustic stimulation in man. It is generally acknowledged that, in many animals, both the stapedius and tensor tympanic muscles exhibit a similar response to acoustic stimulation (Borg, 1972a,b; Carmel and Starr, 1963; Kato, 1913; Kobrak, 1938; Møller, 1965). However, in man, acoustic impedance measurement of the tensor tympanic muscle response has rarely been reported (Weiss et al., 1962). For the most part, when implied by acoustic impedance change, the response to acoustic stimulation appears to be confined to the stapedius muscle (Djupesland, 1964, 1967; Feldman, 1967b; Jepsen, 1955; Klockhoff, 1961; Møller, 1961; Terkildsen, 1960). Activity of the tensor tympani in response to high sound levels has been reported by means of electromyographic recordings (Djupesland, 1967; Salomon and Starr, 1963) and also by manometric or pres-

sure transducer recordings (Liden *et al.*, 1970b; Terkildsen, 1957; Yonovitz and Harris, 1972). Acoustically elicited eardrum displacement attributed to action of the tensor tympani muscle, recorded with a pressure transducer, occurs at a much higher intensity than simultaneous
acoustic impedance changes attributed to the stapedius muscle.

In clinical practice, acoustic impedance changes caused by contraction of the intraaural muscles have been viewed as being either present
or absent, with little regard given to other characteristics of the reflex.
In general, responses are elicited with acoustic or nonacoustic stimulation and, with electroacoustic impedance instruments, can be monitored
as a meter deflection or recorded on a strip-chart recorder.

1. Acoustic Stimulation. The normal-ear threshold for acoustic elicitation of the stapedius reflex has been studied by a number of investigators (Deutsch, 1972; Franzen and Lilly, 1970; Fulton and Lamb, 1964;
Jepsen, 1951; Metz, 1952; Peterson and Liden, 1972; Robertson *et al.*,
1968; Weiss *et al.*, 1962). It is generally accepted that the normal threshold for the reflex ranges between 75- to 95-dB SL re audiometric zero
and about 20 to 30 dB less than that for broad and narrow band noises
(Deutsch, 1972; Franzen, 1970; Niemeyer and Sesterhenn, 1972). Although the reflex is considered to be a protective response to loudness,
the relationship between pure tone and noise thresholds would suggest
that the explanation of the response is more complicated. It is generally
acknowledged, however, that a reduction of the reflex SL implies cochlear pathology and is an indirect test of loudness recruitment (Metz,
1952; Thomsen, 1955b; Djupesland and Flottorp, 1970). The predominant clinical application of the stapedius reflex has been in the differential diagnosis of middle-ear disorders. Tests for the reflex should always be performed with pressure in the ear canal set at the peak amplitude pressure of the tympanogram.

(a) Evaluation of conductive loss. With the sole exception of ossicular interruption at the level of the stapedius crus, the presence of a
stapedial reflex implies an intact and mobile ossicular chain. Hearing
loss that exists as a consequence of middle-ear pathology does not always
eliminate the reflex. The general principle would appear to be that, if
contraction of the stapedius muscle can further increase the acoustic
impedance, the contraction will be evident. Ears with poor Eustachian-
tube ventilation, adhesions, resolving middle-ear effusion, and crural
interruption will generally demonstrate an acoustic reflex if a stimulus
with an effective SL can be delivered to the contralateral ear. Opposed
to these conditions, ears with otosclerosis, ossicular interruption peripheral to the insertion of the stapedial tendon, and acute serous otitis
media will fail to elicit the reflex. Distinctions between these latter path-

ologies are possible with static acoustic impedance and tympanometry.

Flottorp and Djupesland (1971) and Terkildsen (1964) have reported a biphasic negative on–off response in otosclerotic ears and speculated that this might be a tensor tympani muscle response. A similar response was reported by McCall (1973) in normal-hearing patients exhibiting spastic dysphonia. And Hung and Dallos (1972) noted that one-half of their normal subjects displayed a brief lowering of impedance that was attributed to a relaxation of the stapedius preceding its contraction. This short, quick drop in impedance prior to stapedius contraction is a common clinical observation and might also represent a momentary incudo–stapedial decoupling as the stapes head is pulled across the incudo–stapedial joint (Feldman and Zwislocki, 1965). The usual clinical observation in otosclerosis is a lack of any kind of intraaural muscle response to acoustic stimulation.

When no reflex is evident until extremely high stimulating SPLs are presented, caution must be applied in interpreting the results. If the eliciting stimulus is too close in frequency to the probe frequency and the signal sufficient to cross the skull to the contralateral ear canal, a false indication of a reflex may appear on the meter. This is a result of cross hearing by the bridge microphone. If the only response noted is for a frequency within an octave of the probe frequency, it should be ignored.

(b) Evaluation of cochlear and neural function.   Another important application of the stapedius reflex measurement relates to the response that is controlled by the ear stimulated with the reflex-eliciting stimulus. The reflex is monitored with an impedance probe in one ear by noting impedance changes in response to contralateral acoustic stimulation. Reduction in SL for the reflex is generally interpreted as an objective indication of cochlear pathology and the presence of recruitment (Beedle and Harford, 1970; Ewertsen et al., 1958; Jepsen, 1963; Kristensen and Jepsen, 1952; Lamb et al., 1968; Metz, 1952; Thomsen, 1955b). Thus, in ears with hearing loss but without evidence of middle-ear pathology, the presence of a reflex at a reduced sensation level re the normal (less than 65 dB) is considered to be an indication of cochlear pathology, as is recruitment. When no conductive loss is present and there is no reflex obtained, the locus of the pathology causing the hearing loss is considered to be retrocochlear. Jerger et al. (1972) have suggested that, in patients with loudness recruitment, the probability of obtaining a stapedial reflex diminishes with increasing hearing loss. The likelihood of obtaining a reflex is 90% with up to a 60-dB loss and diminishes from 50% with an 85-dB loss, to 5–10% with as much as a 100-dB loss.

Anderson et al. (1970) have suggested a further application of this test. They noted that patients with VIIIth nerve tumors demonstrated abnormal decay of the reflex (exceeding 50%) at a 10–dB reflex SL for 1000 Hz and below. Presentation of the eliciting stimulus to the ear with the tumor results in an initial response that rapidly decays as the stimulated nerve adapts. Other applications include tests for the reflex in Bell's palsy (Ramsey Hunt syndrome), herpes zoster oticus, and traumatic facial paralysis (Dieroff, 1965; Djupesland, 1969a; Feldman, 1964; Jepsen, 1955; Klockhoff, 1961). In these patients, when hearing is normal, a reflex in the uninvolved stapedius muscle will be obtained from the paralyzed side, but the reverse may not be true. Monitoring progression or recovery of acute conditions is greatly facilitated with this test.

There has been evidence also offered in support of the application of the acoustic reflex test in the evaluation of brainstem tumors. As Jerger (1973) has noted, lesions of the central auditory system often reflect the elaborate crossed pathway network of the auditory system in such a manner as to produce symptoms in the ear opposite to the affected side of the brain. While most clinical tests of the acoustic reflex are from the contralateral side, it is possible with electroacoustic instruments to introduce the eliciting stimulus through the pressure capillary tube in order to ipsilaterally test for the reflex. Greisen and Rasmussen (1970) reported on two patients with brainstem tumors who demonstrated normal ipsilaterally induced reflexes, which were absent when stimulation was from the contralateral ear. Similar results were noted by Steinberg and Lenhardt (1972), who reported reflexes absent from the ear contralateral to space-occupying lesions in four patients who had normal ipsilateral responses.

While reflex amplitude growth has not been fully documented, gross differences may be evident in pathologies. Peterson and Liden (1972) did note what appeared to be an abnormally small growth in reflex amplitude in relation to increasing contralateral stimulus amplitude in one patient with a lesion in the corpus callosum.

Most clinicians who have performed stapedius reflex tests have encountered the interesting, but at the same time impossible, phenomenon of a patient who demonstrates a stapedius reflex at better hearing levels (HL) than the threshold measured by pure-tone audiometry (Lamb and Peterson, 1967; Lamb et al., 1968; Thomsen, 1955a). This observation convincingly supports the presence of a functional hearing loss. The stapedius-reflex test is an objective indication of the validity of a hearing loss. While it is not possible completely to predict audiometric threshold for pure tones from reflex thresholds, only in rare instances will the reflex SL be as little as 15 dB. When the pure-tone audiometric threshold is better than the reflex threshold, it acts only as supporting evidence of either a functional hearing loss or a cochlear impairment. These findings should be interpreted in the context of the total battery of other audiological measures.

Various recent reports (Jerger *et al.*, 1974; Niemeyer and Sesterhenn, 1972; Olivier, 1972) have suggested techniques by which the threshold for the stapedius reflex may be used to predict pure-tone audiometry thresholds. It is still too early to evaluate whether or not these techniques will prove to be effective clinical procedure. The essential problem is related to the variability of the stapedius-reflex threshold in a normal population. The most promising approach may be that advocated by Jerger *et al.* (1974), who modified the Niemeyer and Sesterhenn approach by categorizing the degree of hearing impairment into three groups: normal, mild to moderate, and severe. Assuming that the normal difference between the broad-band noise and the pure-tone average of 500–2000 Hz elicited stapedial reflex threshold is 30 dB, then a reduction of this difference would place the loss in one of the two latter categories. When a difference of 20 to 30 dB exists, the degree of loss would be placed within normal limits. If the difference is reduced from 10 to 20 dB, a loss of mild to moderate degree is postulated. If less than a 10-dB difference is measured between the acoustic reflex threshold for the broad-band noise and pure tones, then a severe loss is postulated. There are a number of modifying criteria; the derivation of the difference is not based solely on the broad-band noise and pure-tone average. It also considers the reflex threshold of the best frequency and 500 Hz alone, as well as the absolute broad-band noise threshold. The slope of a hearing loss is determined by comparing the reflex threshold for two broad bands of noise, one a low pass up to 2600 Hz and the other a high pass above 2600 Hz. If the reflex threshold for each band is similar, then the pure-tone threshold configuration is presumed to be flat or gradual in slope. A difference in excess of 5 dB implies a steeper slope to the loss.

The observation that loudness discomfort levels for pure tones relates closely to reflex thresholds for pure tones has been the basis for the suggestion that the stapedius reflex threshold be used as a guide for establishing maximum power output of hearing aids (McCandless and Miller, 1972). However, until the relationships are better established between the reflex and pure tones, complex signals, and signal durations, specific parameters for such recommendations should be considered tentative. While it is probably not reasonable to infer discomfort for speech directly from reflex thresholds for pure tones, a reduced SL for the reflex should be considered supportive evidence of a lowered discomfort level for speech. This reduction should be considered when specifying the gain and maximum power output (MPO) of hearing aids.

For patients with a hearing loss, but with reflex thresholds within normal SPL ranges, the hearing aid output and gain should be kept at a minimum.

2. *Nonacoustic Stimulation of the Intraaural Muscles.* Failure to elicit a stapedius reflex does not necessarily imply the presence of middle-ear pathology. Not only is the reflex present in certain conductive pathologies, but other factors may be acting independently to inhibit a response. In both normal and pathological ears, the inability to generate the response may be due to (1) an inability to generate a sufficiently loud reflex-eliciting stimulus, (2) a paralysis of the stapedius muscle, or (3) an absence of the stapedius muscle. The most common of these is, of course, the first, whereby either a conductive or retrocochlear hearing loss effectively attenuates the loudness of the reflex-eliciting stimulus. Furthermore, tests for contraction of the tensor tympani muscle, as revealed by an acoustic impedance change, are usually unsuccessful with acoustic stimuli but may be detected with various nonacoustic stimuli (Djupesland, 1964, 1967, 1969a,b; Klockhoff, 1961; Terkildsen, 1960).

Certain precautions must be taken in nonacoustic stimulation, and these relate to minimizing artifacts. Head movement relative to the probe in the ear and contact with the probe will both result in meter-needle deflection that will appear similar to the muscle response. Most nonacoustic stimuli, and, hence, most consequent reflex responses, are of short duration and are difficult to differentiate from artifact responses. The failure to elicit a response is often more informative than the presence of an apparent response.

(*a*) *Stapedius muscle responses.* Failure to elicit an acoustic stapedius reflex should be followed by tests using nonacoustic stimuli to attempt to establish the mobility of the middle-ear system under examination. Klockhoff (1961) advocated ipsilateral electrical stimulation of the ear canal. This was achieved by placing a foil electrode on the ear-canal probe tip, using a train of electrical pulses with a frequency of 50 cps and 1 msec duration. Djupesland (1964, 1967) reported contralateral stimulation to be effective either when the skin in the canal or on the surface of the face and head around the aurical was stimulated by a blast of air from a Politzer bag, or when the same area was touched with a piece of cotton wool. When a change in impedance is recorded in conjunction with this type of nonacoustic stimulation, one may infer a contraction of the stapedius muscle, presuming there was no artifact-inducing movement of the head.

(*b*) *Tensor tympani muscle responses.* This reflex appears to be more a startle-generated reflex than an acoustic reflex. When a stapedius reflex has not been recorded, both Klockhoff (1961) and Djupesland (1964,

1967, 1969a,b) have reported successful elicitation by stimulation of the orbital region. An air jet directed toward this region, or a lifting of the patient's eyebrows, will elicit a response in those ears in which any of the previous tests directed at a stapedius muscle reflex were unsuccessful. The response is particularly exaggerated in instances of ossicular discontinuity peripheral to the insertion of the stapedial tendon. In the presence of a normal stapedius reflex, it is not possible to specify what portion of the response to nonacoustic stimulation may be controlled by a tensor contraction. Table VII provides a delineation of common middle-ear clinical entities and their probable effect on the various measurements in the battery of acoustic impedance measurements.

3. *Age Limitations of Reflex and Tympanometric Measurements.* Application of the impedance measurement battery is not limited by an age factor. Keith (1973) reported that successful measurements were obtained from a group of newborns ranging from 36 to 151 hours old. The study reported quite normal findings with the exception of a "W" pattern that occurred in the tympanograms of seven of the 40 infants. Stapedial reflex testing was also contaminated in 44% of the subjects by their susceptibility to behavioral response to loud signals. In general, the results of the study would support the use of impedance measurements as an objective procedure to evaluate middle-ear function in newborns.

VI. TESTS OF EUSTACHIAN-TUBE FUNCTION

Under normal conditions, equalization of air pressure between the middle-ear space and the ear canal is accomplished by passage of air between the nasopharynx and the middle ear through an actively functioning Eustachian tube. It has already been noted (Feldman, 1973; Holmquist, 1972a) that the range of middle-ear pressure relative to the ear canal is ±25 mm H_2O, and deviations from this range are suggestive of either some stage of middle-ear pathology or Eustachian-tube malfunction.

Tests for patency and function of the Eustachian tube can be performed with open and closed tympanic membranes, using an electro-acoustic impedance device (Holmquist, 1969, 1972a,b,c). The testing involves observation of (*1*) deviations in tympanogram peak pressure point, (*2*) changes in the tympanogram peak pressure point associated with swallowing, after artifically induced pressure changes have been generated by Valsalva, Toynbee, or Politzer maneuvers or by a device

TABLE VII

EFFECT OF MIDDLE-EAR PATHOLOGIES ON STATIC AND DYNAMIC IMPEDANCE

Middle-ear condition	Static impedance	Pressure point peak of tympanogram	Shape of tympanogram	Acoustic reflex	Nonacoustic reflex
Normal ear	Normal	Atmospheric pressure	Normal	Present	Present
Otosclerosis	High	Atmospheric pressure	Normal	Absent	Probably absent
Adhesive otitis	High to very high	Negative pressure	Normal or "W" for high frequency probe—may have sharp peak	Usually present at peak amplitude of tympanogram	Usually present at peak amplitude of tympanogram
Acute otitis	High to very high	Starts positive—may shift negative	Normal	Usually absent early stages	Usually absent early stages
Healed TM	Low normal to low	Atmospheric pressure, but can be negative if other pathology exists, such as adhesions	Normal or sharply peaked with low frequency probe tone—peaked sharp notched (W) with higher frequency probe tone	Present	Present
Glomus tumor	Very high	Usually absent	Flat with vascular perturbations	Absent	Absent
Interruption crus	Very low	Atmospheric pressure	Normal or peaked with lower frequency probe tone—deep broad notch with higher frequency probe tone	Present	Present
Interruption incudo-stapedial or incus	Very low	Atmospheric pressure	Same as for interruption of crus	Absent	Present for orbital air jet, but (?) not for tactile

138

Serous otitis	Very high	None or extreme negative with shift to less negative as condition resolves	Flat, but becomes normal as condition resolves—high and low frequency tympanograms converge as pressure becomes negative	Absent with flat tympanogram—returns as system becomes more mobile	Absent with flat tympanogram—returns as system becomes more mobile
Blocked Eustachian tube	High	Negative pressure	Normal	Present at peak of tympanogram—may be absent at ambient pressure	Present at peak of tympanogram—may be absent at ambient pressure
Open TM	Cannot obtain	None	Flat, but elevated from baseline	Absent	Absent

to generate negative pressure (Holmquist, 1969), or (3) in the case of open tympanic membranes, the ability to sustain artificially induced negative- and positive-pressure buildups without swallowing.

A. Tests with an Intact Tympanic Membrane

As has been noted, the negative peaking of a tympanogram (more than -30 mm H_2O) relative to ambient atmospheric pressure is consistent with inadequate function of the Eustachian tube. It is, however, only an indication of the status at that point in time, and may not be a true indication of the potential tubal function.

Tests of function involve the ability to equalize pressure after artificially induced changes have been generated by introducing positive or negative pressure to the middle-ear space through the Eustachian tube. Repeated tympanograms before and after a pressure change from successive swallows show a shifting of the tympanogram peak, as displayed in Figure 27. It is more difficult to artificially generate a negative

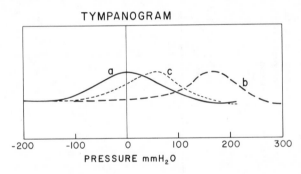

Figure 27   Normal tympanogram (a) shifted to a large positive pressure peak following Valsalva maneuver (b) and reverting toward normal pressure with several swallows (c).

pressure from the nasopharynx, yet this would be the more significant measure because the physiology of the system is such that adequacy of tubal function can be implied more accurately from negative than from positive stress (Holmquist, 1969). Inability to equalize pressure with three or four swallows implies poor tubal function.

A pressure swallow test (psw) that can be performed in the course of routine tympanometry has been described by Williams (1974). After running a standard tympanogram, the pressure in the ear canal is elevated to a $+400$ mm/H_2O level and the patient is asked to swallow. This can be done by taking a few swallows of water. A tympanogram is then repeated, recording in the same direction as the original tympanogram. In the presence of a functioning tube, the second tympanogram peak will be displaced in a negative direction, possibly with a peak elevation. After swallowing a second time at the point of the original peak to again equalize the pressure, the swallow procedure is repeated with a -400 mm/H_2O pressure in the ear canal. A third tympanogram, again run in the original direction, will reveal a peak displaced in positive direction. Normal Eustachian-tube function generally results in peak displacement of 10–25 mm/H_2O, while in poor functioning tubes, the three tympanograms are superimposed.

B. Tests with an Open Tympanic Membrane

With an open perforation or a patent pressure equalization (p.e.) tube in the eardrum, several observations may be made by means of an electro-acoustic impedance device. First, the volume of the initial measurement will be extremely large, implying that the measurement is of the middle-ear space in addition to the ear canal. This immediately verifies the presence of a perforation or the patency of the p.e. tube. Second, application of positive pressure will be difficult beyond $+150$ to $+200$ mm H_2O, because the Eustachian tube will open spontaneously, implying patency. This is a measure of its patency, not of its function. If a tube does not open under positive pressure, as revealed by a drop on the pressure meter, it can be considered nonpatent. Furthermore, if positive pressure does not evacuate with swallowing, it is an additional indication of poor function. Finally, application of negative pressure generally will not be a measure of patency, since the negative pressure should not allow for leakage through the Eustachian tube. Thus, in this condition, the examiner observes pressure meter stability and reductions associated with swallowing. Inability to equalize from a negative pressure of up to -150 mm H_2O implies poor tubal function.

VII. SUMMARY

This chapter has dealt with the development and current status of acoustic impedance–admittance measurements. The battery of tests provides an objective procedure for the evaluation of both the middle ear and some aspects of sensorineural function that will assist in the differential diagnosis of auditory disorders. Present clinical instrumentation provides for measurement of (1) some of the absolute parameters of static acoustic impedance–admittance at the eardrum, (2) changing characteristics of the flow of energy through the middle ear in relation to a changing air-pressure gradient across the eardrum, (3) the presence and effect of intraaural muscle response to auditory and nonauditory stimulation, and (4) the patency and function of the Eustachian tube.

While the isolated measurements within this battery of tests may sometimes fail to provide the examiner with definitive diagnostic information about the middle-ear or sensorineural status, the combined battery of static and dynamic acoustic impedance measurements constitute the fastest and most effective means at our disposal for this determination. The short battery of tests completely eliminates the need for bone-conduction audiometry in cases of pure sensorineural losses, and lends objective support to the examination of the auditory system medial to the middle ear. Although it does not supplant much of the traditional audiological battery, it may reasonably substitute for some procedures and provide a substantial reinforcement for other clinically obtained data.

REFERENCES

Alberti, P. W., and Jerger, J. (1974). *Arch. Otolaryngol.* **99**, 206.
Anderson, H., Barr, B., and Wedenberg, V. (1970). *Acta Oto-Laryngol. Suppl.* **263**, 232.
Beedle, R. K., and Harford, E. R. (1970). *Asha* **12**, 435.
Bicknell, M. R., and Morgan, N. V. (1968). *J. Laryngol. Otol.* **82**, 673.
Bluestone, C. D., Berry, Q. C., and Paradise, J. L. (1973). *Laryngoscope* **83**, 594.
Borg, E. (1972a). *Acta Oto-Laryngol.* **74**, 173.
Borg, E. (1972b). *Acta Physiol. Scand.* **85**, 374.
Brooks, D. N. (1968). *Int. Audiol.* **7**, 280.
Brooks, D. N. (1969). *Int. Audiol.* **8**, 563.
Brooks, D. N. (1971). *J. Speech Hear. Res.* **14**, 247.
Burke, K. S. (1972). *Asha* **14**, 655.
Burke, K. S., Shults, R. E., and Milo, A. P. (1967). *J. Acoust. Soc. Amer.* **41**, 1364.
Burke, K. S., Nilges, T. C., and Henry, G. B. (1970a). *J. Speech Hear. Res.* **13**, 317.
Burke, K. S., Herer, G. R., and McPherson, D. (1970b). *Acta Oto-Laryngol.* **70**, 29.
Carmel, P. W., and Starr, A. (1963). *J. Neurophysiol,* **26**, 598.
Dallos, P. J. (1964). *J. Acoust. Soc. Amer.* **36**, 2175.
Deutsch, L. J. (1968). Rep. No. 546. Bur. Med. & Surg., U.S. Navy Dept., Washington, D. C.
Deutsch, L. J. (1972). *Acta Oto-Laryngol.* **74**, 248.
Dieroff, H. G. (1965). *Int. Audiol.* **4**, 32.
Dishoeck, H. A. E. von (1938). *Arch Ohren. Nasan. Kehlkopfheilkd.* **53**, 22.
Djupesland, G. (1962). *Acta Oto-Laryngol.* **54**, 143.
Djupesland, G. (1964). *Acta Oto-Laryngol. Suppl.* **188**, 287.
Djupesland, G. (1965). *Int. Audiol.* **4**, 34.
Djupesland, G. (1967). *Norw. Monogr. Med. Sci.* (No vol. no.)
Djupesland, G. (1969a). *Acta Oto-Laryngol.* **68**, 1.

Djupesland, G. (1969b). *Int. Audiol.* **8,** 570.

Djupesland, G., and Flottorp, G. (1970). *Int. Audiol.* **9,** 156.

Eagles, E. L., Wishik, S. M., and Doerfler, L. G. (1967). *Laryngoscope Suppl.* 1.

Ewertsen, H., Filling, S., Terkildsen, K., and Thomsen, K. A. (1958). *Acta Oto-Laryngol. Suppl.* **140,** 116.

Feldman, A. S. (1963). *J. Speech Hear. Res.* **6,** 315.

Feldman, A. S. (1964). *Int. Audiol.* **3,** 156.

Feldman, A. S. (1967a). *J. Speech Hear. Res.* **10,** 165.

Feldman, A. S. (1967b). *J. Speech Hear. Res.* **10,** 616.

Feldman, A. S. (1969). *Laryngoscope* **79,** 1132.

Feldman, A. S. (1971). *Maico Aud. Lib. Ser.* **9,** No. 8.

Feldman, A. S. (1973). A Report of Acoustic Admittance Parameters in Normal Ears. Paper given before the Acoust. Soc. of Amer., Los Angeles, California.

Feldman, A. S. (1974). *Arch. Otolaryngol.* **99,** 211.

Feldman, A. S., and Zwislocki, J. (1965). *J. Speech Hear. Res.* **8,** 213.

Feldman, A. S., Djupesland, G., and Grimes, C. (1971). *Arch. Otolaryngol.* **93,** 416.

Flottorp, G., and Djupesland, G. (1971). *Acta Oto-Laryngol. Suppl.* **263,** 200.

Franzen, R. L. (1970). Threshold of the Acoustic Reflex for Pure Tones. Doctoral dissertation, Univ. of Iowa City, Iowa.

Franzen, R. L., and Lilly, D. J. (1970). *Asha* **12,** 435.

Fulton, R. T., and Lamb, L. (1964). Rep. No. 1. Parsons Res. Center, Parsons, Kansas.

Greisen, O., and Rasmussen, P. E. (1970). *Acta Oto-Laryngol.* **70,** 366.

Holmquist, J. (1969). *Acta Oto-Laryngol.* **68,** 501.

Holmquist, J. (1972a). Handout from a short course given by Donaldson and Holmquist, Amer. Acad. Ophthalmol. and Otolaryngol., Dallas, Texas.

Holmquist, J. (1972b). Handout from a short course given by Donaldson and Holmquist, Amer. Acad. Ophthalmol. and Otolaryngol., Dallas, Texas.

Holmquist, J. (1972c). *Audiol. J. Audit. Commun.* **2,** 209.

Hung, I. J., and Dallos, P. (1972). *J. Acoust. Soc. Amer.* **52,** 1168.

Jepsen, O. (1951). *Acta Oto-Laryngol.* **39,** 406.

Jepsen, O. (1953). *Acta Oto-Laryngol. Suppl.* **109,** 61.

Jepsen, O. (1955). Studies of the Acoustic Stapedius Reflex in Man. Doctoral dissertation, Univ. of Aarhus, Aarhus, Denmark.

Jepsen, O. (1963). *In* "Modern Developments in Audiology" (J. Jerger, ed.), pp. 193–239. Academic Press, New York.

Jerger, J. (1970). *Arch. Otolaryngol.* **92,** 311.

Jerger, J. (1972). *Arch. Otolaryngol.* **96,** 1.

Jerger, J. (1973). *In* "Modern Developments in Audiology" (J. Jerger ed.), 2nd ed., pp. 75–115. Academic Press, New York.

Jerger, J., Jerger, S., and Mauldin, L. (1972). *Arch. Otolaryngol.* **96,** 513.

Jerger, J., Burney, P., Mauldin, L., and Crump, B. (1974). *J. Speech Hear. Dis.* **39,** 11.

Kato, F. (1913). *Arch. Ges. Physiol.* **150,** 569.

Keith, R. W. (1973). *Arch. Otolaryngol.* **97,** 465.

Klockhoff, I. (1961). *Acta Oto-Laryngol. Suppl.* **164,** 1.

Kobrak, H. (1938). *Ann. Otolaryngol. (Paris)* **47,** 166.

Kristensen, H. K., and Jepsen, O. (1952). *Acta Oto-Laryngol.* **42,** 553.

Lamb, L., and Norris, T. W. (1969). *In* "Audiometry for the Retarded" (R. Fulton and L. Lloyd, eds.), pp. 164–209. Williams and Wilkins, Baltimore, Maryland.

Lamb, L. E., and Peterson, J. L. (1967). *J. Speech Hear. Disord.* 32, 46.

Lamb, L. E., Peterson, J. L., and Hansen, S. (1968). *Int. Audiol.* 7, 188.

Liden, G., Peterson, J. L., and Bjorkman, G. (1970a). *Arch. Otolaryngol.* 92.

Liden, G., Peterson, J. L., and Harford, E. R. (1970b). *Acta Oto-Laryngol. Suppl.* 263, 208.

Lilly, D. (1964). *J. Acoust. Soc. Amer.* 36, 2007.

Lilly, D. J. (1970). *Asha* 12, 441.

Lilly, D. J. (1972). In "Handbook of Clinical Audiology" (J. Katz, ed.), pp. 434–469. Williams and Wilkins, Baltimore, Maryland.

Lilly, D. J. (1973). In "Modern Developments in Audiology" (J. Jerger, ed.), pp. 345–406. Academic Press, New York.

Lilly, D. J., and Shepherd, D. C. (1964). *Asha* 6, 380.

Lilly, D. J., Sherman, D., Compton, A. J., Fisher, C. G., and Carney, P. J. (1968). *J. Speech Hear. Disord.* 33, 307.

McCall, G. N. (1973). *J. Speech Hear. Disord.* 38, 250.

McCandless, G. A., and Miller, D. L. (1972). *Nat. Hear. Aid J.* 25, 7.

Metz, O. (1946). *Acta Oto-Laryngol. Suppl.* 63, 1.

Metz, O. (1952). *Arch. Otolaryngol.* 55, 536.

Møller, A. R. (1960). *J. Acoust. Soc. Amer.* 32, 250.

Møller, A. R. (1961). *Ann. Otol. Rhinol. Laryngol.* 70, 735.

Møller, A. R. (1962). *J. Acoust. Soc. Amer.* 34, 1524.

Møller, A. R. (1963). *J. Acoust. Soc. Amer.* 35, 1526.

Møller, A. R. (1965). *Acta Oto-Laryngol.* 60, 129.

Newman, B. T., and Fanger, D. M. (1973). "Otoadmittance Handbook #2." Grason Stadler Co., Concord, Massachusetts.

Niemeyer, W., and Sesterhenn, G. (1972). *Audiol. J. Commun.* (*Abstr. Suppl.*) 84.

Nilges, T. C., Northern, J. L., and Burke, K. S. (1969). *Arch. Otolaryngol.* 89, 727.

Olivier, J. C. (1972). *Audiol. J. Audit. Commun.* (*Abstr. Suppl.*) 85.

Onchi, Y. (1949). *J. Acoust. Soc. Amer.* 21, 404.

Onchi, Y. (1961). *J. Acoust. Soc. Amer.* 33, 794.

Peterson, J. L., and Liden, G. (1970). *Arch. Otolaryngol.* 92, 258.

Peterson, J. L., and Liden, G. (1972). *Audiol. J. Audit. Commun.* 11, 97.

Pinto, L. H., and Dallos, P. J. (1968). *IEEE Trans. Biomed. Eng.* 15, 10.

Porter, T. A. (1972). Personal communication.

Priede, V. M. (1970). *Int. Audiol.* 9, 127.

Richards, G. B., and Kartye, J. P. (1973). *Arch. Otolaryngol.* 88, 162.

Robertson, E. O., Peterson, J. L., and Lamb, L. E. (1968). *Arch. Otolaryngol.* 88, 162.

Rock, E. H. (1972). Impedance Newsletter. Madsen Electromedics Corp., 3, 1.

Rose, D. (1973). Cited in "Otoadmittance Handbook #2." Grason Stadler Co., Concord, Massachusetts.

Salomon, G., and Starr, A. (1963). *Acta Neurol. Scand.* 39, 161.

Schuster, K. (1934). *Phys. Z.* 35, 408.

Steinberg, D., and Lenhardt, E. (1972). *Z. Laryngol. Rhinol. Otol.* 51, 693.

Stone, G. M., and Feldman, A. S. (1971). A Comparison of Impedance Measurements in Normal and Pathological Ears. Paper given before the Amer. College of Surgeons, Atlantic City, New Jersey.

Terkildsen, K. (1957). *Arch. Otolaryngol.* 66, 484.

Terkildsen, K. (1960). *Acta Oto-Laryngol. Suppl.* 158, 230.

Terkildsen, K. (1962). Akustike Impedancsmalinger og Mellemørets Funktin. Doctoral dissertation, Københaven Univ., Copenhagen, Denmark.
Terkildsen, K. (1964). *Int. Audiol.* 3, 147.
Terkildsen, K., and Scott Nielsen, S. (1960). *Arch. Otolaryngol.* 72, 339.
Terkildsen, K., and Thomsen, K. A. (1959). *J. Laryngol.* 73, 409.
Thomsen, K. A. (1955a). *Acta Oto-Laryngol.* 45, 82.
Thomsen, K. A. (1955b). *Acta Oto-Laryngol.* 45, 544.
Thomsen, K. A. (1958). *Acta Oto-Laryngol. Suppl.* 140, 269.
von Békésy, G. (1932). *Ann. Physiol.* 13, 111.
Weiss, H. S., Mundie, J. R., Jr., Cashin, J. L., and Shinabarger, E. W. (1962). *Acta Oto-Laryngol.* 55, 505.
Wilber, L. A. (1971). Static Acoustic Impedance in Differential Diagnosis of Auditory Disorders. Paper given before the Amer. Speech and Hearing Assoc., Chicago, Illinois.
Wilber, L. A. (1972). *Impedance Symp.* (D. Rose and L. Keating, eds.), pp. 109–125. Mayo Clinic—Mayo Foundation, Rochester, Minnesota.
Wilber, L. A., Goodhill, V. G., and Hogue, A. C. (1969). *Asha* 11, 417.
Wilber, L. A., Goodhill, V. G., and Hogue, A. C. (1970). *Asha* 12, 435.
Williams, P. S. (1974). Submitted for publication to Ann. Otol. Rhinol. Laryngol.
Yonovitz, A., and Harris, J. D. (1972). Rep. #723. Naval Submarine Med. Res. Lab., Groton, Connecticut.
Zwislocki, J. (1957a). *J. Acoust. Soc. Amer.* 29, 349.
Zwislocki, J. (1957b). *J. Acoust. Soc. Amer.* 29, 1312.
Zwislocki, J. (1961). Ann. Otol. Rhinol. Laryngol. 70, 599.
Zwislocki, J. (1962). *J. Acoust. Soc. Amer.* 34, 1514.
Zwislocki, J. (1963a). *In* Middle Ear Function Seminar (J. L. Fletcher, ed.), Rep. No. 576. U.S. Army Med. Res. Lab., Ft. Knox, Kentucky.
Zwislocki, J. (1963b). *J. Speech Hear. Res.* 6, 304.
Zwislocki, J. (1968). *Acta Oto-Laryngol.* 65, 86.
Zwislocki, J., and Feldman, A. S. (1963). *J. Acoust. Soc. Amer.* 35, 104.
Zwislocki, J., and Feldman, A. S. (1970). *Asha Monogr. No. 15,* 1.

Chapter Five

Electrocochleography

F. Blair Simmons[1] and Theodore J. Glattke[1]

I. INTRODUCTION

Observation of electrical potentials recorded from the vicinity of the cochlea has become an important clinical tool for determining the integrity of the peripheral auditory mechanism. The techniques required to study these potentials carefully have been adopted by clinical investigators, and experience with more than 500 patients has been presented in the literature. From these studies, one can easily conclude that the auditory nerve response to transient stimuli is the most sensitive objective indicator of end-organ function in those patients who cannot be evaluated by conventional audiometry.

Several approaches to electrocochleography have been developed over the past 10 years. Common to all of these are:

1. the use of repetitive acoustic stimuli of a type that causes a large number of auditory nerve fibers to discharge synchronously;
2. the use of an averaging computer to decrease the effects of background electrical noise; and
3. the use of recording electrodes placed somewhere between the earlobe and the cochlea.

Procedural differences that have been advocated have dealt largely with the location of the recording electrode. Some of these sites are illustrated in Figure 1. In general, electrodes closest to the cochlea provide the

[1] Division of Otolaryngology, Stanford University School of Medicine, Stanford, California.

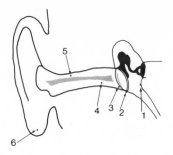

Figure 1 Examples of recording locations used in cochleography. These have included the promontory and round window (1); the annulus and posterior–inferior quadrant of the tympanic membrane (2); the posterior canal wall (3, 4, 5); and the earlobe (6). Representative studies based on these sites are: Aran (1971), Portmann and Aran (1971), Yoshie and Ohashi (1969) for the round window or promontory; Cullen *et al.* (1972) and Yoshie (1968) for the tympanic membrane; Coats and Dickey (1970) and Yoshie (1968) for the external canal; Moore (1971) and Sohmer and Feinmesser (1967) for the earlobe. Site comparison data include those of Simmons (1972) and Yoshie and Ohashi (1969).

clearest records, but they also require penetrating the tympanic membrane. Electrodes placed in the ear canal or on the tympanic membrane or earlobe need not perforate the skin, but yield recordings with greatly reduced amplitudes. As such, these "noninvasive" techniques often give equivocal results with respect to threshold measurements. They are of very limited use in supplementing either behavioral audiometric findings or other equivocal physiological findings. These limits will be described in more detail in a later section of this chapter.

While electrocochleography is extremely sensitive in comparison to other physiological measures of human hearing, no authoritative set of tables or descriptions of all varieties of normal and abnormal electrical responses exists at this time. Consequently, the interpretation of patients' cochleograms, detection of artifacts, and so on, rest upon four decades of animal studies which are entirely compatible with human responses. Some of these data will be reviewed in this section, both as background material and as entries into the extensive literature for the interested reader.

A. Electrical Activity near the Cochlea

The output of a recording electrode placed in the vicinity of the cochlea may show at least three electrical events that are stimulus-dependent. These are the *cochlear potential* (CP), the *summating potential* (SP), and the *compound action potential* (AP) of the auditory

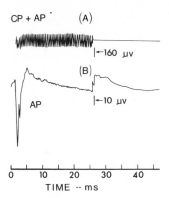

Figure 2 Examples of the cochlear potential (CP) and compound action potential (AP) recorded for a tone burst of about 60-dB SPL at 2 kHz. Tracing (A) is the mean of 32 samples of data gathered when the tonal stimulus was switched on and off at exactly the same phase for each sample. The AP presence in the top tracing is shown by the irregularities in the onset and offset of the (principally CP) response. The bottom tracing was obtained for 32 samples of the same tone, but the phase of the stimulus was allowed to vary randomly with respect to the point in time at which it was turned on. The mean of those samples approaches zero for the CP component, and the AP component may be seen clearly. Note that the recording sensitivity was increased for the bottom tracing, and that the AP response is much smaller than the CP.

nerve. Figure 2 shows examples of the CP and AP responses to a 2000-Hertz (2 kHz) tone pip. Both the CP and AP are present in tracing A of the figure, and tracing B shows the AP corresponding to the onset and offset of the tone. The techniques used to extract the individual responses are described in the figure legend.

The CP is often referred to as the "cochlear microphonic" (Wever, 1966) because its wave-form reflects the acoustic stimulus wave-form over a considerable frequency and intensity range. In this manner, it is much like the output of a microphone. It is the earliest (shortest latency) of the three potentials, occurring nearly instantaneously after a stimulus reaches the cochlea. The CP disappears or is greatly diminished when there is damage to the organ of Corti, particularly hair cells, or when there is diffuse damage secondary to metabolic changes or aging. (See Perlman *et al.*, 1951; Butler, *et al.*, 1962; Wever, 1966; Dallos, 1973, for original data or reviews of this area.)

The CP has been used extensively as a monitor of cochlear integrity and function in laboratory animals. The use of the CP in human clinical cochleography, either as an index of auditory thresholds or site of lesion is extremely risky, though it has been suggested (Ruben, 1967). The reason that it is risky is that very strong evidence from several sources has demonstrated that the CP recorded from outside the cochlea, including the round window, is generated from a small segment of the organ of Corti no further than a few millimeters along the basal turn (Misrahy et al., 1958; Simmons and Beatty, 1962). In humans, this region probably corresponds to frequencies above 10 kHz as far as perceptual thresholds are concerned. Therefore, even though low-frequency stimulation may be used, CP activity recorded from outside the cochlea is a poor indicator of cochlear viability in the upper apical regions, which are of greater clinical interest. In order properly to measure CP relevant to lower frequencies, it is necessary to place electrodes within the cochlea, using much more sophisticated techniques than clinical cochleography would permit (Dallos, 1969, 1973).

The SP is a *dc* shift which occurs during the presentation of a stimulus (von Békésy, 1960). The magnitude and polarity of that shift are dependent on the recording site, stimulus frequency, and stimulus intensity (Dallos, 1973). The SP component cannot be seen in Figure 2 because it is very small relative to the other potentials and because its effects were reduced by filters on the recording apparatus. The SP is not in contention as an index of normal cochlear function in humans.

The auditory nerve AP is the useful electrical response in cochleography. It results from the near-simultaneous discharge of many individual nerve fibers. While it is clear that this response derives from activity in the auditory nerve, the exact electrical location of its origin is unknown. The electrical events that classically produce the AP have been thought to originate in the internal auditory canal as the fibers from the spiral ganglion twist together to form a compact bundle (Teas et al., 1962; Dallos, 1973). However, Derbyshire and Davis (1935) suggested that the AP recorded from the round window and its surroundings comes from nerve fibers in the bony spiral lamina. The individual nerve fibers produce unitary "spike" discharges of constant amplitude and duration in this region. The AP is apparently the sum of these spike potentials. It does not appear to be made up of successive fast spikes because the bone, fluid, and tissue, as well as the recording electrode itself, filter or smooth out the discrete spike effects.

B. Action Potential Characteristics

In the normal and abnormal ear, detection of the AP rests upon using an acoustic stimulus that causes a great many individual nerve fibers to discharge within a time period of a few hundred microseconds. Clicks, abrupt tone bursts, or bursts of noise are effective if their rise time is sufficiently short (Goldstein and Kiang, 1958). Figure 3 shows the AP response detail for a click stimulus. The principal component of the AP is a large negative-going peak, which is often followed by a second peak. These are labeled N_1 and N_2, respectively. Additional negative-going peaks are sometimes seen, and are labeled N_3, N_4, and so on. Most of the descriptive data in cochleography have been derived from measurements of the N_1 component, namely its peak amplitude and latency (as indicated in Figure 3) and occasionally its onset latency.

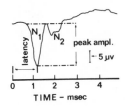

Figure 3   Compound action potential (AP) of the auditory nerve. The action potential characteristically is composed of one or more negative-going peaks. These are labeled N_1, N_2, and so on, in order of their appearance after the onset of the stimulus. The specific origin of the individual components has been the object of much speculation (Dallos, 1973). At moderate- and high-stimulus intensities, at least, the multiple components of the response all seem to derive from neurons innervating the basal portion of the cochlea rather than reflecting neural activity at more apical regions.

The origin, growth, and latency of the AP response may be appreciated by an examination of Figure 4. The responses shown in part A are means of 32 samples of data obtained from an electrode placed on the promontory. Each mean was obtained at the stimulus intensity (dB re normal adult perceptual threshold for the same stimulus) shown at the beginning of each tracing. The responses near threshold occur with a relatively long latency (to about 4 msec), and the AP wave-form is distributed over a long (1–1.5 msec) time period. As the stimulus intensity is increased, the responses become more succinct, grow in amplitude, and occur with shorter latency.

The reasons for the changes in shape, amplitude, and latency appear to be as follows. At stimulus intensities near threshold, transmission of the click through the middle-ear mechanism will emphasize a band of frequencies around the resonant point of the ear, from 2 kHz to about 4 kHz. Nerve fibers which are located in the upper portion of the basal turn are maximally responsive to this frequency region, and their discharges will form the major component of the AP response. As the click intensity is increased, its high-frequency energy becomes effective in stimulating more basalward portions of the cochlea. The latency and shape of the response to low-intensity stimuli are probably reflections of

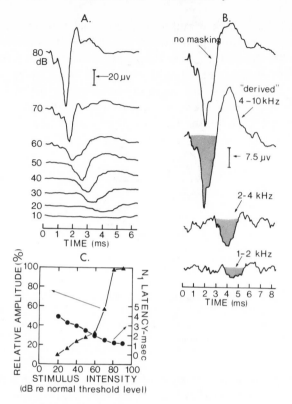

Figure 4 (A) Auditory nerve responses, (B) derived responses, and (C) a cochleogram from a normal-hearing individual. The auditory nerve responses (A) were obtained from click stimuli at the stimulus intensity indicated to the left of each tracing. The "derived" responses (B) were obtained according to the method of Teas *et al.* (1962), as described in the text. Shading of the derived responses was done for emphasis of the N_1 component of each (after Glattke, 1972). Stimulus intensity for the derived responses was 70 dB. The cochleogram (C) for the responses shown in (A) is a plot of the latency and the relative amplitude of the N_1 component of the responses. It is within normal limits in terms of rate of growth of the responses and rate of latency change.

(*1*) the time delay related to the cochlear traveling wave and (*2*) the temporal spread of stimulation over a relatively long time period. At higher intensities, an earlier succinct N_1 response occurs as a result of (*1*) less travel time to the region being stimulated and (*2*) more abrupt local stimulation. The overall amplitude growth of a response is due to two principal factors: More single units are responding to the stimulus, and those units which do respond do so with better synchrony for high-intensity stimulation.

At stimulus levels more than about 60 dB relative to normal human perceptual thresholds, the basalward fibers come to dominate the response. Even though the fibers innervating the middle- and low-frequency portions of the cochlea are still responding, their contribution cannot easily be detected in the composite response, because the large amplitude basal response obscures them. These hidden components of the AP response can be demonstrated by more sophisticated stimulus programming and computer-derived analysis (Teas *et al.*, 1962). In broad terms, the technique uses the computer not only as an averager, but also to subtract one group of AP responses from a second group collected under different stimulus conditions. The results of one such analysis are shown in Figure 4B.

First, a regular click-evoked AP response is obtained at a given stimulus intensity. It is stored for later use. Then, a known band of noise is introduced to the test ear, and the same click stimulus is presented against this noise background. The notion here is that the nerve fibers already being stimulated by the noise band cannot respond to the click also, and will not be part of the AP. Finally, the computer obtains the difference between the normal AP and the AP obtained with the click presented with the noise. The difference is assumed to be due to those nerve fibers masked by the band of noise, and is considered to be a "derived" response for those fibers. The three lower tracings in Figure 4B are examples of these derived APs for three different bands of masking noise: 4–10 kHz; 2–4 + 4–10 kHz; and 1–2 + 2–4 + 4–10 kHz. The AP component removed by the 4–10 kHz noise is shown as the "derived" 4–10 kHz response. The additional AP removed by the extension of the noise to 2 kHz is shown as the 2–4 kHz response, and the 1–2 kHz component is that which was removed by extending the noise to 1 kHz.

The AP that was removed by the 4–10 kHz noise resembles the unmasked AP response most closely. It has a large positive-going peak following the N_1, which was not present in the unmasked AP response to the same degree. Examination of the 2–4 kHz and 1–2 kHz responses reveals why, for they occurred at about 3–5 msec, or about the same time as the positive component. Since these latter two were negative-going, they summed to reduce the effects of the large positive component. It should also be noted that the general shape, amplitude, and latency of the low-frequency "derived" responses are quite similar to the unmasked responses shown in column A for low-intensity stimulation.

The three principal characteristics—latency, amplitude, and shape— of the AP response might be described in the following manner. The *latency* of the AP response is a clue to the frequency region of the cochlea contributing to the response. The *amplitude* of the AP response is a reflection of the number of active elements contributing to it and the synchrony of their discharges. The *shape* of the AP response is the result of a compromise between the electrical fields of neurons which have discharged and are refractory, and neurons which are discharging at a given moment.

Abnormal growth and latency functions, and elevated thresholds, provide the first clues to atypical cochlear function. The plot of the N_1 peak latency and relative amplitude shown in Figure 4C is the cochleogram for the individual from whom the recordings were taken. In a completely normal ear, these measurements are adequate to describe the AP. They are not totally adequate to describe all types of abnormal results, and this problem will be described in a later section.

Three general characteristics of normal cochleograms are:

1. The threshold of detection of the AP response is within 10 dB of the individual's perceptual threshold for tonal stimuli in the 2–4 kHz region.
2. While the absolute amplitude of the AP may vary over two or three orders of magnitude among recording situations and individuals, the rate of change in amplitude with changes in stimulus intensity will remain fairly constant. This will be 0.5–1.0% per dB for stimuli up to about 60-dB sensation level (in normals) and 1.0–3.0% per dB above this point. This change in rate of growth corresponds to Yoshie's (1968) L and H portions of the amplitude growth functions —relatively slow or flat near threshold, and steep at high intensities.
3. The peak latency of the N_1 component of the AP response is dependent on the intensity of the stimulus. In normal subjects, it will be in the region of 4 msec at threshold, and it will decrease to less than 1.5 msec at 90 dB re threshold.

Because the shape, growth, and latency of the AP response are of interest clinically, it is important that recordings are not unduly influenced by other electrical potentials. In particular, it is imperative that the CP not contaminate the AP recordings, because the CP grows at a different rate than the AP and because the CP latency does not change appreciably with changes in stimulus intensity. Figure 5 shows a means by which the CP may be removed from responses to click stimuli when the AP is the response of interest. Tracing A shows the mean response to eight clicks presented in a condensation phase (earphone diaphragm moves toward the tympanic membrane). Tracing B shows the response to clicks presented in a rarefaction phase (earphone diaphragm moves away from the tympanic membrane). This stimulus phase-reversal is mirrored exactly in the reversal of the phase of the CP (Derbyshire and Davis, 1935).

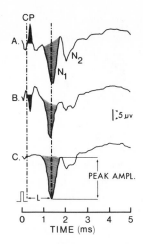

Figure 5 Examples of cancellation of the CP component. Tracing A is the mean response to eight click stimuli presented in a condensation phase. Tracing B is the mean for eight click stimuli presented in a rarefaction phase. Tracing C is the mean of the upper two tracings. The CP, which is the earliest shaded portion of tracings A and B, reverses phase when the stimulus phase is reversed. The AP preserves its general N_1–N_2 wave-form, but its latency (L) shifts. The response shown in C is free from CP influence and represents a compromise between the neural responses in A and B.

The AP component does not change phase, but does show a slight latency shift and change in shape. The latency shift occurs because neurons discharge during the period of upward displacement of the basilar membrane; this occurs earlier for the rarefaction pulse than for the condensasation pulse (Peak and Kiang, 1962; Kiang, 1965; Pfeiffer and Kim, 1972). The mean of tracings A and B is shown in tracing C. Since the CP component followed the stimulus phase, it was eliminated. The AP response which remains in the tracing is not exactly like that for either the condensation or rarefaction pulses, but it is a compromise between them. Since the latency shift caused by reversing the stimulus polarity amounts to about one-half of the period of the stimulus pulse (or about 50 μsec), it is not important clinically.

The use of phase reversal of the stimulus to cancel the CP will be satisfactory only if the CP has a constant amplitude when the stimulus phase is reversed. This will not be the case for high-intensity stimuli, because amplitude distortion of the CP will occur. Consequently, some caution must be exercised when this technique is used. An alternative to the phase-reversal procedure is the use of low-pass electrical filters, which attenuate the CP component (relatively high-frequency) and pass the AP. This technique must be used carefully as well, because the non-judicious use of filters may affect the wave-form and apparent latency of the AP component. All of the response characteristics that influence clinical judgments of the AP recordings may also be contaminated by improper placement of the recording electrodes. Some of these problems will be considered in the next section.

C. Effects of Electrode Placement

Good quality AP recordings from normal ears have been reported from all of the recording sites indicated in Figure 1. However, it becomes very difficult to judge the normalcy of a response as recordings are taken from points removed from the promontory or round window. Only a limited amount of comparative data exists, but the results from Simmons (1972) and Yoshie and Ohashi (1969) show how devastating the amplitude reduction caused by moving the electrode site may be. Figure 6, for

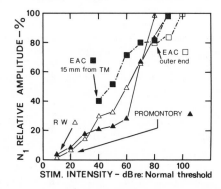

Figure 6 The growth of responses obtained from four recording sites. The relative-amplitude measures for a given site are taken as a percentage of the response of greatest amplitude recorded from that site. External auditory canal (EAC) recordings reduce the range of the growth function by at least 30 dB, and often more. They are not useful for determination of threshold. Round window (RW) and promontory recordings generally are 10 to 100 times greater in amplitude (of the AP response) than those from the EAC; and thresholds for the AP activity obtained from those sites are within 10 dB of the individual's perceptual threshold for the same stimulus. The data in this figure are redrawn from Yoshie and Ohashi (1969) for RW and EAC, and from Simmons (1972) for promontory recordings.

example, shows the relative growth of AP recordings from normal-hearing individuals when the electrode site was moved from the round window (RW) to the outer end of the external auditory canal (EAC). The RW and EAC curves are based on eight normal individuals studied by Yoshie and Ohashi (1969). The promontory recordings are based on six normal individuals in Simmons' (1972) study. The growth functions for the EAC recordings are abbreviated, with threshold normally no better than 40 dB re perceptual threshold for the click. Because of this threshold elevation, the range over which response can be observed is seriously reduced. The growth from no response to maximum response actually follows a pattern similar to that seen for some cases of sensorineural hearing loss. This problem was also addressed by Cullen *et al.* (1972) for responses obtained from an electrode placed near the tympanic membrane. All individuals in their population of 28 ears demonstrated responses presumed to be AP at 60-dB sensation level, but only 54% did so for stimuli at 50-dB sensation level. These investigators, therefore, suggested that the AP growth and threshold be abandoned in considering clinical subjects when recordings are made from the ear canal near the tympanic membrane, and that only response latency be considered.

The AP response becomes vulnerable to several kinds of artifacts when recordings are taken from the tympanic membrane and EAC sites. Because of this, consideration of latency alone may also be seriously impaired. Figure 7 shows an example of this type of problem. Tracing A

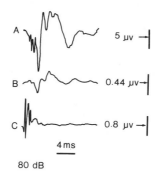

Figure 7 Examples of recording from three sites. Tracing A is from the promontory; tracing B is from the annulus of the tympanic membrane; and tracing C is from the posterior–inferior quadrant of the tympanic membrane. All recordings were taken for click stimuli at 80 dB re perceptual threshold for normal-hearing individuals, and all recordings were taken from the same individual.

is a recording from the promontory; tracing B from the annulus of the tympanic membrane; and tracing C from the posterior–inferior quadrant of the tympanic membrane. All records were based on the same patient and identical stimulus conditions. Initially, the order-of-magnitude sensitivity differences between the promontory and other recordings may be noted. Further, there is a clear differentiation between the CP and AP components in the promontory recordings. The annulus recording, while

clear of the CP, is only about 3% of the absolute amplitude of the promontory recording, and would fall to an undetectable level with a 20-dB
change in stimulus intensity. The tympanic membrane record is uninter-
pretable because of the presence of a microphone-like artifact. This was
probably due to motion of the tympanic membrane relative to the electrode tip. It would be well to consider for a moment the consequence of
misdiagnosis of a profoundly deaf child on the basis of artifacts of this
type.

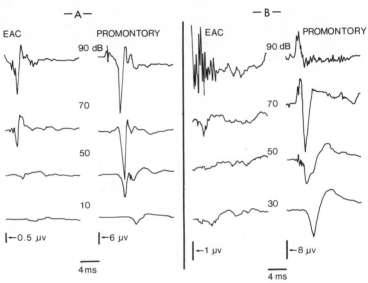

Figure 8 Examples of EAC and promontory recordings from two subjects (A)
and (B). The recordings in (A) were taken from an individual who showed remarkable sensitivity at both recording locations. Those in (B) are more typical, in the
sense that EAC thresholds were elevated and high-intensity stimulation resulted in
serious contamination of the response with microphone-like artifacts. Stimulus levels
are shown in dB re normal perceptual threshold for the click stimulus. (After
Simmons, 1972.)

The recordings in Figure 8 underscore this notion. The tracings in
part A are from one individual in Simmons' (1972) study who showed
the best comparison between EAC and promontory recording sites, in
terms of response sensitivity. The promontory responses are present unequivocally at all levels above 10 dB re perceptual threshold, but the
same cannot be said for EAC recordings, though some activity was obtained near threshold. The tracings in part B are from a subject who was
more typical of Simmons' group of subjects. In this case, the EAC recordings showed no evidence of AP activity until moderate stimulus intensi-

ties were reached. At high intensities, the AP activity was obscured by microphone-like artifacts. The unusual nature of the promontory response (principally positive-going) was completely lost in the EAC recordings.

Because of the problems associated with recording sites outside of the middle ear, some investigators have suggested that rather heroic computer analysis may be substituted for highly sensitive recordings, in order to salvage them for clinical use. Keidel (1971), for example, has used an autocorrelation analysis of recordings obtained from electrodes placed upon the hard palate. Charlet de Sauvage et al. (1973) have suggested that cross-correlation measures taken between a "master" AP response (for high-intensity stimulation) and other responses from the same individual may be useful. The fact is that not all electrode sites are useful in clinical cochleography, even though a selected normal can yield sensitive responses from several locations. If equivocal findings from other sources must be reckoned with, poor cochlear recordings are of little value. Prior to consideration of clinical results, a brief history of these techniques will be reviewed.

II. CLINICAL APPLICATIONS

A. Development of Electrocochleography as a Clinical Technique

The possibility of using human cochlear electrical activity as both a research and a clinical procedure has been explored intermittently since shortly after these potentials were discovered in animals. Andreev et al. (1939) published records of CP responses from humans about a decade after Wever and Bray (1930) made the first successful recordings of combined CP and AP responses from laboratory animals. Considering the infancy of the state of the electronics and display media at that time, they produced remarkable input–output functions relating CP amplitude to stimulus intensity. Their recordings were taken in the vicinity of the RW on patients with perforations of the tympanic membrane. Perlman and Case (1941) obtained similar findings in patients with perforations, but failed to obtain usable recordings when the electrode was placed against the tympanic membrane. Lempert et al. (1947, 1950) produced discouraging reports on attempts to record CP in humans, and cautioned against overinterpretation of auditory function based on that type of recording.

Ruben et al. (1960) presented data on both CP and AP obtained from the region near the RW in humans at the time of surgery. Most of their work is summarized by Ruben (1967), who suggested means of differentiating conductive, cochlear, and neural lesions on the basis of CP and AP responses. (As we have suggested previously, the CP does not appear to be useful in clinical studies.) At about this same time, Ronis (1966) coupled the surgically placed electrodes with electronic response-averaging equipment. Since that time, two additional reports have reviewed data gathered during surgical procedures (Flach and Seidel, 1968; Finck *et al.*, 1969).

The clinical application of these early attempts at cochleography was frustrated by the comparatively high electrical-noise background and the very low-voltage responses recordable from outside the cochlea. The RW measurements were mandatory because of this problem, but even then the responses from abnormal cochleas were indeterminant because of the conductive hearing losses temporarily produced by elevating the tympanic membrane. In addition, procedural variability undoubtedly obscured trends in the data. The application of the averaging computer made the measurement of these potentials practical. Further, this instrument made it possible to detect cochlear potentials at considerable distances from the RW, through an intact tympanic membrane.

The regular use of computer averaging of AP responses to many sequential transients was developed independently by two groups of investigators. Yoshie and Ohashi (1967, 1969, 1971) have made extensive recordings from both the RW and EAC. Portmann *et al.* (1967) began measuring the AP responses, using a tympanotomy approach, but they have changed to a procedure in which the electrode is passed through the tympanic membrane (Portmann and Aran, 1971, 1972; Portmann *et al.*, 1973).

In current practice, a local anesthetic is always required for the transtympanic method or for placement of a needle electrode in the canal skin. An anesthetic is not required for electrodes placed in the EAC or on the earlobe. The possible disadvantages of the use of anesthesia or of damage to the middle ear or cochlea resulting from the transtympanic electrode, and the additional personnel required, are heavily outweighed by the advantages of recording clarity and sensitivity. As such, the transtympanic membrane approach appears to be the method of choice, and the clinical data which will be reviewed are based on that recording method.

B.   Clinical Findings in Electrocochleography

The most important clinical application of cochleography in this decade is as a physiological test of cochlear function in individuals who cannot be tested by conventional audiometry and whose responses to other electrophysiological tests are equivocal. In the extreme case, where no AP response occurs at any stimulus intensity, there is no real problem in interpretation. The cochlea is nonfunctional for hearing.

In most instances, however, at least some AP will be measurable, and an input–output function, viz., a cochleogram, may be constructed. Interpreting this abnormal cochleogram into probable audiometric thresholds is an imprecise adventure at this moment in the development of the technique. Yoshie and Portmann and their associates have begun preliminary attempts, and we shall borrow heavily from the latter group's material in describing some features of abnormal findings.

The gross relation between AP threshold and audiometric thresholds has been analyzed by Aran (1971) for 106 clinical cases. He compared the AP threshold for clicks with the average of all pure-tone thresholds between 0.25 and 8 kHz. In 50% of the cases, the audiometric average was within 10 dB of the AP threshold. Eighty-one percent were within 20 dB, and 93% were within 30 dB, of the AP threshold. The best single frequency correlation was at 2 kHz, where the average AP threshold was within *1.5 dB*, and the interquartile range was ±8 dB. These averaged data from a large group of patients support a generally good correlation between the audiometric and cochleographic findings.

Such averaged data cannot, however, be applied to interpreting individual patient cochleograms because some very major discrepancies can exist. AP thresholds depend not only on the severity of the hearing loss, but also on the slope of the audiometric configuration. Recall that the reasoning presented in the first section of this chapter suggested that responses observed for low-intensity stimuli were probably from the 2–4 kHz region of the cochlea, and that basal-turn dominance accompanies high-intensity stimuli. With this in mind, consider Figure 9. As the AP recording is influenced by the spread of activity toward the base of the cochlea, *thresholds* for AP responses corresponding to 10, 30, 50, or 70 dB re normal thresholds might be expected to derive from regions of the cochlea responsive to the shaded areas on the audiogram at these intensities. Therefore, a threshold response occurring for a 50-dB stimulus may be due to activity in a cochlear region extending from a region normally responsive to 2 kHz through a region responsive to 8 kHz. At 70 dB, a threshold response might be derived from an even wider region. The hearing loss outside this band of frequencies can vary widely without affecting threshold of the AP, as is the case in the two extremes, A and B, shown in the figure. Stated another way, it is only necessary that one frequency region within the shaded range be functioning at that intensity for a threshold AP to be recorded. This example should be taken as a theoretical illustration only. The principle is correct, but con-

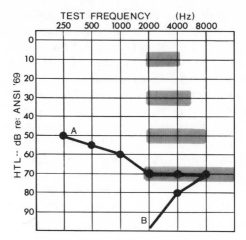

Figure 9 Frequency regions corresponding to click-stimulus excitation. The shaded areas in the audiogram are representative of theoretical frequency regions which correspond to AP thresholds obtained at the intensities indicated on the ordinate. Hearing within normal limits would give rise to an AP response threshold in the 10–20 dB region, and this would most likely correspond to excitation of the cochlea in the regions most commonly associated with 2 to 4 kHz stimuli. Threshold elevations to 50 or 70 dB would result in an AP response based on a much broader region of the cochlea. It would be possible, for example, for individuals with the pure-tone thresholds shown in A and B to produce the same AP-response threshold because of spread of excitation in the cochlea. Thus, audiometric configuration cannot always be deduced from the AP-response threshold.

siderable additional clinical material needs to be analyzed before exact numerical correlations and variations can be described.

The suprathreshold characteristics of the abnormal AP can give further information about cochlear function. While they, too, are worked out only incompletely, some definite trends are appearing. The following information roughly describes these trends.

1. Conductive hearing losses. Cochleograms obtained from individuals with conductive hearing losses are identical in configuration to those from normals, except that they are shifted to a higher intensity. Thus, once threshold is reached, a normal-appearing growth and latency function will occur.

2. Sensorineural hearing losses. The most common AP response configuration with sensorineural hearing losses is the *recruiting* cochleogram (Portmann *et al.*, 1973). An example of this type of finding is shown in Figure 10. Part A of the figure shows responses to stimuli presented at 20 through 100 dB in 20-dB steps. Part B shows the cochleogram result-

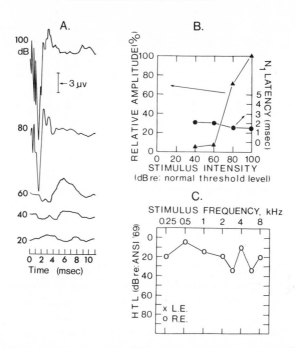

Figure 10 Examples of the "recruiting" response pattern. Tracings shown in A are AP responses at the indicated intensities. This individual's cochleogram is shown in B, and the audiogram for the test ear is shown in C. Characteristically, as soon as threshold is reached, the response appears with a very short latency. With further increments in stimulus intensity, the rate of growth of the response is rapid, generally at 3% or more per dB. The response wave-forms are not dissimilar to the normal case.

ing from those responses, and part C shows the audiogram for the ear from which the responses were obtained. As may be observed in the figure, the threshold is elevated, but the AP peak latency at threshold is as short as it might have been had no hearing loss been present and had the stimulus been delivered at the same intensity (40 dB re normal thresholds). In addition to this, since the latency is so short at threshold, it changes only a minimal amount over a 60-dB range of stimulus intensities.

The growth of the AP is also unusual, and this is the "recruiting" aspect of the response pattern. Rather than rising gradually over a 40–60-dB range, it climbs abruptly only 20 dB above threshold. For a hearing loss more severe than that shown in this example, the lower portion of the growth function curve may not be apparent at all, according to both Yoshie (1971) and Portmann *et al.* (1973). It has been suggested by these workers that the change in slope in the growth rate function, which normally occurs at around 60 dB re threshold, reflects a transition between outer hair cells (which are presumed to have low thresholds of excitability) and inner hair cells (presumed to come into play at moderate stimulus intensities). Therefore, a cochleogram that shows only the growth pattern normally associated with responses 60 dB or more above threshold (Yoshie's "H" portion of the curve) is thought by these investigators to reflect damage to the outer hair cells.

The AP recruiting response must not be confused with auditory loudness recruitment, which is a perceptual phenomenon. The recruiting cochleogram may coexist with loudness recruitment, but it also occurs in persons whose loudness recruitment studies are totally negative. In addition, the classical concept of inner and outer hair-cell loudness and recruitment phenomena is inadequate to encompass both the AP and audiometric findings (Simmons, 1966).

A second general type of abnormal cochleogram is the double-peaked or *disassociated* pattern. An example of this type of response is shown in Figure 11. It is associated with hearing loss of cochlear origin which is not uniformly distributed along the cochlea. Thus, the audiogram (C) may show abrupt peaks and dips of great magnitude, usually in the higher frequencies. The characteristic features of this type of cochleogram (B) are: (*1*) a threshold that may be normal or moderately elevated; (*2*) a normal or slower than normal amplitude growth immediately above threshold; (*3*) an abrupt change in both the wave-form and latency of the AP as the stimulus intensity is increased further; and (*4*) a response amplitude maximum that may be less than normal. The example in Figure 11 shows the first three of these features. The threshold is reached by 30 dB, and as the stimulus intensity is raised, the change in latency and amplitude appears to be reasonably normal until the disassociated response appears at 60 dB. (See "d" in the response tracings (A) and cochleogram (B).) Above this level, the response growth and latency appear much like the recruiting response pattern. The 60-dB AP is reflecting the 6-kHz hole (dissassociation) or notch in the audiogram; that is, there are two N_1's, one coming from cochlear regions below the audiometric notch and the other from regions above it.

Using the rationale described previously (see Figure 9), the relative normalcy of the low-intensity portion of the response patterns appears to correlate well with normal hearing sensitivity in the 2-kHz region. As the stimulus intensity is increased, the AP becomes larger, but at a rate somewhat slower than normal. Then, at 30 dB above this individual's threshold for the AP, the earlier N_1 appears, and the amplitude and

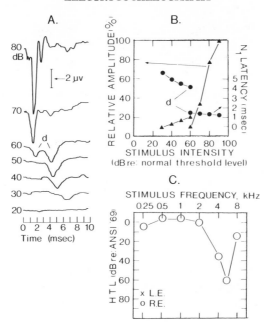

Figure 11 Examples of the "disassociated" response pattern. The disassociated (d) response is apparent in the AP responses (A) for stimuli at 60 dB, and in the abrupt changes in the cochleogram (B). These are often associated with high-frequency notched audiometric configurations. There may not be a marked threshold elevation for the AP, particularly if the hearing loss is restricted to 4 kHz and above. Initially, the response latency appears to progress normally, and its growth is normal or slower than normal. With further increases in stimulus intensity, an early component appears (d), and two responses coexist. Finally, the earlier response comes to dominate the AP. This disjuncture is noted in the marked latency and amplitude shifts shown at 60 dB in this example.

latency of each of the negative components may be plotted. The shorter latency component originates from excitation of the extreme basalward region of the cochlea, and the hole in the AP response (and in the cochleogram) corresponds to the loss of sensitivity between 2 and 8 kHz. Basal-turn dominance then causes the later peak to disappear as the click intensity increases further.

All disassociated or double-peaked AP-response wave-forms are not as clear-cut as the example shown in Figure 11. Other response wave-forms, in which the contour of the audiogram is smoother and the high-frequency hearing thresholds are much poorer than those for low frequencies (no sharp notch), may show less distinct double or disassociated peaks. Some wave-forms may show only a flattening or broadening of a single N_1. This broadening of the AP may correspond in some instances to the Portmann and Aran (1972) description of their "complex" response in sensorineural hearing losses. This general response category is somewhat elusive. The "larges" (broad) responses which they have observed have occurred in persons later diagnosed as having retrocochlear lesions of several varieties. One key element in a broadened AP, even to high-intensity stimulation, must be that neurons are not discharging in their normal synchrony. This may occur secondarily to neural metabolic changes, but it may also occur if the region of the cochlea normally responsive to high-frequency stimulation has a severe deficit, and if that deficit does not coexist in the apical turns.

Finally, a very unusual AP configuration described by Aran (1971) has an initial positive-going component present before the conventional N_1 component. This "abnormal" response has been recorded from patients having an VIIIth-nerve neuronoma, nuclear icterus, complex neurological disturbance, and vertebral artery compression. It is Aran's impression that this type of AP wave-form may represent a combined cochlear disorder and a more general brain pathology.

C.   Suggestions for Further Exploration

Although clicks are the most efficient means of producing an AP response, clicks passed through narrow-band filters to produce tone pips may have some advantage in identifying the location of cochlear lesions. The presumption in using tone pips is, of course, that if the stimulating frequency range can be limited, the resulting AP response will also be limited to those nerve fibers normally responsive to that range. Figure 12 shows examples of CP and AP activity based on Yoshie's (1971) findings. At first glance, the neural responses that are shown (note shaded N_1's) appear to behave according to this presumption. The response to the 8-kHz stimulus (A) would be expected to have a shorter latency than that for the 2-kHz (C) stimulus, because the fibers contributing to the 8-kHz response are closer to the basal end of the cochlea. Indeed, there is a regular progression of response latency as the tone pip varies from 8 through 2 kHz. Secondly, as the stimulus frequency is lowered, one might expect the temporal dispersion of discharges to increase, and a broader N_1–N_2 complex might be anticipated. This, too, can be observed in the tracings.

However, there is another very good explanation for the neural latency and wave-form effects. As the CP tracings show, the lowering of the frequency of the filter passband is accompanied by changes in the rate at which the tonal stimulus rises to its maximum. The latency shifts could be explained partly on this basis, rather than by eliminating basal-turn

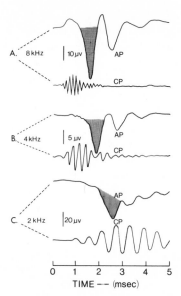

Figure 12 Examples of AP and CP responses to tone pips at approximately 90-dB SPL. Responses are shown for three frequencies: (A) 8 kHz, (B) 4 kHz, and (C) 2 kHz. The N_1 component of the AP response is shaded for emphasis. The higher frequencies (A) and (B) give rise to a "classic" AP-response wave-form. At 2 kHz and below, the AP response appears to follow individual cycles of the stimulus by showing small individual negative-going peaks, which occur at time intervals appropriate to the stimulus period. (After Yoshie, 1971.)

dominance from the response. It is possible that the lower-frequency (slower) stimuli are simply driving the basal neurons to respond at progressively later times relative to the onset of the stimulus. In addition, since the lower frequency tonal stimuli have relatively broad maxima and minima in comparison with high frequencies, the temporal dispersion resulting in a broader neural response could also be based simply on the way basal fibers are excited.

It should be noted that Yoshie (1971) did find generally good agreement between hearing threshold levels and thresholds for AP responses as a function of test frequency. In addition, he was able to demonstrate gross response shape differences for APs in response to tone pips among his sensorineural patients. Finally, Yoshie suggested that the response growth patterns could be demonstrated to be markedly different from normal patterns, but only if the response growth were plotted as a function of an individual's own sensation level. Since this requires knowing his audiometric threshold configuration prior to analysis of the AP responses, it does not appear to be a useful substitute for the audiogram. The general probe into frequency-selective AP evaluation should be continued, using these stimuli or modifications of them.

Another approach to frequency-selective measurement of the AP involves the technique developed by Teas *et al.* (1962). Generally, this technique involves presenting steady background-masking noise to desynchronize nerve fibers in known and controlled regions of the cochlea while obtaining AP responses to clicks. The AP responses to the clicks are presumed to be obtained from those nerve fibers not affected by the masking noise. Some results from this type of approach are shown in Figure 4. This approach has been used with humans only to a limited extent (Glattke, 1972). The general finding has been that high-pass bands of noise that progressively extend to lower cutoff frequencies can be used to obtain derived responses that evolve from progressivly more apical cochlear regions. These findings in humans were entirely in agreement with those of Teas *et al.* (1962) in laboratory animals. Test conditions utilizing high-pass bands of noise should definitely be explored further.

The majority of clinical investigations dealing with AP responses have attempted to describe relationships between conventional audiometric threshold configurations and the AP-response thresholds or growth patterns. Except for the a posteriori discovery of abnormal growth patterns, little has been done to study suprathreshold AP behavior. Yet, this area may be as useful as conventional suprathreshold audiometry in defining the site of lesion. For example, it is well-known that stimulation of the ear with clicks or pulses at low-stimulus rates (less than 10 per sec) will produce AP responses that follow the stimulus repetition rate faithfully. The time period (100 msec or more) between the clicks is sufficient to allow enough neurons to recover from their discharge in response to the prior click, to produce AP responses to the succeeding clicks (Derbyshire and Davis, 1935; Peak *et al.*, 1962). At rates higher than about 10 per sec, the responses that succeed the first (or "on" response) become smaller. While some rate-following behavior may exist for pulses up to 2 kHz or more (see tracing C in Figure 12), the amplitude of these responses is seriously reduced relative to the first response. Aberrations of this rate-following behavior may be indications of abnormal auditory nerve function. Yoshie and Ohashi (1971) have explored this possibility with one patient, and it is likely that this general approach will be very promising. Similarly, the recovery of the AP response from prior stimulation, by means of either transients or other stimuli, may be a valuable supplementary test, even if audiograms can be obtained (Simmons and Glattke, 1972).

III. TECHNICAL CONSIDERATIONS

This section is addressed to readers who may be considering the development of electrocochleography as a diagnostic and research technique, but whose experience with recording auditory potentials is limited. We have not had experience with all possible permutations of recording sites, transducers, or computers, and will limit our comments to those techniques which we know will work, without prejudice to others which we have not used.

A. Stimulus Parameters and Hardware

Good click stimuli are produced by single rectangular electrical pulses passed (after suitable control for intensity) to good quality transducers with excellent high-frequency response. The click duration should be kept very short in order to optimize the transducer performance; we have used 100 μsec satisfactorily. The pulse generator may be driven by an external synchronizing pulse or by its own time base. In either case, the stimulus rate should not exceed about 10 pulses per sec, for to do so would cause an artifactual reduction in the AP response amplitude due to neuronal recovery characteristics. (See previous section.)

Specification of the click stimulus spectrum and overall sound pressure level is difficult, and requires sophisticated analysis. However, Cullen *et al.* (1972) have described a technique that produces repeatable results in terms of obtaining an approximation of sound pressure level. A microphone is placed in the test environment in a location normally corresponding to the position of the patient's ear. The click stimulus is presented as usual, and the output of the microphone is monitored visually on an oscilloscope. The peak amplitude of this output is noted, and the click stimulus is replaced with a 4-kHz sine wave. The level of the sinusoid is adjusted to obtain a peak output from the microphone equal to that observed for the click. Then, the peak sound pressure level (dB re 0.0002 μbar) is computed for that sinusoid and is taken as the peak sound pressure level of the click stimulus. (Also see Yoshie and Ohashi, 1969.)

Because it is more meaningful clinically, we express the stimulus intensity in terms of the level necessary for perceptual threshold in normal-hearing young adults. This is analogous to the hearing threshold level in audiograms, and, in our experience, "0 dB" (no loss) corresponds to a click peak sound pressure level of approximately 14.5-dB SPL.

Since the distance between the transducer and patient affects the stimulus level reaching the patient's ear and the stimulus travel time, it is imperative that this distance be constant from patient to patient. Carelessness here can result in elevated thresholds. If a transducer is moved during the evaluation of a single patient, peculiar latency results may be obtained. For example, changing the transducer–patient distance by 6 inches will result in an approximate 0.5-msec change in travel time.

The most accurate latency measurements are probably made on the basis of the recordings themselves. When it can be observed, we use the onset of the CP as the reference for computing AP peak latency. In this manner, the patient is, in a sense, carrying his time reference around in his ear. In many instances, a true CP will not appear, even at high stimulus levels. In those cases, careful specification of transducer–patient distance is mandatory.

An averaging device of some type is required. We use a small general-purpose computer (Digital Equipment Corporation (DEC) PDP-8/I) with an analog-to-digital converter (DEC 138E) and a digital-to-analog converter (DEC VC-8/I), both as a time base and analysis device, and to provide control over display media. Other devices would be suitable so long as their sampling rate is fast enough to capture details of the AP responses. Generally, in order to *detect* an event, one must sample at least at twice the rate of the event. For N_1 recordings, this should be a sampling rate of 4 kHz. In order to display details of the recording, the rate should be increased markedly. In our clinic, individual samples are taken at 50- or 100-μsec intervals (10 to 20 kHz) during a given stimulus epoch.

The individual samples are converted to digital form and summed in the computer memory prior to computation of the arithmetic mean (and occasionally, the variance). They are then stored on magnetic tape in digital form for later recall and observation. The data may also be stored in their analog form on a good quality ¼-inch tape recorder, with a frequency response sufficiently low to obtain the slow portions of the response. This is usually accomplished by FM recording techniques. The FM technique also preserves the relative phase of the AP-response components, which is important in determining normalcy of wave-form. Data stored in analog form may be submitted to computer analysis after the recording session is completed. While simple averaging computers (dedicated) are satisfactory for obtaining mean and variance data, a true general-purpose machine should be sought if programming skills are available. The flexibility of the general-purpose device makes it more desirable, particularly in efforts involving display and later analysis of data.

Our mean data are displayed on an oscilloscope when the computer is used to automatically extract latency and amplitude data. The data are stored permanently by writing them on magnetic tape in digital form or on an X–Y plotter using standard graph paper. In this manner, they may be preserved indefinitely and are available for scrutiny at any time.

A final comment on hardware is based on concern over the acoustic environment in which a patient is tested. It is well-known that background acoustic noise is a very effective means by which AP responses may be masked. With this in mind, extreme care should be exercised in selection of a test environment. Ideally, this would be a conventional audiometric test facility, meeting ANSI requirements for threshold testing. If these requirements cannot be met, for example, in the operating room of a hospital, care should be taken to eliminate as much ambient noise as possible, and to maintain a *constant acoustic environment* during a single test and among tests on different patients. A sound level survey of a nontreated test environment should be carried out prior to any clinical evaluation.

Sound trauma must also be considered when studying the AP responses of clinical patients. Intense stimuli can cause a temporary reduction in the normal, and probably in the abnormal, AP. This phenomenon is similar in concept to a perceptual TTS and occurs at about the same stimulus magnitudes (Rosenblith *et al.*, 1950). These traumatic stimulus intensities are within the range normally used for cochleography. In clinical application, it is wise to do all low-intensity stimulation initially, reserving stimulation at more than 85 dB for the last portion of the procedure.

B. Electrodes and Recording Techniques

We have found it technically much easier to pass an electrode through the tympanic membrane and onto the promontory than to place a bare wire, or one tipped with saline-soaked cotton, onto the canal skin. Unless the canal electrode is exactly placed and fixed with glue or by some other method, induced motion will cause the APs recorded thereby to be of poor quality. Markedly elevated, erroneous thresholds may result without proper caution.

On a few occasions, we have also tried to use needle electrodes placed in the skin of the canal, but found the sensitivity to be no better than with a well-placed fixed-surface electrode. In clinical applications, such transdermal electrodes seem to offer no advantage over canal skin surface electrodes, and in addition, require a local anesthetic and yield more post-recording discomfort.

In contrast with our difficulties with canal electrodes, the first and every subsequent transtympanic-membrane promontory recording has been completely satisfactory. Our methods are essentially those of Portmann and Aran (1971). A local infiltrative anesthetic is used. (See Simmons *et al.*, 1973, for one early complication of this technique.) The electrode is introduced, using a nasal speculum rather than an indwelling ear canal speculum to dilate the ear canal. We measure the approximate length of required electrode beforehand to ensure that the outer end pushes against an elastic-band retainer, with the minimum pressure necessary to sustain the tip on the promontory. Almost no discomfort is felt by the patient. He is aware of the arrival of the electrode at the promontory, but the sensation felt at the moment of contact is not seriously uncomfortable, and it subsides within seconds. The greatest distraction at this time is caused by handling the electrode to secure it after placement is effected. The sound from this is equivalent to about 50-dB sensation level.

The transtympanic electrodes are made from segments of #22 spinal needles which are insulated by several coats of varnish (Formvar, General Electric Co.), except at the tip and butt end. The elastic retainer is fitted with a metal cup to hold the butt end, and the active lead is attached to this cup. A reference electrode is a short segment of needle placed in the earlobe, and a silver EEG-disc electrode is placed on the forehead as a ground.

These electrodes are connected through a short-shielded cable to a low-level differential amplifier, with filters set from 0.9 Hz through 10 kHz. Total gain in the amplification circuit is 10,000 to 100,000, in order to provide levels adequate for computer processing.

We have not attempted "chronic" electrodes of the type referred to by Yoshie (1971), because the clinical measures obtained thus far have been entirely satisfactory at the first attempt for each. It may also be noted that the relatively large promontory responses require much fewer stimulus samples in order to obtain useful data than do the EAC-based recordings. Since not more than 32 samples are required (and often only 8), an entire input–output function may be generated for click stimuli in *less than* 30 sec! The usual procedure, with measures obtained for both ears and with suitable replications, requires less than 1 hour from introduction of anesthesia to plotting of data in permanent form.

IV. CONCLUSIONS

If one counts pages, it is obvious that we have devoted the majority of this chapter to basic facts about normal auditory nerve responses, and a comparatively small amount of space to their clinical application. In itself, this distribution of words is a between-the-lines comment on the state of the art at this moment. We know a great deal about normal responses after many years of animal research, which, for a pleasant change, is directly applicable to humans. Clearly, the cochleogram, in the infancy of its clinical application, is the most powerful electrophysiological index of cochlear integrity yet applied to the damaged ear. In fact, we are aware of no other method by which it is possible to know with reasonable certainty that, when a response is present, there is at least some residual hearing at the end-organ, and that, when there is no response, there is no residual hearing at the frequencies tested. Making that distinction *is* today's clinical application.

Tomorrow's clinical application is equally certain: the not-too-difficult jump to predicting, with perhaps 10-dB accuracy, the contour of the threshold audiogram and some suprathreshold hearing characteristics of damaged ears. The information is present in the wave-form and latencies of the N_1–N_2 action potential. Slightly more sophisticated analysis is capable of extracting it. In fact, this is already possible for certain kinds of hearing losses. The number of patients with whom we must resort to any electrophysiological test will, however, be quite limited. Cochleography is not about to replace the audiometer.

The most important long-term application of cochleography is in clinical hearing research. The ability actually to measure the VIIIth nerve response to sounds directly, immediately, and with microsecond precision is a powerful new procedure for the dynamic understanding of hearing impairment. Forty years ago, the electrocardiogram was at a similar stage in its evolution. We are confident that 10 years from now the cochleogram will emerge as a diagnostic tool of comparable importance in a more limited field. In the meantime, there are problems of application and philosophy concerning human patients, problems that are not quite the same as those involved in electrocardiography. A needle through the tympanic membrane is not the same as electrodes pasted on the skin. The patient with a hearing loss must assume a slight additional risk, and the first few hundred (or thousand) patients who undergo cochleography will not benefit themselves most of the time. Yet, until we can fill the gaps in our knowledge about how different hearing losses are reflected in AP responses, we remain in the usual dilemma between research and clinical application. Some of these problems can easily be solved via animal research because the AP response in other species is immediately and directly applicable to humans. Thus, those hearing losses that can be produced in the laboratory (sound damage and trauma, ototoxicity, senility) ought to be reviewed for their relevance to humans.

Other pathological conditions without animal models (Meniere's syndrome, membrane breaks, tumors, hereditary–degenerative, etc.) can only be approached by experiments with humans. Until now, we have been limited to observations on temporal bones made long after the fact of the hearing loss. In contrast, cochleography is a technique that gives at least a little peek into the ongoing dynamic processes of a hearing impairment.

REFERENCES

Andreev, A. M., Arapova, A. A., and Gersuni, S. V. (1939). *J. Physiol. USSR.* **26**, 205.

Aran, J-M. (1971). *Arch. Klin. Exp. Ohren. Nasen. Kehlkopfheilk.* **198**, 128.

Butler, R. A., Honrubia, V., Johnstone, B. M., and Fernandez, C. (1962). *Ann. Otol. Rhinol. Laryngol.* **71**, 648.

Charlet de Sauvage, R., Anderson, D. J., and Pugh, J. E. (1973). A Digital Signal Processing Technique Applied to the Analysis of Cochlear Nerve Potentials. Paper given before the Acoust. Soc. of Amer., Boston, Massachusetts.

Coats, A. C. and Dickey, J. R. (1970). *Ann. Otol. Rhinol. Laryngol.* **79**, 844.

Cullen, J. K., Jr., Ellis, M. S., Berlin, C. I., and Lousteau, R. J. (1972). *Acta Oto-Laryngol.* **74**, 15.

Dallos, P. (1969). *J. Acoust. Soc. Amer.* **45**, 999.

Dallos, P. (1973). "The Auditory Periphery." Academic Press, New York.

Derbyshire, A. J., and Davis, H. (1935). *Amer. J. Physiol.* **113**, 476.

Finck, A., Ronis, M. L., and Rosenberg, P. E. (1969). *J. Speech Hear. Res.* **12**, 156.

Flach, M., and Seidel, P. (1968). *Arch. Klin. Exp. Ohren Nasen Kehlkopfheilk.* **190**, 229.

Glattke, T. J. (1972). Human Auditory Nerve Responses Obtained in the Presence of Band-limited Noise. Paper given before the Amer. Speech and Hearing Ass. San Francisco, California.

Goldstein, M. H., Jr., and Kiang, N. Y-S. (1958). *J. Acoust. Soc. Amer.* **30**, 107.

Keidel, W. D. (1971). *Rev. Laryngol. Otol. Rhinol. Suppl.* **92**, 709.

Kiang, N. Y-S. (1965). Discharge Patterns in Single Fibers in the Cat's Auditory Nerve. *Res. Monogr. No.* **35**. MIT Press, Cambridge, Massachusetts.

Lempert, J., Wever, E. G., and Lawrence, M. (1947). *Arch. Otolaryngol.* **45**, 61.

Lempert, J., Meltzer, P. E., Wever, E. G., and Lawrence, M. (1950). *Arch. Otolaryngol.* **51**, 307.

Misrahy, G. A., Hildreth, K. M., Shinabarger, E. A., and Gannon, W. J. (1958). *Amer. J. Physiol.* **194**, 396.

Moore, E. J. (1971). Human Cochlear Microphonics and Auditory Nerve Action Potentials from Surface Electrodes. Doctoral thesis, Univ. of Wisconsin, Madison, Wisconsin.

Peak, W. T., and Kiang, N. Y-S. (1962). *Biophys. J.* **2**, 23.

Peak, W. T., Goldstein, M. H., Jr., and Kiang, N. Y-S. (1962). *J. Acoust. Soc. Amer.* **34**, 562.

Perlman, H. G., and Case, T. J. (1941). *Arch. Otolaryngol.* **34**, 710.

Perlman, H. G., Kimura, R., and Fernandez, C. (1951). *Laryngoscope* **69**, 591.

Pfeiffer, R. R., and Kim, D. O. (1972). *J. Acoust. Soc. Amer.* **52**, 1669.

Portmann, M., and Aran, J-M. (1971). *Laryngoscope* **81**, 399.

Portmann, M., and Aran, J-M. (1972). *Acta Oto-Laryngol.* **73**, 190.

Portmann, M., LeBert, G., and Aran, J-M. (1967). *Rev. Laryngol. Otol. Rhinol.* **88**, 157.

Portmann, M., Aran J-M., and Lagourgue, P. (1973). *Ann. Otol. Rhinol. Laryngol.* **82**, 36.

Ronis, B. J. (1966). *Laryngoscope* **76**, 212.

Rosenblith, W., Galambos, R., and Hirsh, I. J. (1950). *Science* **111**, 569.

Ruben, R. J. (1967). *In* "Sensorineural Hearing Processes and Disorders" (A. B. Graham, ed.), pp. 313–337. Little, Brown, Boston, Massachusetts.

Ruben, R. J., Sekula, J., Bordley, J. E., Knickerbocker, G. G., Nager, G. T., and Fisch, U. (1960). *Ann. Otol. Rhinol. Laryngol.* **69**, 459.

Simmons, F. B. (1966). *Arch. Otolaryngol.* **83**, 449.

Simmons, F. B. (1972). Human Auditory Nerve Responses: a Comparison of Three Commonly Used Recording Sites. Thesis submitted to the Amer. Laryngol., Rhinol. and Otol. Soc.

Simmons, F. B., and Beatty, D. L. (1962). *Ann. Otolaryngol.* **71**, 767.

Simmons, F. B., and Glattke, T. J. (1972). *Ann. Otol. Rhinol. Laryngol.* **81**, 731.

Simmons, F. B., Glattke, T. J., and Downie, D. B. (1973). *Arch. Otolaryngol.* **98**, 42.

Sohmer, H., and Feinmesser, L. (1967). *Ann. Otol. Rhinol. Laryngol.* **76**, 427.

Teas, D. C., Eldredge, D., and Davis, H. (1962). *J. Acoust. Soc. Amer.* **34**, 1438.

von Békésy, G. (1960). "Experiments in Hearing." McGraw-Hill, New York.

Wever, E. G. (1966). *Physiol. Rev.* **46**, 102.

Wever, E. G., and Bray, C. (1930). *Proc. Nat. Acad. Sci. U.S.* **16**, 344.

Yoshie, N. (1968). *Laryngoscope* **78**, 198.

Yoshie, N. (1971). *Rev. Laryngol. Otol. Rhinol. Suppl.* **92**, 646.

Yoshie, N., and Ohashi, T. (1967). *J. Otolaryngol. Jap.* **70**, 920.

Yoshie, N., and Ohashi, T. (1969). *Acta Oto-Laryngol. Suppl.* **252**, 71.

Yoshie, N., and Ohashi, T. (1971). *Rev. Laryngol. Otol. Rhinol. Suppl.* **92**, 673.

SUPPLEMENTARY READINGS

Aran, J-M. (1973). *Adv. Otorhinolaryngol.* **20**, 374–394.

Beagley, H. A. (1973). *Audiology* **12**, 470–480.

Eggermont, J. J., and Odenthal, D. W. (1974). *Audiology* **13**, 1–22.

Hecox, K., and Galambos, R. (1974). *Arch. Otolaryngol.* **99**, 30–33.

Lev, A., and Sohmer, H. (1972). *Arch. Ohr. Nas. u. Hehlk-Heilk.* **201**, 79–90.

Moushegian, G., Rupert, A., and Stillman, R. D. (1973). *Electroencephalogr. Clin. Neurophysiol.* **35**, 665–667.

Picton, T. W., Hillyard, S. A., Krausz, R. I., and Galambos, R. (1974). *Electroencephalogr. Clin. Neurophysiol.* **36**, 179–190.

Yoshie, N. (1973). *Audiology* **12**, 504–539.

Chapter Six

Reflex and Conditioning Audiometry

William G. Hardy[1]

I. BACKGROUND

Within the past decade, there has come about a tremendous burgeoning of concern with various measures and functions of the auditory system, especially as this system operates in the infant and very young child. No doubt, much of this interest comes into focus with a general social commitment to *earliness*—the earlier a potentially handicapped child can be found, the earlier his problems can be detected, mitigated so far as possible, and well-managed if not mitigated. Therefore, the earlier he can be tested, and found wanting or not wanting, the better off both he and society will be. Some of the efforts undertaken to these ends have scientific merit; others are apt to be hopeful expressions of desire and need, without much relation to basic requirements of scientific method. All are humanitarian.

Lest this be considered ultramodern and radical thinking, it might be well to turn back nearly a quarter of a century:

> We have been considering . . . three basic concepts related to . . . young children with severely impaired hearing. First, . . . the communicative disorder centering around the hearing loss is a disturbance that affects the whole behavioral complex of the child. Second, emphasis has been given to the idea of a multilateral approach to the problems of these children; this is not a matter for the physician alone, nor for the educator

[1] The Johns Hopkins University School of Hygiene and Public Health, The Johns Hopkins University School of Medicine, and The Johns Hopkins Hospital, Baltimore, Maryland.

alone; it needs the best that can be made available in the entire aggregate of professional interest. Third is the idea that treatment and training should be begun as early as possible in a child's life; this is a concept that has only recently been put into practice in a very limited fashion in some communities, and one that has already proved to be of great value [Hardy, W. G., et al., 1951, p. 86].

At that time, what we know now as valuable instrumental tests were in their experimental infancy; and much that we take for granted by way of reflex and conditioned testing was only at very early developmental stages. Fifteen years ago, there was general concern about early detection of auditory problems among school children. The observations and measurements of these problems have now moved down the developmental scale to include the preschool-age child, in the kindergarten, the nursery, the dayschool; the very young child (under 3 years); the infant, the newborn, and finally, indeed, the foetus. This chapter undertakes to outline current philosophies and procedures directly related to the development and use of reflex and conditioning audiometry (exclusive of specialized instrumental procedures discussed in other chapters of this book), in an attempt to bring behavioral and physiological aspects of acoustic responses into some accord.

II. GENERAL CONSIDERATIONS

In order to avoid some of the homiletic bents that tend to force attention on the goodness of doing good, and in order to concentrate on some of the practical problems of early testing and the interpretation of responses, it seems wise to begin with a few broad guidelines.

The first of these is so obvious that it is frequently overlooked—the very young infant is quite immature. He comes with much potential (particularly relative to hearing, inasmuch as the cochlea, at least, is quite fully developed by 26–28 weeks of term), but can rarely put all this to immediate use. In general, "the newborn animal is primarily a 'brain-stem individual'. . . . At some early stage of our development we are functioning primarily at the hippocampal level [Hawke, 1965, p. 219]." Apparently, the degree of plasticity in the very young brain varies considerably with the area. If it is kept in mind that hearing is largely a function of the brain—not the ear—it follows that, as the brain matures, the child's capacity to hear is rapidly incremental. In the course of the opening remarks of an important conference on "The Young Deaf Child" that took place some years ago, there was considerable discussion about pressing needs for early detection, which the chairman summarized when he said:

> Out of all this comes the suggestion that until a certain degree of maturation has occurred in the cortex it will probably not make much difference whether there is sensory deprivation or enrichment. What we need to know is exactly when it is necessary to move in and provide sensory input: in other words, to know when the developing brain is ready to take advantage of the input. At the present we rely entirely on intuition; and for the present perhaps that is the best we can do. Perhaps clinical. evidence will give us some additional insight [Davis, 1965, p. 219].

In very large part, this chapter reports what has been accomplished in these terms within the past decade.

A second need for some structured thinking centers in the fact that both mass screening programs and more extensive and definitive measurements have been undertaken with very little regard for normal developmental features of the newborn and young infants. It is only in quite recent years that sufficient normative information has been available to make possible really thoughtful appraisals of behavior relative to various kinds of responses to acoustic stimuli. It is clear now that even newborns are capable of responding with a considerable amount of differentiation among various levels of frequency, intensity, and acoustic quality (Eisenberg et al., 1964; Eisenberg, 1970b; Goldstein and Tait, 1971; Hoverstein and Moncur, 1969, and others). As development continues, these responses become more refined, and clearly reflect the infant's interest in, and capacity to learn from, acoustic cues. Some of the details of this development will be considered step by step as this discussion proceeds from younger to older infants and young children.

Further, in this regard, it is apparent that the ear is the sense organ with the widest array of connections within the central nervous system. Although the details are not matters exclusively for this chapter, it has been made amply clear that the broad spectrum of behavioral responses to sound, both reflex and learned, is only a foreshortened reflection of the brain's capacities that are demonstrated in electroencephalic responses to sound. Regardless of the placement of electrodes, there are clear responses to acoustic stimuli of even moderate intensity. These are rather obvious observations about the very young brain. Its potentials most readily come to fruition in the development, within the first few months, of a changeover from perception to learning. The effect of these developmental features is apparent in the infant's responses to acoustic cues—in his progression from reflexive activity to orientation in his environment. In terms of testing his responses to sound, it is apparent that, the more time he has spent in listening (training?), with the resultant increments in learning, the better is the possibility of achieving some valid observations about his capacity to hear and his capacity to use his hearing. Throughout the various developmental phases of the first year of life, it becomes apparent that the infant as a whole represents much more than the sum of his parts.

The relationships between responses to acoustic stimuli and the receptive development of what will become language have only quite recently been seriously addressed in some detail. It is clear that language development is a direct derivation from hearing. What needs much more study are the relations among listening, attention to those sounds in the environment that become increasingly important (like the sounds of speech), and the connections between these experiences and the general process of phonologic and linguistic development. Much of the implication of these experiences for the infant's capacity to learn the rules of language has been expressed very succinctly:

> Whether the capability is innate or learned (if, indeed, that distinction is valid) babies do acquire the ability to recognize speech as they become increasingly sophisticated at deriving relatively constant properties of highly variable acoustic signals. By some process of selecting, rejecting, filtering, and transforming inputs which are often very crude and indistinct, babies make the transition from receiving acoustical sounds to perceiving informational language.
>
> It is hard to imagine any aspect of subsequent linguistic and psychological development more formidable than that [Friedlander, 1972a, p. 2].

How are the early stages of these phenomena accessible for observation?

In addressing ways and means of ascertaining what is going on between the infant and sounds in his environment—more particularly, in testing his responses to various sounds—we must try to distinguish between the functions and objectives of a program of mass screening and those of a detailed study of responses under carefully controlled circumstances. The failure to recognize and maintain such a distinction has caused much professional and parental anguish in recent years. The two approaches are by no means "the same thing." This matter is perhaps one of the most important aspects of our guidelines. Implicit here is the point that there are very considerable differences between both procedures and goals of the mass screening of newborns with a single-frequency signal in the hands of observer-volunteers, and the kinds of careful studies that are being made in a relatively few laboratories. The one is almost casual, relative to the knowable details of early infantile behavior; the other is a form of scientific effort from which much can be learned.

III. GUIDELINES

This kind of thinking forces attention on some of the variables that are implicit and explicit in any study of infant behavior. A few of these are worth special attention.

A wide variety of sources of sound is, or may be, available. Included here in work with infants in the first year of life are simple noisemakers (horns, bells, whistles, clackers, tonettes, xylophones, and so forth); various specific acoustic signals, electronically generated and controlled in frequency and intensity; and, perhaps most important, the human voice (for purposes of validation of responses, this is best done with recorded material). With some imagination, one can think of many variations that might have become part of a baby's daily experiences by 6–9 months of age—barks, mews, coos, moos, growls, and various mechanical, percussion sounds.

Reflex or startle responses are observable very early in the baby's life: The Moro (named after a German pediatrician) offers a galvanized extension of the peripheral musculature; the eye-blink is common (acoustopalpebral reflex, APR): the auditory orienting reflex (AOR) is clearly discernible after about 4 months of age; the so-called "conditioned orienting reflex or response" (COR) has been found useful in the range between 12 and 24+ months; various changes in respiration and in heart rate (both increase and decrease) have been associated with auditory responses; and there are other responses, such as cessation of sucking, awakening, and so forth, that are part and parcel of the infant's daily activity. For the most part, in the early months, these are general muscular or physiological responses—largely in terms of preorientation to sound. It must be emphasized that such responses offer qualitative, rather than quantitative, information (Frisina, 1963; Hardy, 1965; Hardy, J. B., et al., 1959; Hardy, W. G., et al., 1962; and many others). By 4–6 months of age, the infant typically shows various aspects of auditory orientation, turning of the head and torso, or the eyes, toward the source of sound. Later, with much further development and learning, many test refinements can be employed (play–audiometry, pure-tone audiometry in general, and measurements with the use of speech signals).

Throughout these developmental stages—the "passing of landmarks"— various questions arise. When does an infant become a child? How does one know? What is the marker?—language development? speech output?

adaptive behavior? cognitive activities? social adjustment? In the present context, it is possible that the answers might contribute much to the understanding of what is appropriate in a test situation, and of the interpretation of responses.

An important aspect of testing all infants and very young children is the presence of the observer in the test environment. This is particularly worthy of careful attention in working with infants. With newborns, for instance, occasional turning of the head may or may not be a response to sound—rather, it may be to the presence of the person. It is important, moreover, to consider the relations between reliability among observers (commonly found to be fairly good within defined limits) and the validity of their judgments. Many times, observers may agree on having seen responses; the problem is to ascertain "responses to what?" The offerings of chance remain at 50–50%. Students of infantile responses to the carefully structured use of acoustic stimulation have expressed this warning over the years (Hardy, J. B., et al., 1959, and many others).

Then there is the obvious matter of the subject's readiness and willingness to respond in various test circumstances. Again, this point was summarized succinctly after a long discussion of various aspects of identification in terms of definitive tests of hearing:

> I wish to emphasize once more the importance of the proper degree of arousal or attention or motivation of the subject. This point has appeared in the discussion of practically every test from Dr. Wedenberg's awakening test and the Ewing method directly on through play–audiometry and the peepshow. The Ewing distraction method and the peepshow were both designed specifically to obtain the proper degree of attention, interest, and cooperation. We shall see that the problem of the degree of arousal appears again in the electrodermal and electroencephalic methods. The condition and attitude of the subject must never be forgotten [Davis, 1965, p. 89].

In very general terms, this question of readiness is one of the principal aspects of maturity, and furnishes a major guideline for the details of procedures, observations, and judgments as these must vary from subject to subject and from one developmental age-status to another (e.g., the baby of normal intelligence may respond at 7 months of age far better and more consistently than the profoundly retarded child at 3 years of age).

Perhaps equally important is the factor of major differences between "testing for hearing" and "observing responses to acoustic stimuli." There has been considerable discussion of this point, to which relatively little attention has been paid (Eisenberg et al., 1964; Eisenberg, 1970a, 1971; Hardy and Hardy, 1963; Hoverstein and Moncur, 1969; and several others). These differences are fundamental in observing the behavior of newborns and young infants. This behavior (or, these behaviors) may— and commonly does—include many false-positive and false-negative responses. And, unfortunately, many of the procedures that are regularly undertaken are geared to some concept or other about *deafness* rather than to the *observation of responses to acoustic stimuli*. Indeed, perhaps because of a basic predilection on the part of observers, any sort of testing that involves an appeal to auditory sensations must necessarily be a test of *hearing or not hearing*. Yet, the most important aspects of responding to sound are functions of the brain, not of the ears alone. Accordingly, anything about the infant that reflects disease, or infection, or even immaturity, in terms of brain functions, will usually show itself in a lack of, or differentness about, responses to acoustic stimuli. At stake here is not the presence or absence of hearing impairment alone, but, as well, the presence or absence of "mental" or "motor" interferences with the capacity to respond to sound. Judgments about the meaning of the presence or absence of responses to sound are extremely complex, not to be made casually, and involve much more than hearing or not hearing.

By way of a summary of concepts, ideas, and needs relating to the testing of infants and young children, attention may be turned again to the conference on "The Young Deaf Child":

> Several types of auditory tests have been developed. They rest upon different classes of physiological or behavioral response. Some are more suitable than others for young children and they vary also in the definiteness of the information which they yield. Many of the tests are quite satisfactory within established limitations, but further research is required. We need to understand more fully the expectations in the normal development of children and we also need to improve our techniques, both for screening and for definitive diagnostic testing. In particular, further analysis in terms of simple reflexes, thalamic and cortical sensory systems, the "second signal system," and conditioned reflexes is needed [Davis, 1965, pp. 16–17].

IV.   PRENATAL TESTING

Wedenberg and his associates in Stockholm have long paid attention to auditory responses of the foetus. They were led into the inquiry because of concern with therapeutic abortion as this might obtain, for instance, in the case of a woman who had had rubella or had been exposed to it early in term. Were it possible to demonstrate responses of the foetus to various sounds introduced in utero, then, the reasoning went, the foetus could be allowed to come to term. (N.B.: Obviously, this kind of thinking was ingenious at the time; later, with the findings from the prenatal rubella epidemic of 1963–1965, many multiple involvements aside from impaired hearing were discovered to be part of the rubella syndrome.)

Various observations were carried out with great care. The signal was a frequency of 3000 Hz, with an SPL of 110 dB (ISO). A phonocardiograph was employed to record muscular changes. Repeated runs demonstrated no responses at 22 weeks of term, but clear responses were typically observed at 26 weeks (too late for therapeutic abortion under Swedish law). In follow-up, it was determined that responses "became increasingly distinct with foetal age." Postnatal tests indicated "normal hearing." These observations have been replicated (Johansson et al., 1964). Aside from this careful study, there have been numerous anecdotal reports of responses to acoustic stimuli in utero, but nothing of comparable scientific order.

V. A HIGH-RISK REGISTER

There long has been deep concern with hereditary factors in the study of deafness. This has been extended and deepened, in recent years, with current findings in genetics. Such concerns inevitably direct attention to the possible variety of causal factors relatable to hearing impairment and communicative disorders in general.

During the conference on "The Young Deaf Child," held in Toronto in 1964, Dr. Janet M. B. Hardy presented the concept of a "High-Risk Register for the Better Identification of Children with Communication Problems." It was her contention, directly related to Dr. Wedenberg's discussion of hereditary and foetal influences, that there are many other sources of pertinent information besides the use of perinatal testing or screening. She expressed the thought that the majority of problems found in very young children can be determined before the perinatal period in terms of familial history, conditions of pregnancy and delivery, and what occurs immediately after delivery.

This registry was published as part of the proceedings of the conference (Davis, 1965, pp. 15–16). It included five major headings— antenatal, complications of labor, neonatal difficulty, factors in early childhood, and possible social factors. Within these five topics are listed 23 subtopics, covering the gamut of direct and indirect causal factors of impaired hearing or relatable disorders. There was ready acceptance of the concept, and extensive discussion among those present at the conference. This general point has been remarkably developed in the relatively few years since this initial statement. Some aspect of the use of a high-risk register appears commonly in audiological and pediatric discussions these days, often as a preparatory or selective step preceding some sort of definitive testing. This was its author's intention, and bears out some afterthoughts of the conference expressed by the chairman–editor:

> The High-Risk Register constitutes a practical recommendation of how to deal with the problem from the point of view of Public Health. It represents a compromise to be sure, but if we can actually succeed in establishing such registers and alerting obstetricians, pediatricians and parents to the possibility of hearing impairment in this group of children and the desirability of detecting it in order to institute proper and helpful management, we shall have made a very significant contribution to the solution of our overall problem [Davis, 1965, p. 70].

VI. NEONATAL TESTING

The matter of testing neonates has been of special concern within the past few years. There are strong proponents and strong opponents, and more than a few "experts" who are rather indifferent. Involved here are some quite complex questions that have to do with efficacy, efficiency of procedures, and need. Clearly, any professional person whose mind is steeped in the problems of this aspect of the field is bound to have some bias. The present writer has, and will do his best—probably without complete success—to present a balanced picture of the state of the art.

There have been expressed many criticisms of neonatal testing, but few critiques. Among the latter are two statements that will be referred to from time to time in this presentation (Goldstein and Tait, 1971; Hoverstein and Moncur, 1969; many related comments are made recurrently). Probably the most exhaustive consideration of the topic (undertaken with some notable biases from all sides) was carried out in a "Conference on Newborn Hearing Screening: Proceedings, Summary, and Recommendations." [2] It is this writer's belief that this conference represents a genuinely mature attempt to get at the core of some difficult matters. The summary and recommendations include important modifications of views previously expressed by some of the participants.

---

[2] Held at the San Francisco Airport, February 23–25, 1971, this conference was convened under the auspices of the Maternal and Child Health Services of the Department of Health, Education, and Welfare and the Bureau of Maternal and Child Health, California State Department of Public Health.

The proceedings include an excellent review of neonatal auditory testing; in fact, this is more an overview than a review. In conclusion, the overviewer observes:

> It seems . . . that in the hands of competent, astute observers, neonatal screening tests may be valid and reliable. The problem which faces us for the immediate future is how to generate either competent, astute observers or techniques or to develop techniques to make the rest of us appear to be competent and astute [Gerber, 1971, p. 31].

For better or worse, these observations—lugubrious as they may be—appear to obtain for all sorts of difficult clinical testing. It is worth noting again, however, that there remain fundamental differences between screening tests and an attempt to derive definitive measurements for each child.

A. Some Pros and Cons

At this stage in the discussion of neonatal auditory testing, it might be well to review some of the reasons commonly offered to support the undertaking, and to refer to some less supportive opinions. The positive points usually involve one aspect or another of the following:

1. The neonatal period is the only time when the infant is fully available: More than 95% of our babies are born in hospitals, and both professional and volunteer staffs are ready at hand; the testing does not take long and does not seriously interrupt schedules.
2. Although those caught in the screen are few in both numbers and proportion, those who are found might have been missed.
3. A check-out at birth is at least a reference point against the later detection of a hearing loss.
4. There is some measure of serendipity, in that lack of responses to sound often serves to alert the staff to the possibility of defects other than hearing.
5. Neonatal testing may provide at least some information about normal development that would not otherwise be obtained.
6. The scheme affords the establishment of good relations with physicians interested in the welfare of the children.

From other viewpoints, there are some genuine reservations:

1. Neonatal testing offers many problems and large numbers of children; mass screening takes in too much ground with procedures that are largely experimental.

2. With presentation levels of the order of 80–100-db SPL, it is impossible to detect the mild–moderate impairments, which far outnumber the profound losses.
3. Many babies with hearing impairments are not discovered, or their problems are confounded by an inordinate number of false-positive and false-negative responses.
4. Little attention is paid to the test environment and to the definition of reliable judgments about the meaning of a baby's behavior.
5. In terms of parental guidance and of information contributory to it, both false-positive and false-negatives can be deleterious.

All this has been recapitulated in considerable detail (Eisenberg, 1970b, 1971; Goldstein and Tait, 1971; Hardy and Hardy, 1963; Hardy *et al.*, 1970).

B. Procedures and Goals

An early approach to a definition of infantile behavior in terms of acoustic stimuli was undertaken at the Karolinska Institute in Stockholm (Wedenberg, 1956). In discussing the background of this work, Wedenberg referred to the use of the acoustopalpebral reflex or response (APR) by Pregorin, 1882, described in a report entitled "Die Seels des Kindes," and to the report of early studies by Ewing and Ewing (1944), which established the fact of the APR in the first 6 months of life, with the warning that thereafter there was apt to be reduction in the response. In an early study, Wedenberg used a cowbell as a stimulus source with 150 babies of 1 to 7 days old. The bell had a frequency range around 750 Hz and an intensity of 125 dB (re acoustic zero). All but one of the newborns responded. The investigator reasoned that the response must be phylogenetically related to some sort of a warning system. A later study centered on 20 normal babies, 1 to 10 days old (Johansson *et al.*, 1964). This study was undertaken with a wide range of pure tones from a loudspeaker, which was lowered over the baby in its crib. There were consistent APRs to tones of the order of 105–115 dB, with awakening down to 75 dB. This was done at the time of the announcement from neurology of much new information about the brain's reticular formation, which controls awakening, or, when the responder is awake, controls alerting. It was considered that the APR was mediated at a higher level than the stapedius reflex to sound. The stapedius reflex is mediated low in the brainstem through the superior olivary structures; the APR involves much more extensive aspects of the reticular system. Long-term follow-up was proposed. Some years later, this was described as an "awakening test," useful for older children; for this purpose, the stimulus consisted of tone pulses of 3000 Hz at 75-dB SPL (Davis, 1965, p. 94).

The conference on "The Young Deaf Child" included a report from Downs based on the findings published in an immediately concurrent article (Downs and Sterritt, 1964). Four cases of impaired hearing were found in a screened aggregate of 5000 newborns. Two signals were employed: a broad band of white noise presented at 70-, 80-, 90-, and 100-dB SPL, and a narrow band of filtered noise peaking at 3000 Hz with an energy band of 2500–3500 Hz, presented at the same levels. "Rating scales and rigid definitions of response categories are applied to the various parameters of the infants' responses so that independent observers can agree on what they have seen when the very complex event of an infant's response takes place [Davis, 1965, p. 41]." This was done with great care, and reported in terms of variables of time, the site of responses, and the intensity of responses. Particular attention was paid to the condition of the infant both in the test environment and relative to his history.

This was the beginning of Downs' current rating scale abetted by the use of aspects of a high-risk register, now modified to "At Risk for Hearing Impairment" (verbal discussion, 1972). In reference, here are nine items in the A B C D's of H E A R:

> Affirmative familial history
> Bilirubin of 20 mgm or less
> Congenital rubella
> Defects at birth
> Small at birth
> Hearing concern
> Ear test normal
> Awakens to sound
> Responses to developmental and communicative scales

This mnemonic device is designed to direct attention to the question which, in Downs' opinion, is the point of screening newborns—"Does he hear or not?"

These approaches are described in detail in two recent articles (Downs, 1970, 1971a). The second of these, included in the San Francisco "Conference on Newborn Hearing Screening," records up-to-date findings on the follow-up of approximately 20,000 newborns. Essentially all who were found to be deaf could have been accounted for in terms of the findings of a high-risk register, even a group "who were identified as deaf and who expired within short periods after birth." A set of proposed guidelines is offered, to which the reader is referred for complete details.

These include: (1) "routine screening tests at birth . . . on every infant on a High Risk Register for deafness"; (2) individual behavioral testing in a quiet room; (3) "selected investigations on newborns who can be monitored developmentally and audiologically for at least a year"; and (4) "recommendations for physicians and all health personnel to attempt to identify the older deaf infant."—this involves recurrent tests "at every health visit [pp. 116–117]."

C.   Some Baselines of Reference

Amid these various points of view regarding the testing of newborns, it might be well to interject some generalizations. First, from the conference in Toronto, with reference to early postnatal tests, we are reminded that:

> The actual percentage of children with significant impairments (neonatal) is very small. . . . Any screening test . . . must be quick, simple, and inexpensive. . . . [It is] poor strategy to apply a screening test until the infant or child is old enough to make the test reliable. . . . We shall have too many false positives, and . . . miss too many cases [Davis, 1965, p. 33].

Second, from the conference in San Francisco:

> Sound is capable of producing changes in any or all portions of the organism. There can be changes in heart rate, peripheral circulation, sweating, respiration, in movement of eyes, face, limbs or entire body, complex acts such as sucking, crying, babbling, may increase or decrease and if one accepts consciousness, sounds reach and modify its states [Derbyshire, 1971, p. 104].

Derbyshire goes on to remind us that what we accept as indicative of a response actually offers our definition of "hearing." This that we call "hearing" is scarcely static. The very complexity of the neural system involved, including the cochlea (with both afferent and efferent connections), suggests highly differentiated functions. "On this basis what each experimenter accepts or rejects does define what 'hearing' he is measuring."

It seems apparent that such warning notes should be sounded recurrently, if only to remind us that good clinical practices usually follow along with good scientific principles. Enthusiasm and desire do not furnish sufficient rationale for mounting massive programs in the interest of public health and welfare.

D. Other Points of View

In quite sharp contrast with the objectives and procedures concerned in the screening of newborns (with which there remains some sharp disagreement), Eisenberg's work for more than 10 years has been focused on normal neonatal capacities relative to responses to sound (Eisenberg et al., 1964). Since this first "preliminary" reckoning, there have been several detailed reports and the expression of fundamental concepts pertinent to neonatal and early infantile development (Eisenberg, 1971; Friedlander, 1970; Goldstein and Tait, 1971; Hoverstein and Moncur, 1969).

As a demonstration of continuing laboratory research in a field of inquiry in which relatively few laboratories are working, the concerns and findings expressed by this group of writers surely warrant some detailed consideration. The original report was based on findings from the study of 170 babies ranging in age from 2 hours to 9 days:

> Four calibrated noisemaker signals, matched approximately for an SPL of 65 dB, were used as stimuli: (1) white noise, 1.3 sec.; (2) white noise, 200 msec.; (3) 500–900 cps band-pass, 300 msec.; and (4) 4000–4500 cps band-pass, 250 msec. Each signal was presented five times, at random intervals in excess of 10 sec., according to a randomized presentation schedule [p. 263].

Three observers returned one of three ratings for each child—positive, questionable, negative—relative to each sequence of sound. Ratings were made on the basis of four behavioral indices:

> (1) motor reflexes; (2) eye reflexes; (3) arousal, that is, any form of arousal behavior involving either a significant increase in activity state or the sudden onset of new activity; and (4) orienting–quiet, that is, any form of primitive attentive behavior involving either a significant increase in activity state or the complete cessation of ongoing activity [p. 263].

The experimenters point out that "the proportion of motor reflexes always varies directly with response-ratio [defined as the number of signals relative to the number of responses]; the strength of such reflexes, as rated on a continuum extending from Moro responses to single segment activity, varies similarly."

Obviously, there are many responses from neonatal subjects; a basic problem is to relate the responses to the signals. Various generalizations in these regards are adduced from the observations (Eisenberg et al., 1964):

1. Noise-bands are more effective than pure tones.
2. Duration of the stimulus is critical.
3. Frequency selection apparently shows important range-dependent effects, e.g., low frequency induces motor responses, while high frequency is related to behavior that can be called "freezing".
4. Importance of repetition rate has not been sufficiently studied (see Hoverstein and Moncur, 1969).
5. Rise-time and decay-time are important only relative to high intensities.
6. SPL follows power law with a systematic increase; an optimal level, used in this experiment, is 65 dB.
7. Habituation is important with a normal subject; there are differences in latency among children in "risk groups."
8. In terms of cardiac responses, boundaries change over several trials (see Crowell et al., 1971).
9. In general, constant stimuli produce nonspecific responses.

There is a wealth of ideas involved in these findings. One should refer to the detail of the summary of this particular study. A few quotations from this source may serve to whet intellectual appetites:

1. Under all conditions, signal variables exert differential effects upon the incidence of response to auditory stimulation (response-ratio), the type of behavior elicited during response (response-pattern), and the intensity of that response (response-strength).
2. Response-ratio varies systematically with activity state in the neonate much as performance levels varies with it in the adult. Response-pattern varies systematically in accordance with an "awake–alert–awake" continuum which has been postulated for the ascending reticular formation. Response-strength varies systematically in accordance with the "law of initial values."
3. The proportion of arousal responses tends to decrease, and the proportion of orienting–quiet responses correspondingly to increase, as the sequence progresses. The reciprocal relation between these two reflexes does not accord with concepts of the orienting reflex as a response to "novel" stimuli.
4. Sequential responses (that is, those in which the appearance of several behavioral components in consecutive order connotes increased response-time) vary linearly with age and must be viewed as an index of maturation [Eisenberg et al., 1964, pp. 263–264].

Additional generalizations pertinent to extended work in the field are available in a later work (Eisenberg, 1970b). First, in terms of a broad picture, "It seems possible . . . that neuronal mechanisms for processing SPL are fully mature at birth." (But see Derbyshire, discussed previously.) It may be splitting hairs, but it does not necessarily follow that these neuronal mechanisms can be *used* without further maturity; how would one find out? Second, response increases in proportion to duration in a range of 300–3000 msec. Third, an interesting set of frequency-related observations has been derived. When the stimulus is below 4000 Hz, there are 2–3 times more responses than when it is above 4000 Hz. Much of behavior in response relates to the state of the subject: High-frequency signals are "best" while the baby is awake; low-frequency stimuli are "best" when he is dozing or in light sleep. Inasmuch as the neonate sleeps approximately 22 hours in every 24, this leaves relatively little time for studies of such contrasts. Low-frequency signals, moreover, are "good" and invoke pleasurable responses in later affect. The reverse is apparently true about high-frequency signals, which, it will be recalled, are related to arousal, alerting, and "freezing." As Eisenberg points out, it is interesting to observe that our burglar alarms and warning alerts in general approach the "shrieking" levels of frequency.

E. Related Observations

Various other reports about neonatal testing are available from many sources. From studying them, one can build up a series of reinforced impressions.

In Israel, for instance, Altman and Shenhau (1971) comment on a study of 2810 babies at risk; 35 were considered to show abnormal responses to sound. Of these, two groups were formed: 12 were thought to have "hearing loss"; 23 were considered to have neuropsychiatric disorders. It was found that work with neonates (2 hours to 4 days of age) was generally unsatisfactory with untrained observers. Infants 7–12 months of age were considered excellent subjects, as they were seen in well-baby clinics. These efforts are new and are not yet fully reported.

In 1970, three investigators in Canada undertook an inquiry into "Stimulus, Response and Observer Variables in the Auditory Screening of Newborn Infants" (Ling *et al.*, 1970). They worked with 144 babies, all considered healthy, with an age range of 1–6 days. Four instrumental sounds were employed with an input of 85-dB SPL at the infant's ear: noise bands down to 3150 and 2000 Hz, and pure tones up and down from 2000–4000 Hz. Both masked (noise in headphones) and unmasked observers were used.

The experimenters found what they called "three intrinsic sources of error"—the infant, the observer, and the stimulus. In their opinion, the infants were not ready for routine testing; there was confusion in the observers' judgments—"Response to what?" was asked over and over again as the complex of the infant's muscular reactions was observed; and they believed that much attention must be paid to the stimulus, that is, the use of narrow-band noises of lower frequencies might well produce more positive results. It is of note that this group did not employ voice, long established as a useful stimulus. They were concerned, as have been many others, about the problems of false-positive and false-negative responses.

Their conclusions were quite definite: "The development of more generally efficient stimulus sounds and testing procedures should have the utmost priority. Without such definitive work, newborn screening programs will continue to be assumption-ridden, time-consuming, and highly inefficient [Ling *et al.*, 1970, p. 17]."

Ling (1972a) undertook to check response validity in testing newborn infants. He stated concern about too many false-positives, and again questioned the validity of the mass procedures presently in use. He suggested that the use of four tones, 1500 Hz and above, be undertaken, and reported better consistency of responses with the use of all four. He further suggested that three responses to every four signals be required. He cited the need to use other signals.

At the conference in Toronto in 1964, Bengt Barr reported on the testing of 12,000 neonates at Eskilstuna Hospital in Sweden (Barr, 1965). A gong was used: 126–133 dB (re acoustic zero), at a distance of 13.5 cm from the pinna; the spectrum was like white noise. There was approximately a 95% response with APRs. Only eight infants were found to be deaf; sooner or later, all the other suspects reacted to the stimulus.

Janet Hardy and associates (1959) have studied auditory responses from neonates and young infants in a variety of circumstances. With the use of a wooden clacker (broad spectrum; approximately 60-dB SPL), 98% responded at 46 hours of age. The others were either prematures (in whom it takes about two weeks for responses to develop), or were stuperous (examined too soon after feeding).

She was particularly concerned about one "miss":

> The child had a severe secondary apnoea a few minutes after birth and required resuscitation. At four months of age he responded fairly normally to the Ewing type of screening but at 12 months he did not respond. In the nursery, he had given good auditory responses but at the age of two years he had not developed language. A thorough-going definitive audiology study revealed a profound sensory–neural type of hearing loss [Davis, 1965, p. 35].

The lesson seems clear: *Follow-up is imperative.*

F. Studies of Heart Rate

Various inquirers have had something to say about the study of heart rate as a response of the newborn to sound. Eisenberg (1971) has suggested the routine use of a cardiotachometer, with or without telemetry, as part of a test battery. Others have reported considerable experience. Cardiac audiometry is discussed in Chapter 10.

Crowell and associates (1971) report a study of 37 babies, 35–60 hours old. All were considered clinically normal, with an average 1-min Apgar score of eight. The group used modulated pure tones and found much variability and trouble in measuring and defining changes. Tones were presented for 4 sec at 500, 1000, 2000, 4000, 6000, and 8000 Hz, with constant modulation at 63 dB and 80 dB. The loudspeaker was positioned at 17.8 cm above the infant's right ear. Ten samples were made per second, with 5.4 sec prestimulus and 8.6 sec poststimulus. The greatest number of responses occurred 1.3 sec after the onset of stimulus; there was "on" response within 1 sec; this peaked at 3 sec. Of the 37 babies, 22 responded to all tones, two to three times the level of chance.

Steinschneider and associates did an interesting experiment, which they reported in 1966:

> Cardiac and motor responsivity [a strain guage connected with the crib was used to observe motor responses] was determined on 9 neonates repetitively and randomly presented with four 5-sec. white noise stimuli (55, 70, 85 and 100 dB) and "control" trials. The results clearly indicated that the percentage of motor responses increased and their latency decreased with increasing intensity of stimulation. There was a progressive increase in the duration and a decrease in the latency of the primary phase of the cardiac rate response as the sound level increased [ambient noise measured 47 dB re acoustic zero]. In addition, the average magnitude of both the primary and return phases of the cardiac response progressively increased. Neonates differed in their ability to respond differentially to changing stimulation (discrimination). All newborns responded to a stimulus intensity of 70 dB or less [p. 233].

G. Overview

What may be concluded, then, from this wealth of material on what is basically reflexive response to sound? Most of the opinions that support mass screening of newborns are based on economy rather than science. And this economy is apt to be of an inflated order: A higher and higher price is paid for less and less return. A very few infants are found not to respond; they are called "deaf." As yet, nobody knows the number of infants who give false-positive responses, who are commonly thought about only as "not deaf." Some very recent efforts have been undertaken to offset these tendencies (Downs, 1970, 1971a), but even with the currently suggested modifications (the concentration on high-risk babies, and much more careful follow-up), there must be many babies overlooked who have impaired hearing but who are not deaf, and perhaps almost as many for whom auditory impairment is only one of several interferences with their development.

Some of the major objections or exceptions to current modes of mass screening can be summarized as follows:

1. A very limited array of signals is employed; for the most part, these are noise bands or high-frequency warbled tones at high levels of intensity; complex sounds, such as speech, are rarely used.
2. The effect of this is that only a few infants called "deaf" are selected by the screen; many others pass through as false-positives.
3. Observers are for the most part relatively untrained volunteers.
4. There is little clearcut definition of a response; personal judgment is employed, with little clear demonstration of the validity of results.
5. In mass screening, relatively little regard is paid to a baby's readiness for testing; in contrast, some of the procedures reported here, wherein neonatal testing is done as a careful audiological appraisal, have particularly emphasized the need for careful timing.
6. Follow-up has been inadequate.
7. There is little to do for or about the newborn—*at the time*—who is found not to respond in the test situation.
8. There is some fairly widespread agreement that, for developmental reasons, testing is better done at 6–9 months of age, with no deleterious results that can be demonstrated from this much delay.

One can now report, however, that most of these objections are better recognized and understood by some of those most dedicated to mass screening of newborns than was true 10 years ago. This is a healthy state of affairs.

VII. INFANT TESTING

It is difficult to be certain about what is meant by the term "infant testing." Obviously, in the present context, it does not include newborns. In terms of later developmental status, it probably does not include children who, without interfering problems like deafness or general retardation, can hold at least a rudimentary conversation with the use of two- to three-word phrases or sentences. In practical terms—both developmental and audiological—the infantile period apparently ranges from 4 months to approximately 20 months. This does not mean that infants should not be studied throughout their development; it means only that this is a critical period, particularly for language development and for the dynamics of behavior in general. With the usual admonition about "everything else being equal," this is the major period for the development of "readiness to listen" and "readiness to talk" (Whetnall and Fry, 1965).

A. Some Landmarks and Definitions

In general, there is clear evidence that most children respond with repeatable and quite consistent orienting responses to many kinds of acoustic stimuli by 3 to 4 months of age. Exceptions are very deaf children, those with severe general retardation, and those with motor problems that obviate their capacity to respond. There are many well-documented studies which demonstrate the validity of these generalizations and others which follow (Bordley and Hardy, 1951a,b,c; Eisenberg, 1970a; Eisenberg et al., 1964; Ewing and Ewing, 1944; Friedlander, 1970; Frisina, 1963; Hardy and Hardy, 1963; Hodgson, 1972; Hoverstein and Moncur, 1969; Liden and Kankkunen, 1969; Lillywhite et al., 1970; Lowell et al., 1956; Mounier–Kuhn et al., 1972; Sheridan, 1969).

By 6 to 9 months, there is clear orienting with distraction techniques; this includes identification and differentiation among many kinds of signals, including the complex patterns of voice. Several careful experimenters have found that by 8 months of age the infant with essentially normal hearing probably responds best to a quiet voice. All the procedures suggested many years ago by the Ewings are workable in the age range of approximately 6 to 15 months. By 10+ months of age, the conditioned orienting reflex or response (COR) is useful (Suzuki and Ogiba, 1961). APRs are available throughout the period of infancy.

A bit later in development (M.A. 30–36 months), good and reliable testing can be done with play audiometry and the peepshow (q.v., following). Obviously, from the neonatal period on in development, various special kinds of instrumental testing are employed—most importantly, evoked cortical response audiometry (see Chapter 11) and electrodermal audiometry (see Chapter 8). Several suggestions for other instruments and special adaptations of procedures have recently been made (Eisenberg, 1971). The upshot is that there are various kinds of tests available for the range of infant development (4–20 months), not the least important of which are reflex and conditioned in mode. Much further systematic study is required to refine useful distinctions between normal and aberrant development.

B. Particular Proceedings and Findings

Every working clinic where large numbers of infants and young children are seen routinely for differential evaluation is apt to employ a variety of procedures. Each undertaking may develop much as a kind of detective story. The first chapter is ordinarily concerned with the details of general and specific development, details of communicative behavior in the home and of general health (because etiology can be extremely important in developing a frame of reference), psychosocial descriptions of the family and of the baby, and observation of the child at play. Thereafter, systematic observations—measurements when possible —are made both in ordinary circumstances and in a controlled sound field. Ultimately, it may be considered necessary to use the full test battery, including highly specialized instrumentation (see Chapters 8, 9, 10, and 11). Rarely can all this be done without repeat visits. Perhaps it is necessary to emphasize that this is a step-by-step procedure; the nature and number of the steps depends on the nature of the problem and the dynamics of the family's situation. It follows that early steps usually involve reflex or conditioned responses to acoustic stimuli: these are clinical examinations. It is never enough to ask, "Does the infant hear or not?" The questions to be answered are much more involved: "To what sounds does he respond?" "To what does he not respond?" "What are the details of the acoustic signals?—Intensity? Frequency range? Simple? Complex?" "How many responses occur relative to numbers of trials?" "Is audition meaningful?" "What about attention? adaptation? consistency of responses? fatigue?" "Reinforcement used? What kind? How often?" There are others, but these can generate a useful set of facts about the performance of an infant in the 4–20-month age range.

C. The Ewing Procedure

Various aspects of these parameters were incorporated in the pioneering work of the Ewings, reported in 1944 and extended in 1947 and 1954. They especially emphasized the importance of the human voice, in their reporting of a series of developmental studies. Much attention was paid to "the human voice as the most outstanding and persistent factor in the normal child's aural environment." They noted some capacity in the infant to discriminate voices within a few weeks after birth. "No other forms of sound demand from him such efforts of attention, such intricate analysis and synthesis, so much remembering [1944]." Within 6 to 11 months, they noted sharp turning to localize the sound. Within this same period, "reflexes give way to learned responses," with obviously developing skill in differentiating complex sounds. Without question, in their minds, voice is the most meaningful input for attention from the infant. Later, through the second year, the marked influence of personality on responses to sound is shown in details about alertness, motor responses in general, walking in particular, imitation (as with building blocks), and emotional attitudes. These are clearly learned responses that relate hearing with the learning of language.

The general procedures employed by the Ewings were adopted with some modifications for use in the so-called Collaborative Cerebral Palsy Project of The National Institute of Neurological Diseases and Stroke (later known as the Perinatal Study). A total of 438 babies were tested; 327 of these were 3 to 52 weeks of age; an additional 111 infants 10 to 29 weeks of age were tested in a follow-up clinic for the project. Various noisemakers, toy sounds, and high-frequency consonants were employed. These stimuli were calibrated within a fairly broad tolerance as to frequency and intensity. Most stimuli were used with an output of 40 dB; one at 50 dB and one at 60 dB. The test circumstances have been described in considerable detail (Hardy, J. B., et al., 1959). Twelve stimuli were employed: responses that were looked for included head turn, APR, Moro, and various others. Of the 130 who ranged from 3 to 14 weeks, "no responses" ranged from 6% (clacker), 16% (voice), to 41% (tissue paper). Of the 218 who were 15 to 30 weeks, "no responses" ranged from .5% (squeaker), 3% (voice), to 27% (low rattle). All other "no responses" were within these ranges.

Of the 438 infants (3 to 52 weeks of age), there were 29 failures (no head turn, no body turn, no APR). Somewhat more than one-half of the failures were passed on a second or third test. A few generalizations may be made from the data: (1) The infant who fails to turn his head at 8 months may have a hearing impairment, or he may be developmentally immature; (2) in the age range of 3 to 30 weeks, the test "appears to be a useful diagnostic and research tool but because of the complexity of the responses obtained probably is not applicable as a screening device on a general pediatric and public health level." (3) With the Ewing test, of 90 infants 30 to 52 weeks of age, four failed the initial test—this is a "simple screening device which can be carried out in a clinic setting by nurses with a modicum of special training." It will be recalled that the procedures involved determining whether or not the child can hear a relatively normal range of quite ordinary sounds, and also whether his development makes suitable responses possible, or, rather, serves as a source of interference.

D.   Conditioned Orienting Reflex (COR) and Related Procedures

In 1961, Suzuki and Sato published a report of a procedure which amounts to a modification of so-called "startle-response audiometry." This involved the use of animal sounds. Expected responses by infants of 3+ months included the APR and head turning. Resulting judgments were fairly elementary: The baby can or cannot hear. The level of intensity was apparently high; responses were apparently judged only to indicate deafness.

Later in the same year, Suzuki and Ogiba (1961) reported a rather more sophisticated test, designed for children under 3 years of age (actually 1 to 3 years, for little success was achieved with infants under 12 months of age). It is called a *conditioned orienting reflex* (COR). "When a strange visual stimulus is presented to a child, the child always looks toward the source of the stimulus. . . . If the reflex can be conditioned with a pure tone, the child will respond as soon as the tone is heard [that is, having heard the tone, he looks for the light]." The writers are insistent that this "is not a learned response but a reflex movement which is inherent is an infant a priori." There is a considerable question about the validity of this point of view, for there are several other possibilities, i.e., the obvious point that the relationship between tone and light does in fact involve learning; and association is set up between tone and light.

In this study, two loudspeakers were employed, one on either side of the subject, within an easy angle of vision. Illumination with dolls served as an unconditioned stimulus (UCS) and reward. Tone (conditioned stimulus) was presented 30–40 dB above "estimated threshold"; tone (1 sec), then doll; tone and light combined take 4 sec. "This procedure, that is, conditioning, being repeated three or four times, the child comes to turn its face toward the direction of the tone before the visual stimulation is given." The tone at ±40 dB was used for reinforcement. In summary, at the outset, the lighted doll was presented, then the tone (attention); this was repeated three or four times; then the tone was given first, and the head should turn in anticipation of the light (conditioning).

In practice, as various professional observers have witnessed, the general idea of COR is useful, but not in the way the report describes and not for the reasons adduced in the report. First, there must be grave doubt that turning to the light is either innate or reflexive. If the light is off to one side, or if the child is dull or stuporous, he will probably not respond. Under any circumstances, it is extremely doubtful that three or four repetitions of UCS–CS has much to do with conditioning. It seems clear that some aspect of learning is involved, and that the connection between sound and light is an association, duly reinforced. Short of complete adaptation, a reflex should not require this much reinforcement (maintained at 100%). In a situation of conditioning, moreover, the CS should be accompanied by the UCS, or should precede it by an interval of probably no more than 500 msec. These differences may be only semantic. On the other hand, it seems quite certain that the infant makes good use of learning after reaching a developmental age of 7 to 8 months, particularly in many of his responses to acoustic stimuli.

Suzuki and Ogiba (1961) added a very useful item with regard to norms for infants relative to responses to pure tones (cf., Hoverstein and Moncur, 1969). Within their reported range of subjects (1 to 3 years), they found only one hard-of-hearing child, who possibly had a sensorineural impairment. For the others, they derived the impressions recorded in Table I about "threshold" responses relative to adult "thresholds." These were averages within the speech-hearing range.

TABLE I

Age in months	Level above adults
Under 12	30+ dB
12–18	20+ dB
18–24	20 dB
24–30	15 dB
30–36	10–15 dB

A relatable procedure has been reported with the title, "visual reinforcement audiometry" (VRA) (Liden and Kankkunen, 1969). Slides with pictures are employed as the UCS. The general scheme is simpler than COR, mainly in that various responses are accepted. A response of "reflexive behavior" is seen, then "investigatory behavior," then "orientation," and finally, "spontaneous responses." No mention is made of reinforcement. This is clearly meant to express learned behavior as a major aspect of the response situation. In recent years, some version of these tests has been utilized commonly in clinical practice, ordinarily with good results.

E. Other Studies

In 1969, Hoverstein and Moncur reported the findings from their study of various stimuli and intensity factors in testing infants. The object was to provide normative data from observations of two groups of subjects: there were 21 3-month-old and 22 8-month-old infants. None was "at risk"; all were developmentally normal. Test conditions, modes and procedures for presentation of stimuli, and response criteria were developed from a pilot study of 75 infants.

Five signals were used (white noise, interrupted 500-Hz and 4000-Hz pure tones, voice, and music); each was presented twice at each of four hearing levels. For the 3-month-old group, hearing levels of 30, 45, 60, and 75 dB were used; for the 8-month-old group, the levels were 15, 30, 45, and 60 dB; each level was calibrated with adult thresholds for each type of signal. Responses were determined by the agreement of two judges that there had been behavioral change from random activity after each presentation; each observer was required to record the same behavioral change, which was then defined as a response. In order to consider chance responses, two periods of silence (3 sec) were included at each intensity level. These were considered control periods, and any behavioral changes were recorded.

Behavioral state and changes were interesting. In general, those in the 3-month-old group were calm and awake; the 8-month-olds needed diversion. Stimulus was usually not presented during undue movement, or restlessness and vocalization. Most of the responses to test stimuli included widening or moving the eyes (APR) or a decrease or cessation of activity on the part of the younger group. The older babies responded by looking at the observer, by change in activity, or by localization. (This general pattern of responses was recorded by Britt, 1963.) The study is notable for the special care taken in reporting response differences relative to type of stimulus, variations among responses, and behavioral changes.

> As expected, percentage of response increased with increased intensity [p. 692]. . . . The three-way analyses of variance confirmed age as a highly significant variable, but a relatively less important source of variation than intensity and stimulus. . . . [Study of the data reveals] voice to be the superior stimulus (that is, securing the largest percentage of response) for both groups at each hearing level (with the exception of the 75 dB HL) [p. 696].

Findings indicated that "type of stimulus is not as important as intensity when stimulus is presented at the highest hearing level [p. 697]." This is not true for lower levels of presentation; these involve some variations. The thresholds for voice are quite comparable with those established by other investigations (Britt, 1963; Ewing and Ewing, 1944; Hardy, J. B., et al., 1959, 1970; Suzuki and Ogiba, 1961). The findings were well-tabulated.

The investigators specify the need for otologic clearance prior to examination and for the use of taped material, especially for voice. It is clear that infants "do not respond at adult threshold intensity levels," and that they do "respond differentially to stimuli and this response is affected by age, intensity, and type of stimulus." The use of any standard of measurement must pay respect to age level of the subjects and intensity of stimuli, and the standard "must be established for each type of stimulus." Few would disagree with the interpretation of the data from this study.

A related investigation was reported on the test findings regarding 45 infants in an age range from 7 to 36 months (Thompson and Thompson, 1972). All were considered normal, and were drawn from a well-baby clinic. Group 1 (N = 15) were 7 to 12 months old; Group 2 (N = 30) were 22 to 36 months old. Each of five live stimuli was presented for 2 sec: (1) white noise, (2) speech, (3) high-pass filtered noise, (4) high-pass filtered voice, and (5) 3000-Hz pure tone. Group 1 was tested at four levels of intensity, always in ascending order of 15-, 30-, 45-, 60-dB SPL. Response criteria were localization (head turned to source of sound) or awareness (eyes turned in direction of sound or up to observer). The greatest number of responses was elicited by speech. Group 2 was tested by COR or by play audiometry; speech also produced the greater number of responses. Play audiometry was considered better than the COR procedure.

An attempt has been made to demonstrate typical sets of stimuli employed in various investigations. It seems clear that the use of voice is indicated, as several researchers have suggested; this might reasonably be anticipated a priori. At least with the younger subjects, however, music, as well, is an extremely useful stimulus (DiCarlo and Bradley, 1961). A recent study having to do with a "statistical abstract of an investigation of hearing of infants" included the use of musical instruments or musically related sounds in a battery of stimuli (Mounier–Kuhn et al., 1972).

This was an extensive study involving three principal groups: 183 premature babies (length of term not reported); 400+ newborns in an age range of 1 to 8 days; and 1644 infants ranging in age from 15 days to two years. The newborns and young infants were all considered normal. Various signals were employed (musical instruments, voice, "noises," and two "low-frequency generators"). Electronic calibration was not undertaken; instead, stimuli were described as "loud" or "soft" in terms of their various qualities. The investigators stressed the need for at least four positive responses to the different sounds, and emphasized that the tester (attitude, consistency, and so forth) and the environment were important. A variety of statistical observations were made, despite the somewhat casual treatment of the psychophysical measurements. Small bells (high and low) and castanets were found useful and produced fairly consistent responses, but the best results in terms of reliability were obtained with the use of voice with those infants approximately 250 days old.

F. The Peepshow Test

Since its introduction by Dix and Hallpike in 1947, there have been several variations of the original mechanics of the peepshow, but all are based on a common principle: The child is rewarded when he hears, and he is not rewarded when he does not hear (respond) or when he makes a false response (no signal). In 1947, as now, there are several practical problems in deriving a good pure-tone audiogram with preschool-age children (3 to 6 years). A later paper (1952) by the same authors presented some refinements of procedure and mechanics. The principles have been outlined by Dix:

> It is designed to avoid the two great difficulties which make conventional pure-tone audiometry impossible with young deaf children. In the first place, otherwise meaningless pure tones are given an arresting significance. In the second place, the need for any explanation of the nature of listening and hearing is completely avoided. The test procedure depends upon the conditioned response of the child to a series of short pure-tone stimuli delivered from a loudspeaker. The pure-tone stimuli are synchronized with the flashes of a signal lamp [Dix, 1965, p. 80].

For the test, the child sits with an attendant. In front of him is a viewing box containing pictures. He must press a button in order to see the pictures. The mechanism works only when the light and sound stimuli are delivered. Pure-tone input is calibrated in terms of normal hearing level. With the child's attention centered on the picture-to-be, the signals are presented and the attendant activates the light. After a few repetitions, the child is encouraged to press the button for the picture as soon as the tone–light combination has been delivered. As soon as he has accomplished this to the tester's satisfaction, and the response is established (this is a learned response, not a simple reflex), the attendant removes the stimulus of the signal light, the tone is followed by the picture when the button is pressed, and "the show is on the road." Intensity and frequency are adjusted until a full "threshold audiogram" has been achieved to the tester's satisfaction.

This procedure has been successfully employed at its place of origin (Queen Square Hospital, London) and throughout the world for many years. It is useful for most "otherwise normal" children down to approximately 30 months of age. The originators persistently emphasize the need to prepare the child well and to work with him warmly and closely. In discussing various comments on their work, they emphasize the point that the peepshow can work as a single-shot procedure, under circumstances where the child cannot be called back for successive examinations.

There have been many users of this procedure, and most of them report success when the circumstances are reasonably good. Some generalizations were made at the Toronto conference of 1964:

> We believe that any hard of hearing child who is actually normal in other respects should be able to perform this test satisfactorily between the ages of two and three. After he becomes accustomed to it using the loudspeaker, we then use earphones to determine audiograms for the two ears individually and we can use bone conduction vibrators as well. In the acoustic field we can compare the improvement of pure-tone thresholds that is obtained by use of a hearing aid [Statten, 1965, p. 83].

G. Play Audiometry

In a way, the peepshow might be considered a form of play audiometry; indeed, this is true of the COR procedures. Learning is involved in all of these. It is interesting that something called an "objective" test is thought to be "better" somehow than other kinds of tests. As yet, there seems to be no clearly "objective" audiometry, for the obvious reason that there is always a tester who must utilize some form of judgment (this must be true, as well, of autoaudiometry). In keeping with this compulsion to seek objectivity is the persistent reliance on the attitude that a reflexive response is somehow "better" than a learned response; in physiological terms, the more refined the test, the closer become reflexive and learned behavior. This is a matter of use and the development of meaning.

There are various historical connections relating to peepshow and play procedures. An early modification of the peepshow suggested the use of a jack-in-the-box instead of pictures (Guilford and Haug, 1952). Years before this, a cogent suggestion had been made by the Ewings. Believing that routine pure-tone audiometry could not be done with very young children, they advocated "toy tests," which involved training the child at play to respond to sound. The child could make a toy jump, when given a hand signal. Later in the session, this signal is replaced by a sound. Then the child learns to respond only to what is heard. The signals are used in an open room; most of the signals are spoken sounds or words. Obviously, the child must be attentive and cooperative (Ewing and Ewing, 1938). Some years later, this idea was modified: after the child has learned to respond to calibrated toy sounds, a pure-tone audiometer is used. As the test proceeds, the child builds with blocks; this, too, requires concentration and cooperation (Utley, 1949). This general approach was adapted and modified by several others, some of whose suggestions preceded Utley's description (Bloomer, 1942; Keaster, 1947; Macfarlane, 1941).

In the words of one who wrote an early generalized analysis of pure-tone audiometry for preschool children: "Play-audiometry, in the stricter sense, consists in principle of a combination of the toy test and pure tone audiometry [Barr, 1955, p. 20]." The principle is stated succinctly. It is necessary that "audiometry for young children . . . be planned so that it will have a meaning for the child and so that the child learns to understand that meaning and to show that he has understood it." In short, he must respond to the test tone "with a conscious activity."

A good one-to-one relationship must be established between examiner and child. The former must be interested and confident in his management. Varied procedure is necessary, with the use of a broad mix of toys. "This demands both imagination and an abundance of understanding." The use of headphones is preferable, although a loudspeaker can be used if the child objects to the headphones. A preliminary estimate of a level of responsiveness is made. Toys may include any array of blocks and marbles: Blocks can be piled or dropped in a box, marbles can be dropped or placed in holes. Pegboards are useful: Toys can be moved; animals can be put into a barnyard, or furniture into a dollhouse. The possibilities are multiple, with due attention paid to the child's tastes and with due regard for fatigue.

The test is time-consuming. In Barr's experience, about one-third of the attempts were unsuccessful, many involving younger children. A bone oscillator may be used. It should go almost without saying that a carefully taken history and a careful appraisal of a child's behavior should precede the test. It is a readier procedure with older children (3+ years): it rarely works with those under 30 months. Children with impairment (mild to severe) require much more time and care than would those with essentially normal hearing. "Threshold determinations," in both initial and follow-up examinations of children who clearly responded to sound, were in close agreement (Barr, 1965, p. 61).

For those who did not initially respond, age was clearly an important factor. The test is possible with most children in the 4–6-year age range. The younger the child, the less possibility there is of successful testing (no better than 50% in the 30–36-month range). Most of these audiograms show a down-dropping curve (ostensibly sensorineural) with few high-frequency responses. Bone-conduction responses seem, for the most part, vibratory. These observations have been made commonly. For children with general retardation (developmental quotient below 70), audiometry with those who responded to sound could not be done under the age of 4 years in Barr's series; it was successful about two-thirds of the time in the 4–6-year range; there was no success better than preliminary estimates for those who did not readily respond to loud sound.

Special attention has been paid to Barr's techniques and findings, largely because they are not often referred to in detail. The fundamental ideas have been tested many times, and the basic findings remain entirely valid.

Similar procedures were carried out by Lowell and associates, reported in 1956. The children were "conditioned" with a drumbeat, then play audiometry using varieties of toys was undertaken for pure-tone measurements. These children were 3½ years old. Successful testing was achieved in half an hour with normals, but deaf children took "much longer." Attention, sustained interest, and good motivation are required of the child; experience and patience, of the tester. A retest at almost 7 years of age was in good agreement with the original findings.

It seems clear that all these techniques involve one or another aspect of what is now known as "operant conditioning"; this generally involves modification of behavior. In 1966, Lloyd addressed the point of behavioral audiometry "based on the general principle of reinforcement." He outlined behavioral procedures, with stress on the use of stimulus control. This is largely a matter of appropriate reinforcement with detailed attention to timing and reinforcement shifts. He observed: "Many of the rather vague clinical qualities considered under the term 'rapport' may also be analyzed in terms of operant principles."

Two years later, 1968, Lloyd and associates presented some interesting observations in "an operant audiometric procedure for difficult-to-test patients." This involved operant conditioning with orienting responses, now familiarly called "TROCA," tangible reinforcement operant conditioning audiometry. A loudspeaker may be used, or headphones, or a bone-conduction oscillator. Stimuli include a 5% warble, and reinforcement is given with a Davis feeder (Davis Universal Feeder, Davis Scientific Instruments, North Hollywood, California) or with pictures. This involved from four to 50 sessions of 10–20 min each. Of the 50 children studied, 42 could be tested. Such a procedure is time-consuming, of course, but it is probably true that most of these children could not be tested at all by usual behavioral techniques.

Finally, there is the version of play audiometry that involves hearing for speech. This might be thought of as "show me the . . ." or "where is the . . ." version of audiometry. This is often called "identification audiometry," wherein the object of the identification is the hearing level for speech. The procedure is simple: The child sits on its mother's lap, facing a loudspeaker at a measured distance; the mother holds a tray that contains 10 or 12 objects (airplane, flower, car, bell, shoes, animals, and so forth) that the child may be expected to know by name; the "show me" game continues as the child responds, with more and more attentuation of the signal. When he stops responding, other things being equal, one may know that a given intensity does not elicit a response, whereas the child has just responded to speech that was louder (say 5 dB above the level of no-response). This cannot be defined as a "threshold"; it can only be said that a given value of input was sufficient for a response. This procedure has been carried out successfully and well with children 20+ months of age who meet ordinary developmental norms and who have no more than a mild–moderate amount of hearing impairment. With a reasonably outgoing child, this kind of testing is easier to use than its counterpart with pure-tone measurements. With a cooperative child, once the test in a sound field is accomplished, headphones may be used, with ear-for-ear differentiation. With a child somewhat older, this can be done with one ear masked. The test does not always work: The child must be cooperative, he must be rewarded with enthusiastic approval, and he must have some useful understanding of speech. All this involves intellectual, and some considerable amount of social, maturity. The procedure cannot always be carried out in one session.

VIII. COMMENTS

Clearly, there is a wide variety of attitudes, beliefs, convictions, opinions, and procedures having to do with one form or another of testing the auditory responses of the infant and very young child. Mention has been made of the point that standard, more or less routine, audiometry is not always dependable, even with children of kindergarten age. More to the point, perhaps, is that "school age" is dropping back to age 2 in many school systems; it has already reached this developmental level in programs of day care. The need for early testing is obviously important, for the capacity for hearing is fundamental to learning and psychosocial development, as is a lack of this capacity an important aspect of learning disability and social retardation.

At the beginning of this chapter, mention was made of a "burgeoning of concern" that is current about all these matters. Perhaps emphasis might be given by attention to some generalizations that were written early in 1950:

> Fundamental to all work with hearing impairment is the ability to make an accurate appraisal of auditory function. The need for accurate measurement of the hearing of infants and young children is obvious, and within the past relatively few years a great deal of attention has been paid to this problem. From this experience, a few basic principles have been demonstrated: (1) that hearing tests should be conducted with auditory stimuli of known values of both frequency and intensity; (2) that a better approach to threshold-measurement is achieved when the test-signals are reasonably meaningful to the child. To these might well be added an idea which is perhaps not so well understood; (3) inasmuch as most children with impaired hearing are not totally deaf, the object of clinical measurement is not to determine whether a child hears something, but to determine his threshold of acuity for certain specified ranges and intensities of sound, discrete or complex. If the young child has some speech, and can be tested by speech audiometry, it is important to determine his speech-hearing function at suprathreshold levels. In short, if measurement is done adequately to satisfy both medical and non-medical requirements for diagnosis, treatment and rehabilitation or education, it involves much more than a black-and-white distinction between hearing and not-hearing [Hardy and Bordley, 1951a, p. 346].

Apparently, various efforts and attitudes are destined for continuity. One would hope, however, for more current attention to hearing and somewhat less to not-hearing, in terms both of procedures and of interpretations. The present reconsiderations of ways, means, and objectives for the screening of infants seem salutary, reflecting as they do relatively more developmental logic and less social enthusiasm. There is no particular reason why the screening of infants, about whom the facts of development give warrant for screening, cannot be carried out with scientific care and, within margins, with accuracy. The "margins" have largely to do with the apparent needs of the child (baby) in terms of prenatal, perinatal, and postnatal history. There seems little warrant for the mass screening of newborns, the vast majority of whom prove to be quite normal in most developmental aspects. As has recently been made quite clear, there are many ways to select from the mass the subgroup of importance, including the babies for whom there is some predilection for trouble with hearing at either or both peripheral and central levels. Here one is searching not only for "the deaf" but for all those whose responses to acoustic stimuli deviate significantly from the norms.

One of the deterrents—which simply must be overcome—is the basic lack of detailed information about what to expect week-by-week as babies develop from birth. Their capacity to demonstrate auditory differentiation—albeit limited, of course—has been clearly shown, not by mass testing but by careful, multiple physiological and behavioral measurements. Such careful observations need to be carried on throughout all developmental stages. It is often assumed that all early responses are reflexive, but there must be grave doubt about how long this continues to be true, in developmental terms. Almost countless observations have been made in the range from birth to, say, 6 to 7 months. Somewhere through these weeks and months, there comes a shift from reflexive to learned responses. This is, no doubt, closely related to increased attention span and shortened reaction time (Hardy and Bordley, 1951b). Equally without doubt, there are close relations among cooing, babbling, and the patterns of intonation and stress in prespeech jargon (whether this means self- or social expression is not readily determinable). There is considerable evidence, moreover, that many responses often described as "conditional reflexes" do indeed reflect nonverbal learning and "thinking"; perhaps the best evidence is negative—babies who cannot learn well do not respond well to sound. Indeed, many can scarcely perform at 3 years of age what the normally developing infant achieves by 6 to 7 months.

For even the young child (20 to 40 months), it is worthwhile to establish, as this is possible, a comparative relationship between pure-tone and speech-hearing responses. Learning capacity and learning disability are aspects of behavior that are deeply associated with communicative accomplishment. Indeed, much of our means to apprehend learning disability resides in observations of "the communicative act," man's most human function. The fact of the meaningfulness of the acoustic stimulus has long been stressed. The meaning of pure tones is only inferential, and derives from the subject's willingness to try to respond, or to continue to respond. Hearing for speech when an understandable word is repeated is self-evident. "Threshold" is another matter—for either set of signals— and is largely a function of various aspects of maturity.

Unfortunately, it is plainly impossible to acknowledge the work and concern of all the experimenters and clinicians who have been associated with these problems. It is perhaps of parenthetical interest that only a few of the various studies reported in this fairly extensive review considered an otologic examination of sufficient importance to insist on the need for it. This is a remarkable oversight. All have contributed to a better understanding of the values and goals of long and arduous attempts to understand the developing infant and young child. Much remains to be done; hopefully, this will be accomplished.

It seems apparent that neither reflexive nor conditioned responses are fully reliable for all purposes and needs—medical, educational, habilitative, or rehabilitative—in working with infants and very young children. To these ends, and as part of a battery of appraisals, various special instrumental procedures are now available. These should be used to whatever extent is reasonable and necessary, so long as behavior relative to acoustic stimuli and responses is unresolved.

REFERENCES

Asterisks (*) indicate supplementary references which are not cited in the text.

Altman, M. M., and Shenhau, R. (1971). *J. Laryngol. Otol.* **85**, 35.
* Anderson, C. V. (1972). *In* "Handbook of Clinical Audiology" (J. Katz, ed.), pp. 520–539. Williams and Wilkins, Baltimore, Maryland.
Barr, B. (1955). *Acta Oto-Laryngol. Suppl.* **121**, 1.
Barr, B. (1965). *In* "The Young Deaf Child: Identification and Management" (H. Davis, ed.). *Acta Oto-Laryngol. Suppl.* **206**, 45.
Bloomer, H. (1942). *J. Speech Hear. Disord.* **7**, 311.
Bordley, J. E., and Hardy, W. G. (1951a). *Acta Oto-Laryngol.* **40**, 72.
Bordley, J. E., and Hardy, W. G. (1951b). *Acta Oto-Laryngol. Spec. Suppl.* **40**, 346.
Bordley, J. E., and Hardy, W. G. (1951c). *Pub. Health Rep.* **66**, 17.
* Bordley, J. E., and Hardy, W. G. and Hardy, M. P. (1962). *Pediatr. Clin. North Amer.* **9**, 1147.
Britt, E. (1963). Development of Hearing and Language in Infancy. Doctoral dissertation, Johns Hopkins Univ., Baltimore, Maryland.
* Callas, J. C., and Callas, E. R. (1970). *Pediatrics* **46**, 938.
* Chun, R., Pawsat, R., and Forster, F. (1960). *J. Nerv. Ment. Dis.* **30**, 472.
Conf. Newborn Hear. Screening: Proc., Summary, Recommendations (1971). Sponsored by Maternal and Child Health Serv., Dept. of Health, Education, and Welfare and Bur. of Maternal and Child Health, California State Dept. of Public Health, Berkeley, California.
Crowell, D. H., Jones, R. H., Nakagawa, J. K., and Kapuriai, L. E. (1971). *Proc. Roy. Soc. Med.* **64**, 472.
* Darley, F. (ed.) (1961). *J. Speech Hear. Disord. Monogr. Suppl.* **9**.
Davis, H. (ed.) (1965). The Young Deaf Child: Identification and Management. *Acta Oto-Laryngol. Suppl.* **206**.
* Denmark, F. G. W. (1950). *J. Laryngol. Otol.* **64**, 357.
Derbyshire, A. J. (1971). In *Conf. Newborn Hear. Screening*, pp. 102–111. Bur. of

Maternal and Child Health, California State Dept. of Pub. Health, Berkeley, California.

* Derbyshire, A. J., and Marcus, R. (1966). *J. Amer. Med. Ass.*, **252**, 473.

DiCarlo, L. M., and Bradley, W. H. (1961). *Laryngoscope* **71**, 628.

Dix, M. R. (1965). The Young Deaf Child: Identification and Management. *Acta Oto-Laryngol. Suppl.* **206**, 79–82.

Dix, M. R., and Hallpike, C. S. (1947). *Brit. Med. J.* **2**, 719.

Dix, M. R., and Hallpike, C. S. (1952). *Brit. Med. J.* **1**, 235.

* Downs, M. P. (1962). *Int. Audiol.* **1**, 268.

Downs, M. P. (1970). *Trans. Amer. Acad. Ophthalmol. Otolaryngol.* **74**, 1208.

Downs, M. P. (1971a). In *Conf. Newborn Hear. Screening*, pp. 112–118. Bur. of Maternal and Child Health, California State Dept. of Pub. Health, Berkeley, California.

* Downs, M. P. (1971b). *Otolaryngol. Clin. North Amer.* **4**, 347.

* Downs, M. P., and Silver, H. K. (1972). *Clin. Pediatr.* **11**, 563.

Downs, M. P., and Sterritt, G. (1964). *J. Aud. Res.* **4**, 69.

Eisenberg, R. B. (1970a). *J. Speech Hear. Res.* **13**, 453.

Eisenberg, R. B. (1970b). *ASHA* **12**, 119.

Eisenberg, R. B. (1971). *J. Aud. Res.* **11**, 148.

Eisenberg, R. B., Griffin, E. J., Coursin, D. B., and Hunter, M. A. (1964). *J. Speech Hear. Res.* **7**, 245.

* Elliott, G. B., and Elliott, K. A. (1964). *Laryngoscope* **74**, 1160.

* Ewertsen, H. W. (1966). *Acta Oto-Laryngol.* **61**, 279.

Ewing, I. R., and Ewing, A. W. G. (1938). "The Handicap of Deafness." Longmans, Green, New York.

Ewing, I. R., and Ewing, A. W. G. (1944). *J. Laryngol. Otol.* **59**, 309.

Ewing, I. R., and Ewing, A. W. G. (1947). "Opportunity and the Deaf Child." Univ. London Press, London.

Ewing, I. R., and Ewing, A. W. G. (1954). "Speech and the Deaf Child." Univ. of Manchester Press, Manchester.

* Field, H., Cocack, P., Derbyshire, A. J., Driessen, G. J., and Marcus, R. E. (1967). *J. Aud. Res.* **7**, 271.

* Fisch, L. (1965). *J. Laryngol. Otol.* **79**, 1077.

* Fisch, L. (1967). *Int. Audiol.* **6**, 121.

Friedlander, B. Z. (1970). *Merrill-Palmer Quart.* **16**, 7.

Friedlander, B. Z. (1972a). The Screening and Assessment of Young Children. Presented before the President's Committee on Mental Retardation, Boston, Massachusetts.

* Friedlander, B. Z. (1972b). Receptive Aspects of Early Language Development. Auspices of Nat. Inst. of Child Health and Human Develop. Mimeograph copy.

Frisina, D. R. (1963). *In* "Modern Developments in Audiology" (J. Jerger, ed.), pp. 126–166. Academic Press, New York.

* Froeschels, E., and Beebe, H. (1946). *Arch. Otolaryngol.* **44**, 710.

Gerber, S. E. (1971). In *Conf. Newborn Hear. Screening: Proc., Summary, and Recommendations*, pp. 15–31. Bur. of Maternal and Child Health, California State Dept. of Pub. Health, Berkeley, California. Same as Derbyshire.

Goldstein, R., and Tait, C. (1971). *J. Speech Hear. Disord.* **36**, 3.

* Goodhill, V. (1954). *Arch. Otolaryngol.* **59**, 176.

* Griffing, T. S., Simonton, K. M., and Hedgecock, L. D. (1967). *Trans. Amer. Acad. Ophthalmol. Otolaryngol.* **71**, 105.

Guilford, F. R., and Haug, C. O. (1952). *Arch. Otolaryngol.* **55**, 101.

Hardy, J. B., Doughtery, A., and Hardy, W. G. (1959). *J. Pediatr.* **55**, 382.

Hardy, J. B., Hardy, W. G., and Hardy, M. P. (1970). *Trans. Amer. Acad. Ophthalmol. Otolaryngol.* **74**, 1229.

Hardy, W. G. (1965). In "Audiometry: Principles and Practices" (A. Glorig, ed.), pp. 207–223. Williams and Wilkins, Baltimore, Maryland.

Hardy, W. G., and Bordley, J. E. (1951a). *Acta Oto-Laryngol.* **40**, 346.

Hardy, W. G., and Bordley, J. E. (1951b). *J. Speech Hear. Disord.* **16**, 122.

* Hardy, W. G., and Bordley, J. E. (1969). In "Otolaryngologic Clinics of North America" (L. R. Boies, ed.), pp. 3–26. Saunders, Philadelphia, Pennsylvania.

Hardy, W. G., and Hardy, J. B. (1963). In *Proc. Int. Conf. Oral Educ. Deaf,* pp. 577–581. Alexander Graham Bell Ass. for the Deaf, Washington, D.C.

Hardy, W. G., Pauls, M. D., and Bordley, J. E. (1951). *Acta Oto-Laryngol.* **40**, 80.

Hardy, W. G., Hardy, J. B., Brinker, C. H., Frazier, T. M., and Doughtery, A. (1962). *Ann. Otol. Rhinol. Laryngol.* **71**, 759.

* Haug, O., Baccard, P., and Guilford, F. R. (1967). *Arch. Otolaryngol.* **84**, 435.

Hawke, W. A. (1965). The young deaf child: Identification and management. *Acta Oto-Laryngol. Suppl.* **206**, 75–76, 187, 208, 218.

Hodgson, W. R. (1972). In "Handbook of Clinical Audiology" (J. Katz, ed.), pp. 498–519. Williams and Wilkins, Baltimore, Maryland.

Hoverstein, G., and Moncur, J. P. (1969). *J. Speech Hear. Res.* **12**, 687.

Johansson, B., Wedenberg, E., and Weston, B. (1964). *Acta Oto-Laryngol.* **57**, 188.

Keaster, J. (1947). *J. Speech Hear. Disord.* **12**, 159.

* Letts, A. (1969). *Med. Officer* **122**, 319.

* Leventhal, A. S., and Lipsitt, L. P. (1964). *Child Develop.* **35**, 759.

Liden, G., and Kankkunen, A. (1969). *Arch. Otolaryngol.* **89**, 865.

Lillywhite, H. S., Young, N. B., and Olmstead, R. N. (1970). "Pediatricians Handbook of Communication Disorders." Lea and Febiger, Philadelphia, Pennsylvania.

Ling, D. (1972a). *J. Speech Hear. Res.* **15**, 567.

* Ling, D. (1972b). *Laryngoscope* **82**, 376.

Ling, D., Ling, A., and Doering, D. (1970). *J. Speech Hear. Res.* **13**, 9.

Lloyd, L. (1966). *J. Speech Hear. Disord.* **31**, 128.

Lloyd, L., Spradlin, J., and Reid, M. (1968). *J. Speech Hear. Disord.* **33**, 236.

Lowell, E. L., Rushford, G., Hoverstein, G., and Stoner, M. (1956). *J. Speech Hear. Disord.* **21**, 292.

Macfarlane, D. (1941). *Hear. News* **8**, 9.

* Mendel, M. T. (1968). *J. Speech Hear. Res.* **11**, 811.

* Miller, M. H. (1971). *Clin. Pediatr.* **10**, 340.

Mounier-Kuhn, P., Morgan, D., and Charchon, C. (1972). *Acta Oto-Laryngol.* **73**, 175.

* Murphy, K. P. (1961). *Hear. News* **29**, 9.

* Pauls, M. D., and Hardy, W. G. (1953). *Laryngoscope* **63**, 534.

* Richmond, J. B., Grossman, H. J., and Lustman, S. L. (1953). *Pediatrics* **11**, 634.

* Roberts, C. J. (1968). *Pub. Health* **82**, 173.

* Rudmose, W. (1967). *J. Acoust. Soc. Amer.* **41**, 868.

* Rupp, R. R., and Wolski, W. (1969). *Clin. Pediatr.* **8**, 263.

* Shepherd, D. C., Price, L. L., and Goldstein, R. (1963). *Volta Rev.* **65**, 486.

Sheridan, M. D. (1969). *Proc. Roy. Soc. Med.* **62**, 999.

* Sommer, F. G., and Ling, D. (1970). *J. Aud. Res.* **10**, 292.

Statten, P. (1965). The young deaf child: Identification and management. *Acta Oto-Laryngol. Suppl.* **206**, pp. 82–83.

* Statten, P., and Wishart, D. E. G. (1956). *Ann. Otol. Rhinol. Laryngol.* **65**, 511.

Steinschneider, G., Lipton, E. L., and Richmond, J. B. (1966). *Child. Develop.* **37**, 233.

Suzuki, T., and Ogiba, Y. (1961). *Arch. Otolaryngol.* **74**, 192.

Suzuki, T., and Sato, I. (1961). *Ann. Otol. Rhinol. Laryngol.* **70**, 997.

* Suzuki, T., Tanaka, Y., and Arayama, T. (1966). *Int. Audiol.* **5**, 74.

* Taylor, I. G. (1964). "Neurological Mechanisms of Hearing and Speech in Children." Univ. of Manchester Press; Volta Bur., Washington, D.C.

Thompson, M., and Thompson, G. (1972). *J. Speech Hear. Res.* **15**, 699.

Utley, J. (1949). *Eye Ear Nose Throat Mon.* **28**, 590.

* VanDenHorst, A. P. J. M., and Kyper, P. (1969). *Pract. Otorhinolaryngol.* **31**, 288.

Wedenberg, E. (1956). *Acta Otol-Laryngol.* **46**, 446.

Whetnall, E., and Fry, D. B. (1965). "The Deaf Child." Heinemann, London.

* Whitehurst, M. W. (1961). *Volta Rev.* **63**, 430.

Chapter Seven

Conditioned Galvanic Skin Response Audiometry

Ira M. Ventry[1]

I. INTRODUCTION

A review of recent volumes of the *Journal of Speech and Hearing Research* reveals an interesting but hardly surprising statistic. In the years 1969–1972, a total of 19 articles were published on evoked cortical response audiometry. The total number of articles on galvanic skin response[2] (GSR) audiometry was *zero*. There is little question but that a review of other sources would lead to the conclusion that scant attention is being devoted currently to GSR audiometry, either in the laboratory or in the clinic. This stands in dramatic contrast to present interest in such techniques as impedance audiometry, the aforementioned evoked cortical response audiometry, and some of the other electrophysiologic procedures described in this book. It also stands in dramatic contrast to the interest focused on electrodermal audiometry (EDA) during the 1950s and early 1960s, when there were numerous reports of research on GSR audiometry, as well as reports detailing the clinical value of the test.

I have outlined briefly elsewhere the reasons for the decline in the

[1] Department of Speech Pathology and Audiology, Teachers College, Columbia University, New York, New York.

[2] Goldstein and Derbyshire (1957) notwithstanding, I continue to prefer galvanic skin response (GSR) audiometry to electrodermal audiometry (EDA). To satisfy both camps, GSR and EDA will be used interchangeably in this chapter.

215

popularity of EDA (Ventry, 1970). To reiterate, the disenchantment with EDA can be attributed to great expectations undiluted by a realistic appreciation of the technique's limitations, and the failure, by clinician and researcher alike, to employ adequate methodology in test administration. To put this view in proper perspective, recall the situation in the late 1940s and early 1950s. There were no so-called "objective" tests although the need for such tests was readily apparent. (We recognize quite clearly now that the objectivity of electrophysiologic measures lies almost solely in the nature and recording of the response, and that this "objectivity" is sorely compromised by procedural variables under the less-than-objective control of the tester or experimenter.) There was need, for example, to confirm behavioral thresholds or to obtain threshold data on the difficult-to-test patient—the mentally retarded child, the aphasic adult, the veteran suspected of having a functional hearing loss. The early reports of Michels and Randt (1947), Bordley et al. (1948), and Bordley and Hardy (1949) gave rise to optimism among audiologists that GSR audiometry might be a useful tool for measuring hearing sensitivity, and for the differential diagnosis of hearing disorders in both children and adults. These early reports, emanating primarily from Johns Hopkins, laid the foundation for subsequent research dealing with a variety of test parameters (Doerfler and McClure, 1954; Meritser and Doerfler, 1954; Stewart, 1954a,b) as well as later research conducted at the University of Wisconsin (Aronson et al., 1958; Hind et al., 1958) and by others (Doerfler and Kramer, 1959; Nober, 1958). The clinical use of EDA with adults received strong impetus in the 1950s, when the Veterans Administration (VA) required GSR audiometry for all veterans whose hearing was being evaluated for compensation purposes.

The major problem during this period, however, seemed to be that the research data coming from laboratories throughout the country were not being translated into *standardized clinical* procedures that could be employed by the clinical audiologist. It is not clear whether the responsibility for this lay with the researcher or clinician, but it is clear that many of the clinical reports dealing with GSR audiometry failed to demonstrate an understanding of the methodological prerequisites for obtaining valid and reliable GSR thresholds. As late as 1961, we stated that "it is unfortunate that the term 'GSR Audiometry' has come to connote a specific test that is used in a standardized manner by audiologists . . . . At this time it appears that neither GSR instrumentation . . . nor methodology . . . approach standardization [Chaiklin et al., 1961, p. 278]." Unfortunately, this statement is still true. Compare, for example, Hopkinson's (1973) or O'Neill and Oyer's (1966) description of methodology with the procedures outlined later. Note, too, the many important differences between the procedures described by Engelberg (1970) and those described later. This despite the fact that Engelberg's procedures, as he acknowledges, are based on procedures developed at the VA Hospital in San Francisco by Chaiklin, Ventry, and other staff members. Thus, it appears that a major reason for the disenchantment with EDA lies in the confusion over methodology, the absence of a standardized procedure, and the failure to incorporate into clinical practice the empirical data and laboratory procedures that are necessary to produce valid and reliable measures of hearing sensitivity.

Another reason for the decline in EDA today is probably related to disillusionment over the diagnostic value of the test. In the 1950s, considerable emphasis was placed on the use of EDA for differential diagnosis of *site of lesion*. It was believed, for instance, that GSR results could help differentiate the child with a central auditory problem from the child with a peripheral hearing loss or that the nature of the response itself was of diagnostic value or that failure to condition had diagnostic implications (Goldstein *et al.*, 1954; Hardy and Pauls, 1959). In 1963, Goldstein summarized the diagnostic aspects of EDA:

> (1) The latency and form of EDR do not differ as a function of the auditory disorder; (2) responsivity and conditionability can differ in groups with particular auditory disorders but the differences are not great enough to be diagnostic in an individual patient; and (3) there is no known correlation between central or peripheral pathology and the latency, form, responsivity, or conditionability of EDR [p. 183].

There are no recent data, as far as I know, to contradict Goldstein's view. The fact that EDA provides only a measure of peripheral hearing sensitivity is probably still not well-understood.

Other aspects of EDA have also served to limit its usefulness. The fact that a noxious shock stimulus is employed has raised concern about the use of the test with children. Special and somewhat costly instrumentation is utilized. A major requirement is that the patient, child or adult, sit reasonably quietly for rather long periods of time, a requirement that many young children have difficulty meeting. A certain percentage of patients may fail to meet the conditioning criterion, thus "wasting" valuable clinic time.

Despite these concerns and objections and despite the reduced research and clinical interest in GSR audiometry, it must be emphasized that, assuming a suitable subject and appropriate methodology, EDA is one of the few electrophysiologic procedures currently available to the audiologist to obtain valid and reliable measures of hearing threshold sensitivity (see following). This observation requires careful consideration before conditioned GSR audiometry is prematurely laid to rest by audiologists.

II. SOME PRINCIPLES OF CONDITIONED GSR AUDIOMETRY

A. Introduction

There is a large body of literature dealing with conditioning and learning phenomena, but the discussion here will focus only on those principles that are applicable to audiometry using the conditioned GSR. Grings *et al.* (1959) have correctly pointed out that the audiologist is not interested in learning as such. What the audiologist does care about, they said, "is that he gets a reliable response to tones which he can differentiate adequately from responses to other nonauditory stimuli [p. 382]." To accomplish this end, the audiologist must utilize optimum conditions to produce and sustain the response, must specify the criteria for defining a response, must provide a way for controlling or evaluating spontaneous or random responses, and must specify the criteria for determining threshold (Grings *et al.*, 1959). It is these issues that will be addressed in the remainder of this section.

B. General Features

The general features of conditioned GSR audiometry closely parallel, but are not identical to, classical conditioning techniques.[3] As McGoech and Irion (1952) describe it, conditioning consists of

> (a) an originally neutral stimulus called a *conditioned stimulus,* (b) a stimulus which has the characteristics of evoking one of the natural reflex responses of the learner, termed an *unconditioned stimulus,* (c) the reflex response to this unconditioned stimulus known as an *unconditioned response,* (d) the pairing together in time of the conditioned and unconditioned stimuli, and (e) the eventual occurrence of a response which closely resembles the unconditioned response, but made in response to the conditioned stimulus, known as a conditioned response [p. 64].

In conditioned GSR audiometry, an electric shock serves as the unconditioned stimulus (UCS), a tone or speech signal serves as the conditioned stimulus (CS), and the unconditioned response (UCR) and

---

[3] Instrumental avoidance conditioning has been used to measure auditory thresholds (Hopkinson *et al.*, 1960; Shepherd, 1964) but will not be treated here because the technique appears to be used rarely in clinical practice.

conditioned response (CR) is a change, a lowering in skin resistance (Féré effect), measured in ohms.

Several other terms need a brief explanation. *Reinforcement* can be defined in different ways, but in EDA, reinforcement is defined operationally as the occasional presentation of a CS–UCS event after the patient has been conditioned. Reinforcement is used to maintain responsivity and to reduce the chances of extinction, that is, the disappearance of the CR. Partial reinforcement is more effective in this regard than 100% reinforcement (Grant *et al.*, 1950; Humphreys, 1940; Meritser and Doerfler, 1954). A number of factors influence the rate of extinction, but perhaps the most important, for our purposes here, is the fact that "extinction occurs most rapidly under massed trials [McGoech and Irion, 1952, p. 66]" *i.e.*, when conditioned stimuli are presented with brief time intervals separating them. As will be seen later, massing of trials in EDA must be carefully avoided if strength of conditioning is to be maintained.

Stimulus generalization refers to the fact that

> a conditioned response which has been established so that it may be elicited by a particular conditioned stimulus may also be elicited by other, similar conditioned stimuli. The magnitude of such a generalized conditioned response depends upon the similarity between the conditioned stimulus used in original training and the stimulus used in the test of generalization [McGoech and Irion, 1952, p. 68].

Stimulus generalization includes both frequency and intensity generalization and is important in EDA because it enables the clinician to test at frequencies and intensities other than those used in the conditioning process. For example, assuming a 1000-Hz tone was used as the CS in conditioning, the expectation is that a 2000-Hz CS would also elicit CRs. Similarly, intensity generalization allows the clinician to test at intensities other than that intensity at which conditioning took place. It should be emphasized, however, that tones significantly different in intensity from the tone used in conditioning will elicit fewer CRs (Giolas and Epstein, 1964; Grant and Schneider, 1949). This fact has important methodological implications.

Three other major stimulus parameters need to be described. The first is the *CS–UCS interval*. There have been a number of studies dealing with this variable (Aronson *et al.*, 1958; Kimble, 1947; Tait *et al.*, 1967). In general, the results of these and other studies support the use of a short (*e.g.*, 500 msec) delay between the onset of the CS and the onset of the UCS (Beecroft, 1966). The CS can overlap the UCS or the UCS can follow the termination of the CS. One advantage of the latter procedure is that if the CS–UCS interval is long (*e.g.*, 4 sec), the presence of a CR can be determined during a CS–UCS event, increasing the efficiency of the procedure. As Tait *et al.* (1967) demonstrated, however, the longer interval causes the CR to extinguish more rapidly, thus mitigating against its use in clinical practice.

A variety of *CS and UCS durations* have been used in GSR audiometry. Although UCS duration has little or no effect on conditioning (Beecroft, 1966), generally the UCS durations have been short (200 to 500 msec). The CS durations have been more variable (1 to 5 sec). Aronson *et al.* (1958) found that short tones produced less variable latencies and stronger conditioning. In addition, it makes good sense clinically to use short tones, since relatively brief tones are used in behavioral audiometry and since short tones reduce the chances of adaptation while serving to elicit maximum on-effect.

Finally, a wide range of *interstimulus intervals* have been employed in EDA. The interstimulus interval, in GSR audiometry, refers to the time elapsed between stimulus events, either CS or CS–UCS events. Interstimulus intervals have ranged from 5 to 100 sec, with 30 to 45 sec used most frequently. The important considerations here are (*1*) that interstimulus intervals be varied in order to maintain anxiety and anticipation; (*2*) that the intervals be of sufficient duration to allow for the return of skin resistance to basal levels; and (*3*) that the intervals between events be of sufficient duration to prevent massing of trials. Intervals ranging from 20 to 60 sec meet these requirements. Figure 1 illustrates some of the relationships.

C. Response Characteristics

The adequate definition of a response is at the heart of successful GSR audiometry. In all likelihood, failure to use appropriate criteria for response definition has led to more errors in GSR audiometry than any other single procedural factor. This is surprising in that the definition of an EDR can be more precisely delineated than any other aspect of EDA.

Three major characteristics of the change in skin resistance have been used to define an EDR. In order of importance, they are latency of the response, response magnitude, and the slope of the response. The latency of the EDR is measured from the onset of the CS to the onset of the response. There is ample evidence to indicate that the latency of the EDR, using short tones, ranges from 1.5 to 3.5 sec in most patients (Chaiklin *et al.*, 1961; Goldstein, 1963; Hind *et al.*, 1958). This is the range of latencies that we have used successfully in both clinical and research work with EDA. Latency decreases somewhat as intensity increases; the more noxious the stimulus, the shorter the latency; and there is little intra-

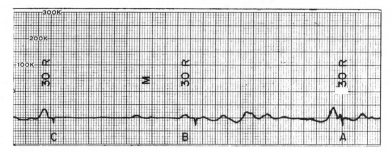

Figure 1   Graphic record depicting several of the stimulus parameters used in EDA. (A) Tone-shock event (CS–UCS) with a 500 msec CS–UCS interval; (B) Tone alone event (CS) producing a minimal (1 mm) change in skin resistance; and (C) CS event producing a response. The interval between events A and B is 58 sec, and the interval between events B and C is 56 sec (paper speed = 1 mm/sec). The clinician has indicated the intensity of the CS (30 dB) and the ear (right) to which the event has been presented. A movement artifact has been labeled "M."

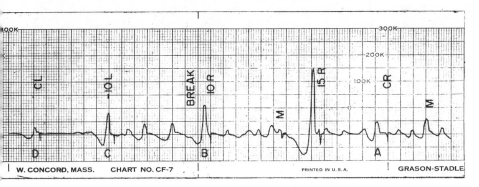

Figure 2   Graphic record depicting different latencies to tonal stimuli (paper speed = 1 mm/sec). (A) A response to a "control" event. The latency is 3 sec. CR is a control (C) presentation during a threshold pass in the right (R) ear. (B) No response to a 10 dB CS event presented to the right ear; latency is too short. (C) Response to a −10-dB CS event presented to the left ear; latency is 2 sec. (D) No response to a "control" event; latency is 1.25 sec. CL means a control presentation during a threshold pass in the left ear.

subject variability in the latency of the response. There are patients, however, who give latencies outside the 1.5–3.5-sec range. If a particular patient produces *consistent* latencies to both CS and CS–UCS events outside the 1.5–3.5-sec range, it may be that his latency is longer or shorter than is typically found. It is unlikely, however, that a patient will have a 2-sec latency to a UCS (or CS–UCS) and a consistent 4-sec latency to CS alone. It is also unlikely that a patient will give a large number of CRs with, say, 2-sec latencies and an occasional "true" response with a

4.5-sec latency. What is likely is some intratest variability in latency, for example, a 2-sec latency to one CS event, a 1.5-sec latency to another CS event, and even perhaps a 2.5-sec latency to still another CS event. It is important to emphasize that *all* of these latencies would meet the latency criterion, while a "response" falling outside of the 1.5–3.5-sec range would not. Figure 2 illustrates some of these points. In event A, the change in skin resistance meets the latency criterion; it has a latency of 3 sec. Thus, despite the fact that this is a control event, a response is recorded. Event B shows a change in skin resistance that, in magnitude and slope, is similar to the response shown in C. This change in skin resistance is a "no response" in that the latency of the change is only 1 sec. Event C is a "response"; there is a 2-sec latency and appropriate magnitude. Event D is a "no response" to a control event; the latency is too short. Although the use of a stringent latency criterion may seem, at first glance, to be overly rigid, the use of such a criterion (*1*) reduces the opportunities for tester bias, (*2*) reduces the number of decisions that the clinician must make during the test, and (*3*) is based on solid clinical and research data. The importance of a strict latency criterion in judging the presence or absence of CRs (or UCRs) cannot be emphasized too strongly.

The second most important response criterion is the magnitude of the change in skin resistance. The magnitude of the response is a function of a number of variables including instrumentation, strength of conditioning, intensity of the CS or UCS, and so forth. With respect to instrumentation, one consideration is the amplification of skin resistance changes. Figure 3 illustrates this point. In the A portion of the record, the sensitivity of the ac amplifier is low, producing a 2-mm change in skin resistance to a CS and minimal background activity. In B, the amplification has been increased, producing a 10-mm change in skin resistance, but also increasing background activity. The signal-to-noise (response-to-background) ratio, however, remains the same. Suffice it to say that amplifier gain is important but is subject to personal preference and to the type of instrumentation employed. My experience has led me to select the low-gain option, minimizing background movement, yet with sufficient amplification to delineate a response if, in fact, a response has occurred. Under these conditions (and with Grason–Stadler Psychogalvanometers), a *1-mm* magnitude criterion has been used successfully in both clinical and research work (Chaiklin *et al.*, 1961; Ventry and Chaiklin, 1965). In clinical practice, we have used a three-category system for judging magnitude: (*1*) 1 mm or greater is a response; (*2*) less than 1 mm but with appropriate latency is a "questionable" response; and (*3*) no change in skin resistance is classified a "no response." The use of the "questionable" category has sometimes assisted in the threshold sampling process

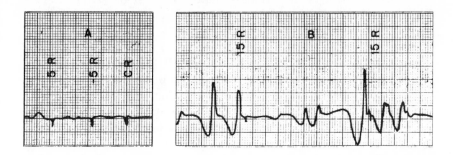

Figure 3   Graphic record illustrating differences in the magnitude of the response as a function of differences in amplification. See text for further details.

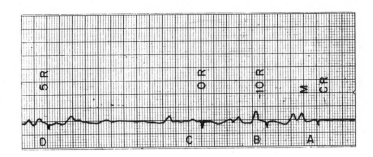

Figure 4   Graphic record showing response interpretation based on the latency and the magnitude of the change in skin resistance (paper speed = 1 mm/sec). (A) Control event presented during threshold pass for the right ear. A "no response" is recorded because latency is too long (5 sec). (B) No response to a —10-dB CS presented to the right ear. Appropriate magnitude (3 mm) but latency is too long (4 sec). (C) A questionable response to a 0-dB CS. Has appropriate latency but magnitude is less than 1 mm. (D) A response to a 5-dB CS; meets both the latency and magnitude criteria.

but has never been used in specifying threshold itself.[4] It is important to note that no matter what the magnitude of change in skin resistance, be it 12 mm or 2 mm, the latency criterion *must* be met first in order to consider the change a response. Figure 4 illustrates some of these points.

---

[4] The clinical procedure could be modified by eliminating the questionable category and by using a 2-mm response criterion rather than a 1-mm criterion. Both of these changes would simplify the decision-making process for the clinician and since the vast majority of responses are greater than 1 mm, the sensitivity of the magnitude criterion would be largely unaffected.

The third, and least important, criterion is the slope of the response. The slope of the response, measured by the angle formed by the intersect of the base line and the leading edge of the response, is usually 45° or more, but depends on instrumentation and chart speed. Figure 1C shows a slope of about 60°, while Figure 3B shows a slope of nearly 90°. Although a slope criterion of 45° or greater has been used in our research, the clinical use of slope as a criterion is much more difficult, in that the judgment of slope during an actual test is not a simple one to make. Thus, the slope criterion assumes lesser importance in the clinical application of EDA.

In summary, GSR audiometry utilizes a modification of classical conditioning techniques whereby tone–shock sequences are used to establish a CR to CS alone. Reinforcement is used following the conditioning sequence to maintain the CR and to prevent extinction. Stimulus generalization allows for the measurement of CRs at tonal intensities and/or frequencies different from the intensity and/or frequency at which conditioning took place. Short tones (1 sec) are used as the CS, brief shocks (.5 sec) are used as the UCS, and the CS–UCS interval is .5 sec. Partial (40%) reinforcement is used throughout, and sufficient time (20 to 60 sec) is allowed between "heard" events to prevent massing of trials. The two major response criteria are a latency of 1.5 to 3.5 sec from the onset of the CS to the onset of the CR, and a magnitude of at least 1 mm (arbitary unit) change in skin resistance. The use of control events, threshold definition, threshold sampling, and other procedural concerns will be described next.

D. Control Events and Threshold Definition

A major confounding variable in EDA is that random or spontaneous changes in skin resistance take the same shape and form as responses to CS events or CS–UCS events. This is illustrated quite clearly in Figure 2, event A. If a random movement happens to occur at the moment a CS event is presented, there is no way of knowing whether the resultant change in skin resistance is a CR or a result of the random movement. The clinician's task, then, is to differentiate random responses from true responses to CS or CS–UCS events. This is done through the use of control events. A control event is merely the simulation of an actual tonal (CS) event; that is, the test conditions are identical to those obtaining when a CS is presented—a stimulus marker marks the graphic record as if a tone has been presented—but no tone is presented. A high rate of responses to control events can invalidate the GSR record simply because the clinician has no way of knowing if the CRs were true responses or random responses.

Although the use of controls can provide a means of specifying the frequency of random responses, two interrelated issues remain unresolved, especially with respect to the clinical application of EDA. The first issue deals with the rate of random responses and the second deals with the relationship between the frequency of random responses to GSR threshold definition. What is an unacceptably high rate of response to control events? Although attention has been devoted to this issue (Goldstein, 1963), I am aware of no definitive answer to the question, at least for the clinical application of EDA. One possible solution is to adopt an arbitrary percentage, e.g., 50%, and if the patient has a 50% or greater response rate to control events, the record is invalidated. The response–no response patterns shown in Table I, which illustrates a relatively

TABLE I
INTERPRETATION OF A GSR RECORD[a]

CS level in dB HL	Threshold pass			
	1	2	3	4
Control	R	N	N	R
0	N			N
5		N	N	
10	N			N
15		N	N	
20	R	R	R	R

[a] See text for explanation. R = response; N = no response.

typical analysis of a GSR record, suggests that this procedure is not altogether adequate. Note that, while the patient gave two responses to four control events, there were no responses at any level below 20–dB HL and a 100% response rate at 20 dB. The GSR threshold would be interpreted quite clearly as 20 dB, but using the abitrary criterion of a 50% response rate to controls would invalidate the record. An arbitrary rate does not seem to be the solution. (A response rate of 50% or greater is not altogether arbitrary, in that threshold definition in behavioral audiometry is frequently, although erroneously, based on a 50% response rate. Thus, if a patient had a 50% response rate to control events, one would conclude that a "threshold" had been obtained for nontonal events).

Another, and perhaps more satisfactory, solution is to relate GSR threshold to the frequency of response to control events. This technique has been used satisfactorily in the past in our study of the reliability of

EDA (Chaiklin *et al.*, 1961). The following technique was employed: If there were no responses to control events ($N = 5$), threshold was the lowest level at which at least two out of four CRs were obtained to the CS; one response to a control required three CRs out of four CS events; two responses to controls required a 100% response rate to the CS; if there were three or more responses to controls, the test was invalidated. The clinical application of this procedure is more complicated, in that the number of control events can vary, as can the number of threshold passes.

Goldstein (1963) has suggested that, if one knows the rate at which a patient is giving random responses, "an acoustic stimulus of a given level should then be judged as threshold or suprathreshold only if it elicits EDRs at a greater-than-chance rate . . . . a clear rationale for what constitutes a greater-than-chance rate in electrodermal audiometry has not been offered [p. 178]." One possible solution is to require at least a 50% *greater* response rate at threshold than to control events, with a minimum of three responses required to CS events, and minimum presentation of four control events. For example, if there were no responses to control events, threshold would be defined as the lowest level at which a 50% or greater response rate was obtained to CS events. If, in another instance, four responses were obtained to nine control events (a 44% rate), threshold would be defined as the lowest level at which a 100% response rate was obtained. If five responses were obtained to nine control events (67%), no threshold could be specified, since the response rate to control events was greater than 50%, thus precluding a threshold response rate that was at least 50% higher than the response rate to control events. I have not employed this specific procedure clinically, but it appears feasible and does represent an attempt to relate random response rate to threshold definition. Regardless of the method employed, it is essential that control events be incorporated routinely in EDA as a means of objectifying the test procedure. Failure to utilize control events represents a serious shortcoming that can lead to invalid and unreliable GSR thresholds.

III. VALIDITY AND RELIABILITY OF GSR AUDIOMETRY

It should be apparent that the validity and reliability of conditioned GSR audiometry is dependent on a number of factors, not the least of which are methodological aspects and population variables, that is, the nature of the patient for whom the test is intended. Be that as it may, it cannot be emphasized too strongly that conditioned pure-tone EDA with adults is a valid and reliable technique, producing results that are in close agreement with behavioral threshold (Burk, 1958; Chaiklin et al., 1961; Doerfler and McClure, 1954; Ventry and Chaiklin, 1965). The problem lies in the use of EDA with a variety of difficult-to-test patients.

In all likelihood, the difficult-to-test patient most suitable for GSR audiometry is the patient with functional hearing loss. Pennington and Martin (1972) report, for example, that EDA has its widest application with this patient population. The VA still requires EDA as part of the test battery used in the evaluation of patients seeking financial compensation for hearing loss. Ventry and Chaiklin (1965), in their long-term study of adults with functional hearing loss, successfully utilized GSR audiometry as the major tool for the identification and classification of subjects. Ruhm and Cooper (1964) employed EDA as the criterion test in their evaluation of delayed auditory feedback (DAF) using key-tapping with patients having a functional hearing loss. There are even some data to suggest that the incidence of functional hearing loss is reduced when EDA is used as the first test of the test battery (Menzel, 1960). The long history of the use of EDA with patients with functional hearing loss (Chaiklin and Ventry, 1963; Hopkinson, 1973), as well as my own clinical and research experience, leads me to suggest that EDA should be ranked first among those electrophysiologic tests currently available for the precise measurement of auditory thresholds in older children and adults suspected of, or having, functional hearing loss. Equipment for cortical evoked response audiometry is far too expensive and complicated for routine clinical use in the evaluation of such patients, while DAF with key-tapping does not seem to have been widely adopted.

GSR audiometry has been less successful with other difficult-to-test populations, especially with the difficult-to-test child. Frisina (1973) has correctly pointed out that "in general, the ability of the research subject or clinical patient to participate in a specified manner is more critical than whether he is adult or a child with respect to chronological or mental age [p. 157]." Many children (and some adults) are poor subjects for EDA because they cannot adequately participate in the test situation. A major requirement of EDA is that the patient or subject remain relatively quiet during the test. The younger the child, the more difficult it is to meet this requirement, especially if the child's communication problem is compounded by other factors such as CNS damage, mental retardation, emotional problems, and the like. The child's difficulty in participating in the EDA test situation, combined with factors related to the test itself—the use of a noxious stimulus, the time-consuming nature of the procedure, the need for conditioning, and so on—mitigate against the successful use of *conditioned* pure-tone GSR audiometry with many difficult-to-test children. In addition, other test procedures are available today that allow the clinician to obtain reasonably precise estimates of a child's hearing sensitivity in most instances. These include the use of the conditioned orienting reflex, operant conditioning, impedance audiometry, and cortical evoked response audiometry, to name just a few. Unfortunately, there is the growing realization that those children who are difficult to evaluate with behavioral techniques are the very same children who are difficult to evaluate with electrophysiologic techniques. It may be that in the final analysis, clinical experience and acumen, persistence, flexibility, and time are the most important tools that the clinician has available to him in the evaluation of these young children. Despite the early studies showing reasonably good agreement between behavioral audiometry and EDA in children (Barr, 1955; Bordley, 1956), EDA is not the method of choice today in evaluating the hearing sensitivity of young children (0 to 5 years). Newby (1972) has correctly pointed out that "the difficulties encountered in GSR testing of young children are so great that many examiners prefer to rely on other techniques for assessing a child's hearing abilities. When it is used in the clinic, conditioned GSR audiometry should be interpreted with great caution and it should be used as an adjunct to—not in place of—other methods of assessment [p. 218]."

A number of studies have been conducted on the use of EDA with retarded children and adults (Fulton, 1962, 1965; Irwin *et al.*, 1957; Lamb and Graham, 1968; Moss *et al.*, 1961, and others). A review of these studies supports Hogan's (1969) conclusion that EDA is clinically feasible with the retarded. But Hogan also concludes that "it seems to be rather common . . . for the test procedure to fail more frequently with retarded subjects than with normals. Some retarded persons are difficult to condition, others are either unwilling or unable to submit to examination, and still others exhibit apparently reduced electrophysiological responsiveness [p. 253]." Again, other test techniques, both behavioral and electrophysiologic, are more suitable than EDA in the evaluation of the mentally retarded patient.

The use of EDA with other difficult-to-test patients has been more limited, and the results equivocal. Several attempts have been made to use EDA in measuring the hearing sensitivity of aphasic adults (Hayes *et. al.*, 1961; Mencher, 1967). In the more recent study, Mencher (1967) reported an 84% siccess rate in conditioning aphasic patients and good EDR test–retest reliability, although the reliability was not as good as that found with conventional pure-tone audiometry. Mencher's study is marred, however, by his failure to describe several important procedural aspects, such as the latency criterion employed and the criteria used for threshold definition. In addition, he failed to look at the relationship between thresholds obtained with behavioral audiometry and EDR thresholds. His conclusion that EDA can be successfully employed with aphasic adults thus awaits further confirmation.

EDA has also been employed in subjects with Rh incompatability (Byers *et al.*, 1955; Goodhill, 1956; Lehrhoff, 1961; Matkin and Carhart, 1968). Although early studies suggested that such patients give unusual EDR results (*e.g.*, difficulty in conditioning, abnormal latencies, erratic responses to shock), Matkin and Carhart (1968) demonstrated quite conclusively that, in Rh cases without multiple involvement, EDA produces results comparable to those found in subjects with peripheral auditory impairment. They were able to condition approximately 80% of their subjects; median latency was 2.0 sec, and the slope and amplitude findings were not atypical. In addition, Matkin and Carhart found that there was good agreement between conventional pure-tone thresholds and GSR thresholds, with the latter somewhat poorer than pure-tone thresholds obtained conventionally. They concluded that

the results do not exhibit the type of abnormal electrodermal behavior which reportedly characterizes the responses of children with aphasia and corticothalamic tract lesions. Thus, the results of this study do not support the view that hearing loss arising from Rh incompatability results in bizarre electrodermal responsiveness which in turn indirectly suggests lesions at high levels in the central auditory system [p. 387].

In summary, the success of conditioned GSR audiometry—and success is defined as the ability to obtain valid and reliable thresholds—is dependent, to very large extent, on both patient and procedural variables. The patient's candidacy for EDA is dependent on a number of factors: age, etiology of hearing loss, conditionability, ability to tolerate the test situation, and CNS integrity, among others. Taken independently or in concert, these factors can have a strong influence on the clinician's ability to obtain adequate results. Currently, EDA seems most suitable for patients with functional hearing loss (as defined by Ventry and Chaiklin, 1962) and least suitable for the young, difficult-to-test child. In addition to patient variables, the success of GSR audiometry is directly related to procedural considerations, and it is to this area that we turn next.

IV. PROCEDURAL CONSIDERATIONS

A. Introduction

Considerable emphasis has been placed, throughout this chapter, on the importance of methodology in GSR audiometry. Audiometry is a procedure and, thus, procedural considerations are of paramount concern if valid and reliable GSR thresholds are to be obtained. The procedures to be described were developed at the San Francisco VA Hospital during the mid- and late 1950s, and have been used successfully in both research and clinic practice.[5] Some details of the procedures have appeared in reports by Chaiklin *et al.* (1961), Engelberg (1970), and Newby (1972); other aspects and modifications appear here for the first time. Although the procedures were designed primarily for use with an adult population, there is no reason why they cannot be used with a child, provided that the child is a reasonably good candidate for EDA. The two basic considerations underlying the development of the methodology were (1) to utilize relevant research to specify stimulus parameters and response criteria; and (2) to reduce, to an absolute minimum, the influence and effects of clinician variables on the outcome of EDA. In a word, the basic goal was to attempt to "objectify" GSR audiometry. What follows, then, is a description of the major methodological considerations involved in pure-tone EDA.[6]

B. Equipment

Either custom-built (Hind *et al.*, 1958; Stewart, 1954a) or commercially manufactured equipment (Maico, Grason–Stadler) is available for performing EDA. All of my experience has been with Grason–Stadler psychogalvanometers connected to a variety of audiometers.[7]

---

[5] Many people contributed to the development of the procedures described here. They include L. Barrett, G. Skalbeck, C. Berlin, I. M. Ventry, and above all, J. B. Chaiklin.

[6] The discussion here deals solely with conditioned pure-tone EDA. GSR audiometry employing speech stimuli has received some research attention (Chaiklin, 1959; Ruhm and Carhart, 1958; Ruhm and Menzel, 1959) but appears to be used infrequently clinically.

[7] Unfortunately, the Grason–Stadler units are no longer manufactured. Decreasing demand necessitated discontinuing production. The clinician, without such equipment on hand, will have to borrow a unit, purchase a used unit, assemble an instrument array, or seek another manufacturer of psychogalvanometers.

The latest model of the Grason–Stadler psychogalvanometer (Model 4) contains the following important features:

1. Presentation of a CS event or CS–UCS event is automatic. The CS duration can be varied from 1 to 4 sec, the UCS duration from .25 to 1 sec, the CS–UCS interval from .25 sec to 3 sec, and the UCS intensity from .25 to 2.0 mA. Thus, a wide variety of options are available to control stimulus parameters. All stimuli can be presented manually as well.

2. Two operating modes permit the recording of the patient's response in arbitrary units (mm), or the response superimposed upon the patient's basal skin resistance (in ohms). The former is preferred because the base line remains relatively constant over time and the interpretation of a response is simplified.

3. A strip-chart recorder employs electrically heated styli on heat sensitive strip-chart paper. A marking device notes the presentation of all stimuli. In the latest model (#4), two styli are employed—one to record the baseline activity (or skin resistance) and changes in baseline activity, and one to mark stimulus events. The older model (E664) utilized one stylus for both purposes. The latter system is preferred, in that the judgment of a response is simplified.

4. A sensitivity control adjusts the sensitivity of the ac amplifier to compensate for patient differences in response amplitude. As noted earlier, the goal here is to adjust the sensitivity to the point at which baseline activity is minimized and response amplitude is maximal.

Pure-tone or speech stimuli are presented by means of an audiometer connected to the GSR unit, and the intensity and/or frequency of the stimuli are controlled at the audiometer. The Grason–Stadler psychogalvanometers have been durable, reliable, and relatively uncomplicated to use. Thus, it is unfortunate that the equipment is no longer manufactured.

C. Instructions

The purpose of the instructions is simply to indicate what is expected of the patient and what the sequence of events will be. The following instructions have been used successfully when testing adults:

> You are going to have a test of your hearing. Before the test starts, I will fasten a disc to two fingers of each of your hands. During the test you will hear tones through the earphones, and with some of the tones you will feel an electric shock on the fingers of your right hand. I will adjust the shock to a point which you report as distinctly unpleasant, but not painful. The test will require you to remain as still as possible. If

it is absolutely necessary for you to move, try to limit such moves to the periods immediately following the shocks. Be certain to settle down quickly after each movement.

It is important that you stay alert during the test. Keep your eyes open and do not let your gaze become fixed too long on one spot. On the other hand, you should not move your head around to change your view or look at me. There will be long periods during which you will hear nothing. You should stay alert during these periods. When I say to you, "The test will begin now," you will not have to give me any further signals when you hear something in the earphones or when you feel a shock. The entire test will last no longer than an hour. At the end of the first half hour, if the test is not complete, I will give you a five-minute break.

Note the major points that are made. First, the patient is told about the shock, and that *he* is to determine when it is unpleasant but not painful. Next, an attempt is made to reduce or limit extraneous movements. If a patient moves immediately after a CS–UCS event, it makes little difference to test interpretation. If a movement occurs at the same time or very shortly after a CS event, there is no way of knowing if the change in skin resistance is a CR or is merely due to the extraneous movement. (It should be noted that, if this occurs, the CS event should be discounted and the graphic record marked with an "M" indicating that a movement took place at the same time a CS event was presented.) Remaining alert is emphasized, since dozing or sleeping can reduce responsivity. Finally, the length of time of the test is described. Breaks can be interspersed more frequently if necessary, but two one-half-hour sessions should be maximum. Spending additional time is usually counterproductive. The patient may become restless, annoyed, and on occasion, hostile. If required, another test session can be scheduled. Questions regarding the test should be answered in a straightforward manner and without elaboration.

D. Patient Preparation

The patient should be seated comfortably in the test suite, the clinician seated in the control room. The patient and clinician should *not* be in the same room. The temperature in the test suite should be comfortable. In most audiometric suites, the temperature will be high enough to insure that the patient perspires. The clinician needs to be seated in such a way that the patient can be monitored visually. In addition, auditory monitoring, utilizing earphones, is essential. Both types of monitoring are required to aid the clinician in identifying movement artifacts.

The patient's fingertips are cleaned with alcohol, and pick-up electrodes are firmly attached to the pads of the index and ring fingers of the left hand; the shock electrodes are placed on the same locations on the other hand.[8] Electrode jelly is used to improve contact between the electrodes and the skin. (See Edelberg and Burch (1962) and Lykken (1959) for a more complete description of the effects of electrodes, electrode placement, and other variables on recording the GSR.)

E.   Shock Adjustment

The purpose of the UCS is not to traumatize or intimidate the patient. On the contrary, shock is used to establish a CR and to prevent extinction of the CR. The major goal in UCS adjustment is to set the UCS at the level that the patient reports is distinctly unpleasant but not painful (Chaiklin *et al.*, 1961; Doerfler and Kramer, 1959). There is no support for Hopkinson's recent suggestion (1973) that "the intensity of the shock should be established on a subjective basis so that the patient 'feels it' [p. 190]." The UCS, to be effective, should be unpleasant. Obviously, this is a subjective judgment on the part of the patient, and thus there is considerable intersubject variability. For example, in the 1961 reliability study (by Chaiklin and associates), shock levels ranged from .58 mA to 4.10 mA, with a mean level of 1.78 mA. The intensity of the UCS should be increased in small steps until the patient emphatically reports that the UCS is unpleasant. Following any rest periods, the clinician should again determine if the UCS is still unpleasant. If it is not, the shock intensity should be readjusted to the "unpleasant" level. It is important to note that obtaining optimum UCS intensity levels in this fashion with the difficult-to-test patient may prove impossible. A retarded child, for example, may be hard pressed to give a verbal report of "unpleasantness." Under these circumstances, the UCS can be adjusted to the point at which significant changes in skin resistance are produced by the UCS. It may very well be that the poorer success rate in conditioning or in testing the difficult-to-test patient is

---

[8] A variety of electrode placement sites have been employed, especially with children. Recording site is not unimportant. Hogan (1969) has pointed out that multichannel recording of electrodermal activity at different sites might improve the sensitivity of EDA. He also points out that "present testing procedure which commonly depends upon a fixed palm or fingertip electrode placement seems to be the result of a compromise between clinical expediency, probable success in detecting responses, and the restriction imposed by the single recording channel of our clinical galvanic skin response equipment" [p. 253].

related, to some degree, to the difficulties involved in establishing an optimum UCS intensity.

F. Voluntary Pure-Tone Threshold Measurements

Following UCS adjustment, pure-tone thresholds are measured in a standard fashion, although a verbal response may have to replace finger-raising, since the electrodes are now attached to the fingers. The measurement of voluntary threshold in EDA is an important component of the test procedure. This apparent contradiction—if one can obtain behavioral thresholds, why does one need EDA?—is explained by recognizing that the patient must hear the CS in order to be conditioned to respond to it. If conditioning is performed at subthreshold level, it is highly unlikely that a CR will result. Thus, some indication of a behavioral threshold is a necessary prerequisite in EDA. Again, the difficulty in utilizing EDA with the difficult-to-test child may be related to the problem of obtaining reasonable estimates of behavioral thresholds. Without such estimates, CS intensity levels used for conditioning may be too high or too low, both of which mitigate against successful conditioning and testing.

G. The Conditioning Process

Perhaps the most critical aspect of EDA is the conditioning process. The success or failure of the test is dependent on successfully conditioning the patient. The essence of EDA is the basic assumption that following conditioning, failure to elicit a CR is caused by the patient's inability to hear the CS (or that the CS is too faint to produce a CR). If the clinician cannot make this assumption—that failure to respond is caused by a failure to hear the CS and not caused by inadequate conditioning—then conditioned EDA will not be successful. Many failures in EDA are probably related to inadequate conditioning of the patient, leading to test results of little value.

There are two essential considerations in the conditioning process: (1) the level at which to condition the patient; and (2) the criterion for determining when the patient has been conditioned. It was noted earlier that knowledge of behavioral thresholds is important in establishing the intensity level at which conditioning should take place. This is important so that conditioning can take place at levels close to threshold in order to make optimal use of intensity generalization. That is, it makes little sense to condition at intensity levels significantly above threshold when most of the CSs, during threshold sampling, will be presented close to or at threshold. Intensity generalization is facilitated, then, by conditioning close to those levels at which the CS will be presented during the test. In our clinical and research work, conditioning trials have been presented at a 10-dB sensation level (SL) re patient's voluntary threshold. This poses no problem when voluntary thresholds are known. When the validity of behavioral thresholds is open to question, as in the case of a patient suspected of having a functional hearing loss, or when behavioral thresholds cannot be measured, as in the case of a difficult-to-test child, the clinician is faced with a major problem regarding the level to be used in conditioning. In the former instance, the problem is easier to resolve, since in most cases of suspected functional loss, behavioral thresholds, though possibly exaggerated, can be measured. Thus, conditioning can take place 10 dB above the patient's behavioral threshold, whatever that may be. The clinician knows the behavioral threshold and, most important, knows that the patient hears the tone during the conditioning sequence.

The patient who gives no behavioral thresholds or whose responses are so erratic as to preclude threshold estimation poses the more difficult case. One typical solution is to present ascending CSs to determine if *consistent UCRs* are obtained at some level. If so, then that intensity level or a level 5 or 10 dB higher, can be used as the level at which conditioning will be attempted.[9] Again, the difficult-to-test child presents special problems. Random movements, for example, can be interpreted as UCRs. In addition, for both child and adult, the UCR may extinguish rapidly, and only one or two UCRs may be elicited. Lastly, not all patients give UCRs to pure-tone stimuli. The critical point, of course, is that the patient must hear the CS in order for conditioning to take place, and the clinician must be as certain as possible, prior to initiating the conditioning sequence, that the patient hears the CS. It should be apparent, too, that to err by presenting the CS at too high a level is less serious than the error of presenting the CS at subthreshold levels.

The second consideration deals with the criterion for determining when the patient has been conditioned. The conditioning criterion that we have employed is three successive responses to CS events following the first five events of the predetermined test schedule. The CRs need

---

[9] Sampling for UCRs at levels below behavioral threshold is an important step for all patients on whom EDA is conducted, and should precede the conditioning process. If consistent UCRs are obtained at a level below behavioral thresholds, then that level, or a level slightly higher, can be used as the CS intensity level. The important point is that the clinician must be reasonably certain that the patient is indeed hearing the CS at these levels.

to be consecutive, but there may be intervening CS–UCS events as well as control events.

To explain, in EDA, there needs to be a test schedule that specifies the order of presentation of CS, CS–UCS, and control events. In some instances, especially for research purposes, the interstimulus intervals can also be specified. The total number of events incorporated in the test schedule is less important than (1) the fact that the order of events is randomized, and (2) that partial reinforcement is utilized. Thus, in a 40-event schedule (exclusive of control events), 16 items will be CS–UCS events (40% reinforcement) and 24 items will be CS events only. The number of control events is more arbitrary but, as indicated earlier, there should be at least one control event for each ascending pass at threshold, with a minimum of four control events for each threshold measurement. A distinction should be made here between "heard" and "nonheard" events. Obviously, all CS–UCS events are "heard" by the patient, while all control events are not heard. The 40-event schedule noted previously includes only *heard* events. For example, there will be many CS events during threshold sampling that will not be heard; the pure tones are presented below threshold and presumably will not elicit a CR. These unheard CS events are not included among the 40 events in the test schedule. Thus, the clinician proceeds to the next event in the test schedule only when the previous event has been heard. Note that a CS at or above threshold is considered a heard event even though it may not elicit a CR. Note, too, that a CS presented below "threshold" is considered a heard event if it elicits a CR. Finally, the interstimulus intervals (ranging from 20 to 60 sec) refer to intervals between "heard" events, and the 40% reinforcement schedule means that 40% of the heard events are CS–UCS events. A portion of a test schedule is shown in Table II.

To recapitulate, the conditioning sequence begins by sampling, below behavioral threshold, for UCRs. If consistent UCRs are not obtained, the predetermined test schedule is initiated at a 10-dB SL re the best estimate of behavioral threshold. The clinician must be certain, during the conditioning sequence, that the patient hears the CS in the CS–UCS sequence and that CS intensity is low. Binaural presentations are used during the conditioning process even when there are known differences between the ears. Monaural stimulation is more time consuming, and behavioral thresholds for both ears may not be known. To avoid premature judgment of conditioning, the first five events are discounted. The patient is considered conditioned when three consecutive CRs are obtained to tone alone. Control events are employed during the conditioning sequence, and the stimulus parameters and response criteria described earlier are used throughout.[10]

H. Threshold Sampling

Once the conditioning criterion has been met, threshold sampling can begin. Several considerations need to be noted here. First, all sampling for threshold is conducted using an ascending sequence of CS presentations. This is consistent with clinical practice in behavioral audiometry. In addition, it makes little sense to present CS events at levels well above the patient's threshold. Second, threshold sampling is conducted monaurally with threshold passes alternating between ears. Third, the clinician's goal is to establish a contrast between response–no response behavior. The clinician must be able to conclude, on the basis of EDA, that the patient did not respond at one level (presumably did not hear the CS) and did respond at another level (presumably did hear the CS). The difference between these levels should generally be no greater than 10 dB. Next, sufficient sampling should be conducted at low levels to insure that the patient is not responding at these levels. It is essential that the hearing threshold level at which reinforcement (CS–UCS) is presented be lowered still further if there is strong indication that the patient has heard the CS at these lower levels. Considerable caution must be exercised here, in that CS–UCS events presented at levels at which the patient does not hear will quickly lead to the extinction of the CR. Finally, threshold definition is, as described earlier, the lowest level at which a minimum 50% response rate is elicited, with threshold definition dependent on the response rate to control events.

As far as I can determine, the literature contains only one brief description of threshold sampling procedures used in the clinical application of EDA (Engelberg, 1970). His description fails, however, to capture the decision-making processes involved in threshold sampling, and contains inaccuracies as well. The following example, then, is presented in an attempt to illustrate the threshold sampling sequence in a relatively uncomplicated case whose GSR record is straightforward and

---

[10] In our work with EDA, the first five events of our test schedule have included both CS and CS–UCS events. It may be that conditioning would be facilitated and the test procedure shortened if the first five events were CS–UCS events (100% reinforcement). The 40% reinforcement schedule would then be initiated after the first five events.

easily interpreted. It should be emphasized that not all GSR tests are as uncomplicated.

In this case, the patient's behavioral threshold at 1000 Hz prior to EDA were 50 dB in the left ear and 20 dB in the right ear. Table II shows a portion of the test schedule used during the test. For brevity, the first 11 events have been omitted from Table II. These events, both CS and CS–UCS events, were used during the conditioning sequence.

TABLE II

PORTION OF A TEST SCHEDULE USED DURING THRESHOLD SAMPLING[a]

Event number	Type of event	Event number	Type of event
12	CS	21	CS–UCS
13	CS	22	CS
14	CS–UCS	23	CS
15	CS	24	CS–UCS
16	CS	25	CS
17	CS–UCS	26	CS–UCS
18	CS–UCS	27	CS
19	CS	28	CS
20	CS		

[a] See text for explanation.

The patient met the conditioning criterion on the eleventh event. The patient was conditioned using a 30-dB signal presented binaurally in that no UCRs were obtained at lower levels. Table III shows the interpretation of the test record during the threshold sampling process at 1000 Hz.

The first pass (event 12), in the right ear, shows no response to a control, a 0-dB, or a 10-dB CS. A 20-dB CS produced a CR, and is so noted. The pass is terminated with this response.

Event 13, a CS, represents the first pass in the poorer ear (left) and consists of pure tones presented in 10-dB steps from 0 dB to 50 dB. No responses are noted for any CS except that presented at 50 dB. Two control events were inserted in the pass, and one response to a control was obtained. It should be recognized that all of the stimuli presented below 20 dB in the right ear and 50 dB in the left are "unheard" events. Thus, the interstimulus interval can be short, 5 to 15 sec. The control events, of course, are "unheard" as well. The interstimulus interval between the two heard events, 20 dB in the right and 50 dB in the left ear, should be separated by a minimum of 20 sec.

TABLE III

INTERPRETATION OF A TEST RECORD OF ELEVEN CS EVENTS DURING THRESHOLD SAMPLING AT 1000 HZ[a]

	Right ear					Left ear						
Threshold pass	1	2	3	4	Response rate	1	2	3	4	5	Response rate
CS event No.	15	16	22	25		19	20	23	27	28	
Control	12				0%	13					29%
	N	N	N-N	N		N-R	N	N	N	N	
	N		N	N		N	N	N	N	N	
	R	R	R	R	75%		N	R	N	N	75%
	R										
										R	
						N			N		
						N		N			
									N	N	
						R					
							R	R	N	R	

CS level in dB HL: Control, 0, 5, 10, 15, 20, 25, 30, 35, 40, 45, 50, 55

[a] See text for explanation. R = response; N = no response.

239

Event 14 is a CS–UCS event. The clinician must now choose the ear in which reinforcement is to take place. This can be at either 30 dB in the right or 60 dB in the left. CS–UCS events have not yet been presented to the left ear. Conditioning took place at 30 dB binaurally, but since the behavioral threshold in the left is 50 dB, the patient has not had a CS–UCS presentation to the left ear. This would be the ear of choice in which to present the CS–UCS called for in the test schedule.

Event 15 is a CS event and constitutes the second pass in the right ear. This pass consists of a control event and 5-dB CS, to which a response is obtained. The question confronting the clinician now is whether this is a random response occurring in appropriate temporal relationship to the onset of the CS, or a true CR to a CS 15 dB lower than the patient's behavioral threshold.[11] In either case, the 5-dB CS must be considered a heard event, and the clinician proceeds to event 16, another CS presentation.

For event 16, the clinician must decide whether to continue sampling in the right ear or to switch to the left ear. In this instance, the clinician decides to continue to explore the right ear but needs to decide at what level the CS should be presented. (Note the decision-making processes involved here. Given these processes, it should be quite clear that the "objectivity" of EDA is almost solely related to the nature and evaluation of the response.) The clinician chooses to present the next CS at 10 dB in the right ear. The reason for this choice is that, if the response at 5 dB was indeed a true CR to the CS, then a 10-dB CS should also elicit a response. If, on the other hand, the response at 5 dB was due to a random movement, then a 10-dB CS will produce no response. A 5-dB presentation level was not chosen, since random fluctuations at threshold may mitigate against another response at the 5-dB level. The 10-dB CS elicited a response supporting the response obtained 5 dB lower. The threshold pass is terminated with the presentation of another control event to which no response is obtained.

The next two events (17 and 18) are reinforced events, one presented at 60 dB in the left and the other at 20 dB in the right ear. The hearing level for reinforcement in the right ear has been lowered to take into account the CRs obtained at 5 and 10 dB.

---

[11] Random movements—sighs, sneezes, coughs, and so on—occurring at the same moment as CS presentations, make it impossible to know if the change in skin resistance is due to a CR or to the random movement. Under these circumstances, the CS event is discounted and the clinician proceeds to the next event if the CS was "heard" or repeats the event if the CS was "unheard." The record should be marked with an "M", indicating the presence of a movement.

Event 19 is a CS event and a second threshold pass is made in the left ear. No responses are obtained at 10 through 40 dB, nor is there a response to a control event. A 50-dB CS produces no response. The clinician, however, must consider this a "heard" event in that the patient's behavioral threshold was 50 dB.

Event 20 calls for another CS and, after an appropriate interval (20 to 60 sec), a CS is presented at 55 dB and elicits a response. A prior control presentation failed to produce a response. There are a number of reasons to account for the absence of a CR at 50 dB, including fluctuations in threshold and the fact that CRs are not always obtained at behavioral threshold. Nevertheless, at the end of event 20, the clinician has some evidence that the patient's behavioral threshold in the left ear is valid and that the behavioral threshold in the right ear may be exaggerated.

Event 21 is a reinforcement and is presented at 20 dB to the right ear. Event 22 calls for a CS, and a third threshold pass is made in the right ear. A control produces no response, nor do CSs at 0 and 5 dB. A 10-dB CS produces another response. Note, again, that both the 0-dB and 5-dB CS events are considered "unheard" events in that no responses were elicited and, thus, there is no evidence that the patient has heard these tones. A control event, to which no response is elicited, terminates the third threshold pass in the right ear.

Event 23 constitutes the third pass in the left ear. Sampling takes place at 10, 20, 45, and 55 dB, with no response except at 55 dB. There is no response to a control event. Sampling is still conducted at low levels to insure that the patient, through intensity generalization, is not now responding at these levels. Note, also, that the threshold pass did not include 50 dB but, rather, used the 10-dB interval, 45 to 55 dB. The reason is that a 50-dB signal may be at threshold, sometimes eliciting a CR, other times not. Continued sampling at 50 dB may prolong the test unnecessarily. The point here is not whether the patient's threshold is 50 or 55 dB but, rather, that there is no evidence, at this time, to suggest that his hearing sensitivity is lower than 50 dB. For efficiency, then, threshold sampling now excludes 50 dB, and the no response–response differentiation utilizes 45 and 55 dB.

Event 24 is a reinforcement and is presented at 20 dB in the right ear. Event 25, a CS event, is also presented to the right ear. Sampling for threshold (pass 4) consists of a control (no response), a 0-dB CS (no response), and a 10-dB CS (response). The test is completed for the right ear. Several salient features should be considered. First, the response rate to control presentations was 0%. Second, there was a 0% response rate at 0 dB and a 75% response rate at 10 dB, clearly differentiating response from no response. Third, an attempt to establish a threshold at 5 dB was abandoned after pass 3 when no response was elicited at that level. Pass 4 could have utilized a presentation at 5 dB, but the clinician chose not to do so, in the interest of time. It is clear that the patient's *conditioned* GSR threshold in the right ear is 10 dB, or 10 dB lower than the behavioral threshold obtained prior to EDA. Retesting following EDA elicited a behavioral threshold of 5 dB.

Sampling continues in the left ear. Event 26 (CS–UCS) is presented at 60 dB and event 27, a CS, is presented at 10, 30, 45, and 55 dB, with no responses obtained at any level. The only response noted is to a control event. There are two possibilities to account for the results of threshold pass 4: The patient's threshold has shifted upward or the CR is extinguished (or extinguishing). Again, the clinician must make a decision. Since the next event (28) is a CS, at what level or levels should this stimulus be presented? It is probably an error to choose 60 dB. A CS of 60 dB is 10 dB higher than the patient's behavioral threshold, and a response here would contribute little information of value. The more reasonable choice is to present the CS at 55 dB preceded by presentations at lower levels. Pass 5 produced no responses at 40 and 45 dB, no response to a control, and a CR to a 55 dB CS. The test is completed. (If a response had not been obtained at 55 dB, the test would continue, but a threshold in the left ear may not have been established.) The salient feature here is that there is a 75% response rate at 55 dB, approximately 50% greater than the 29% response rate to control events. Note, too, that no responses were obtained below 50 dB, lending strong support to the use of a 75% threshold criterion in this example. The post-EDA behavioral threshold was 55 dB.

Considerable space has been devoted to this straightforward and uncomplicated example in an attempt to illustrate some of the procedural concerns and decision-making processes involved in the clinical application of EDA. Not all of the problems have been illustrated by the example. Nonetheless, it should be clear that EDA is not simple to administer, it is not objective, and considerable skill and experience are required if valid and reliable results are to be obtained. At the same time, it is important to stress that EDA is not an art form and that the procedure, as described above, lends itself nicely to instructional purposes. For example, the progress of students and junior clinicians can be monitored quite simply by carefully reviewing both the GSR graphic record and the data analysis sheet. Correct interpretation of GSRs, use of appropriate interstimulus intervals, whether or not the student followed the test schedule, and the decisions made during the test, can all be evaluated by the instructor. The only prerequisites are that all events are clearly labeled on the record (see Fig. 2) and that an analysis sheet, similar to that shown in Table III, is employed during the test.

I. Other Procedural Considerations

Although the clinician obviously has to make ongoing interpretations of the test record during EDA, it is imperative that the clinician not only reanalyze the record following the test, but that the tape be analyzed *independently* by a second clinician. EDA is fraught with procedural complexities. During the test itself, decisions have to be made, the graphic record analyzed, the patient observed, dials turned, buttons pushed, and so forth. As a result, errors can easily arise, especially in the interpretation of a response. For example, it may be difficult to determine, at the time of test, whether the latency of a particular response was 1.3 sec or 1.5 sec, the former a "no response," the latter a "response." Thus, in reevaluating the record after the test, the clinician has an opportunity to analyze the record under less demanding circumstances.

The analysis of the record by a second clinician is another attempt to control tester bias and to increase objectivity. Goldstein (1963) has suggested labeling each event with a code number so that "the person who reads the record after the test will then also be ignorant of the intensity and frequency of a tone and which ear is being stimulated when a stimulus is presented [p. 179]." Although this procedure may be appropriate in research applications (see Chaiklin *et al.*, 1961), I see no simple way it can be utilized clinically. The best that can be done is to have the record analyzed independently by another clinician who has no knowledge of the patient's behavioral thresholds. It is possible, of course, that subsequent analysis of the record will produce an outcome different from that noted during the test proper. For example, a GSR considered a CR by the tester during the test may, on closer inspection, fail to meet the response criteria. A "threshold" may not be a threshold upon subsequent analysis. These differences in interpretation are not due to differences in criteria but due, rather, to the fact that the tester must make on-line decisions under trying test conditions. Errors in judgment occur and can be identified only through subsequent analysis of the record. Most important, of course, is that errors be identified and rectified prior to the final judgment about thresholds or about the adequacy of the GSR record.

It is important to note that there are several different outcomes of EDA. Thresholds may be obtained at several different frequencies in each ear during a single test session or, at the other extreme, the patient may not meet the conditioning criterion. Thresholds may be obtained in one ear but not the other. The CR may extinguish at some point during the test and the clinician may be able only to offer a qualified interpretation of the GSR record. A conservative interpretation of the record is to be preferred to a more liberal interpretation that can be supported only with difficulty.

A word needs to be said about the use of masking in EDA. Masking can and should be employed when necessary. In the example presented earlier, the patient failed to respond behaviorally to pure-tone stimuli presented to the left ear when the right ear was masked. The question is whether this is a valid response or whether the masked threshold is exaggerated or elevated. Masking should be employed during EDA to answer this question. It is important to emphasize that the absence of a CR with masking in the right ear may be due to the failure of the patient to hear the CS presented to the left ear *or* the CR may have extinguished. The clinician can check this by removing the masking from the masked ear and then presenting a CS to the test ear at an intensity level that had been sufficient to elicit a CR in the unmasked condition. Failure to elicit a response under these circumstances would suggest that the response has extinguished, whereas the presence of a response, without masking, would indicate that the patient's threshold had shifted with masking of the nontest ear.

V. THE FUTURE OF GSR AUDIOMETRY

Although it is difficult to predict the future of EDA, I am not optimistic about its resurgence or its widespread clinical use with patients other than those with functional hearing loss. The shift away from EDA has been too widespread and too dramatic, and the disenchantment too great.

I am still firmly convinced, however, that conditioned GSR pure-tone audiometry is the method of choice in the electrophysiologic measurement of older children and adults with, or suspected of having, functional hearing loss. It has had a long and successful history with this population and, barring widespread use of cortical evoked response audiometry or delayed auditory feedback with keytapping, I see no change in EDA's status here. The importance of EDA with this population should not be underestimated, since increasing concern over noise-induced hearing loss and increasing compensation claims may very well lead to an "outbreak" of functional hearing loss in this rather sizable population of adults.

The outlook is bleak for the use of EDA with difficult-to-test children, at least in its traditional form, modeled after classical conditioning procedures. The noxious shock, the long test sessions, the conditioning procedures, and so on, all mitigate, in my opinion, against the widespread use of EDA with children. It is possible, of course, that some major breakthrough is in the offing here. Perhaps computer averaging techniques, such as those used with cortical evoked response audiometry, could be successfully employed in EDA, thus eliminating the need for conditioning (Fulton, 1965). Averaging techniques combined with multi-channel monitoring of electrodermal activity at several recording sites (Hogan, 1969) may be a means of improving the efficiency and sensitivity of EDA with children. I think, though, that the apparent lack of research interest in EDA, combined with the negative set, among many clinicians, toward EDA will continue to limit the use of EDA with children.

In conclusion, EDA has had a long and checkered history in the audiology clinic. The procedure has been misunderstood, abused, and misapplied by researcher and clinician alike. Despite this and despite its limitations, taken for what it is—*a valid and reliable electrophysiologic measure of peripheral hearing sensitivity when used with appropriate procedures and applied to suitable candidates*—EDA still has an important place in the audiologist's armamentarium.

ACKNOWLEDGMENTS

This chapter would not have been possible were it not for my long association, both as a colleague and as a friend, with Joseph B. Chaiklin. Many of the procedural aspects described in the chapter were developed by Professor Chaiklin alone or in concert with me and other staff members at the San Francisco Veterans Administration Hospital. The list is too long to include here, but my appreciation is extended to Professor Chaiklin and the others who, because of their concern about good patient care and management, contributed to the EDA procedures described here. Errors in the description of procedures, important omissions, and modifications are solely my responsibility.

REFERENCES

Aronson, A. E., Hind, J. E., and Irwin, J. V. (1958). *J. Speech Hear. Res.* 1, 211.

Barr, B. (1955). *Acta Oto-Laryngol. Suppl.* 121, 1.

Beecroft, R. S. (1966). "Classical Conditioning." Psychonomic Press, Goleta, California.

Bordley, J. E. (1956). *Laryngoscope* 56, 1162.

Bordley, J. E., and Hardy, W. G. (1949). *Ann. Otol. Rhinol. Laryngol.* **58**, 751.

Bordley, J. E., Hardy, W. G., and Richter, C. P. (1948). *Bull. Johns Hopkins Hosp.* **82**, 569.

Burk, K. W. (1958). *J. Speech Hear. Res.* **1**, 275.

Byers, R. K., Paine, R. S., and Crothers, B. (1955). *Pediatrics* **15**, 248.

Chaiklin, J. B. (1959). *J. Speech Hear. Res.* **2**, 229.

Chaiklin, J. B., and Ventry, I. M. (1963). *In* "Modern Developments in Audiology" (J. Jerger, ed.), 1st ed., Chapter 3. Academic Press, New York.

Chaiklin, J. B., Ventry, I. M., and Barrett, L. S. (1961). *J. Speech Hear. Res.* **4**, 269.

Doerfler, L. G., and McClure, C. T. (1954). *J. Speech Hear. Disord.* **19**, 184.

Doerfler, L. G., and Kramer, J. C. (1959). *J. Speech Hear. Res.* **2**, 184.

Edelberg, R., and Burch, N. R. (1962). *Arch. Gen. Psychiat.* **7**, 163.

Engelberg, M. W. (1970). "Audiological Evaluation for Exaggerated Hearing Level." Chapter 7. Thomas, Springfield, Illinois.

Frisina, D. R. (1973). *In* "Modern Developments in Audiology" (J. Jerger, ed.), 2nd ed., Chapter 5. Academic Press, New York.

Fulton, R. T. (1962). Psychogalvanic Skin Response and Conditioned Orientation Reflex Audiometry with Mentally Retarded Children. Doctoral thesis, Purdue Univ., Lafayette, Indiana.

Fulton, R. T. (1965). *In* "The Audiologic Assessment of the Mentally Retarded" (L. L. Lloyd and D. R. Frisina, eds.), pp. 213–237. Speech and Hear. Dept., Parsons State Hosp. and Training Center, Parsons, Kansas.

Giolas, M. H., and Epstein, A. (1964). *J. Speech Hear. Res.* **7**, 47.

Goldstein, R. (1963). *In* "Modern Developments in Audiology" (J. Jerger, ed.), 1st ed., Chapter 5. Academic Press, New York.

Goldstein, R., and Derbyshire, A. J. (1957). *J. Speech Hear. Disord.* **22**, 696.

Goldstein, R., Ludwig, H., and Naunton, R. F. (1954). *Acta Oto-Laryngol.* **44**, 67.

Goodhill, V. (1956). *J. Speech Hear. Disord.* **21**, 407.

Grant, D. A., and Schneider, D. E. (1949). *J. Exp. Psychol.* **39**, 35.

Grant, D. A., Meyer, D. R., and Hake, H. W. (1950). *J. Gen. Psychol.* **42**, 97.

Grings, W. W., Lowell, E. L., and Rushford, G. M. (1959). *J. Speech Hear. Disord.* **24**, 380.

Hardy, W. G., and Pauls, M. (1959). *J. Speech Hear. Disord.* **24**, 123.

Hayes, C., Kavanaugh, J., and Irwin, J. V. (1961). *Asha* **3**, 324. (Abstr.)

Hind, J. E., Aronson, A. E., and Irwin, J. V. (1958). *J. Speech Hear. Res.* **1**, 220.

Hogan, D. D. (1969). *In* "Audiometry for the Retarded" (R. T. Fulton and L. L. Lloyd, eds.), Chapter 8. Williams and Wilkins, Baltimore, Maryland.

Hopkinson, N. T. (1973). *In* "Modern Developments in Audiology" (J. Jerger, ed.), 2nd ed., Chapter 6. Academic Press, New York.

Hopkinson, N. T., Katz, J., and Schill, H. (1960). *J. Speech Hear. Disord.* **25**, 349.

Humphreys, L. G. (1940). *J. Exp. Psychol.* **27**, 71.

Irwin, J. V., Hind, J. E., and Aronson, A. E. (1957). *Train. School Bull.* **54**, 26.

Kimble, G. A. (1947). *J. Exp. Psychol.* **37**, 1.

Lamb, N. L., and Graham, J. T. (1968). *Amer. J. Ment. Defic.* **72**, 721.

Lehrhoff, I. (1961). *Ann. Otol. Rhinol. Laryngol.* **70**, 234.

Lykken, D. T. (1959). *J. Comp. Physiol. Psychol.* **52**, 629.

Matkin, N. D., and Carhart, R. (1968). *Arch. Otolaryngol.* **87**, 383.

McGeoch, J. A., and Irion, A. L. (1952). "The Psychology of Human Learning," 2nd ed. Chapter 3. Longmans, Green, New York.

Mencher, G. (1967). *J. Speech Hear. Res.* **10**, 328.

Menzel, O. (1960). *J. Speech Hear. Disord.* **25**, 49.
Meritser, C. L., and Doerfler, L. G. (1954). *J. Speech Hear. Disord.* **29**, 350.
Michels, M. W., and Randt, C. T. (1947). *Arch. Otolaryngol.* **45**, 302.
Moss, J. W., Moss, M., and Tizard, J. (1961). *J. Speech Hear. Res.* **4**, 41.
Newby, H. A. (1972). "Audiology," 3rd ed. Appleton, New York.
Nober, E. H. (1958). *J. Speech Hear. Res.* **1**, 316.
O'Neill, J. J., and Oyer, H. J. (1966). "Applied Audiometry," Chapter 8. Dodd, Mead, New York.
Pennington, C. D., and Martin, F. N. (1972). *Asha* **14**, 199.
Ruhm, H., and Carhart, R. (1958). *J. Speech Hear. Res.* **1**, 169.
Ruhm, H., and Menzel, O. (1959). *Arch. Otolaryngol.* **69**, 212.
Ruhm, H., and Cooper, W., Jr. (1964). *J. Speech Hear. Disord.* **29**, 448.
Shepherd, D. C. (1964). *J. Speech Hear. Res.* **7**, 55.
Stewart, K. C. (1954a). *J. Speech Hear. Disord.* **19**, 169.
Stewart, K. C. (1954b). *J. Speech Hear. Disord.* **19**, 174.
Tait, C. A., Dixon, R. F., and Chaiklin, J. B. (1967). *J. Speech Hear. Res.* **10**, 570.
Ventry, I. M. (1970). *J. Speech Hear. Disord.* **35**, 96.
Ventry, I. M., and Chaiklin, J. B. (1962). *Asha* **4**, 251.
Ventry, I. M., and Chaiklin, J. B. (Eds.) (1965). Multidiscipline study of functional hearing loss. *J. Aud. Res.* **5**, 179.

SUPPLEMENTAL READINGS

The following are two excellent review articles on basic electrodermal phenomena.

Fowles, D. C. (1974). Mechanisms of electrodermal activity. *In* "Bioelectric Recording Techniques. Part C. Receptor and Effector Processes" (R. F. Thompson and M. M. Patterson, eds.), Academic Press, New York.
Grings, W. W. (1974). Recording of electrodermal phenomena. *In* "Bioelectric Recording Techniques. Part C. Receptor and Effector Processes" (R. F. Thompson and M. M. Patterson, eds.), Academic Press, New York.

Chapter Eight
Respiration Audiometry
Larry J. Bradford [1]

I. INTRODUCTION

It has been known for close to 100 years that visual, gustatory, cuta-neous, olfactory, psychic, and auditory stimuli alter the rate and amplitude of respiration. Howell (1928) wrote that "stimulation of any of the sensory nerves of the body may affect the rate or the amplitude of respiratory movements" and that "the rate may be changed together with an increased or decreased amplitude [pp. 699–700]." Recording of res-piration was initially of interest to physiologists in understanding breath-ing as a vital life-maintaining function and, later, in the understanding of emotions. Alterations of breathing patterns are known to occur in emo-tional states, and became an integral part of the "lie detection" test when Benussi (1914) introduced their recordings as another method of detect-ing deception about criminal guilt. The clinical use of respiration altera-tions has been limited to lie detection examinations that measure blood pressure, pulse rate, skin resistance, and respiration. In physiology and psychology clinics in Europe and the United States, a considerable amount of research on the respiration process has been conducted while pneumo-graphically recording respiration during the presentation of a variety of stimuli, including sound.

Although breathing pattern alterations have been observed following sound presentations, it has only been in recent years that measurement

---

[1] Children's Division of the Menninger Clinic, The Menninger Foundation, Topeka, Kansas.

of these alterations has been used to quantify hearing sensitivity. Since the 1960s, research reports on the use of respiration changes as an indirect measure of hearing sensitivity have appeared from Germany, Japan, South Africa, and the United States. The procedure developed in the United States has been termed "respiration audiometry" by Bradford and Rousey (1972).

This chapter will offer some tentative theoretical explanations for respiration alterations to sound, and will review some of the extensive research with respiration patterning and alterations. The equipment and procedures used in respiration audiometry at The Menninger Foundation will be presented. Case studies employing the procedure with difficult-to-test persons will be offered to emphasize the clinical usefulness of the method. A final section will discuss psychogenic deafness and offer clinical examples of the practicability of respiration audiometry in detecting psychogenic hearing losses.

II. RHYTHMS AND MODIFICATIONS OF RESPIRATION

Respiration includes external respiration (the ventilation of the lungs and the aeration of the blood) and internal respiration (the exchange of gas between blood and the tissues of the lungs). The regulation of breathing is accomplished by neural and chemical control and by the medullary respiration center. It is beyond the scope of this paper to discuss the complex regulation of respiration, but interested readers may find detailed discussions elsewhere (Oberholzer and Tofani, 1960; Pitts, 1946; Severinghaus, 1962; Wyss, 1963).

The term "respiration" will be restricted in this chapter to mean external respiration as recorded by pneumographic tracings of thoracic movements during inspiration and expiration. During inspiration, the thoracic cavity actively expands, drawing air into the lungs; whereas during expiration, it passively contracts, forcing air out of the lungs. Normal respiratory patterns, according to Braatoy (1947), are as follows:

> Recorded with pneumographic curves . . . the respiration curve of normal subjects in a relaxed, supine position will run as a "sinus curve." The respiration curve runs as a recumbent S. From the peak of inspiration, the curve runs smooth and well rounded by the downhill expiratory curve in order to oscillate equally smooth in a new, upward turn, and so the curve continues with steady, even crescentric oscillations above and below its middle course [p. 230].

Since only 15% of the expansion capacity of the chest is used during quiet respiration, respiration patterning can vary greatly beyond the basic need for oxygen consumption (Wade, 1954).

A. Respiration Patterns

Respiratory ventilation results from movement of the rib cage and diaphragm by thoracic or costal, abdominal or diaphragmatic, and unisonal types of breathing. Ventilation in thoracic breathing is achieved by the lifting and sinking of the rib cage. The contraction–relaxation of the diaphragm and abdominal walls constitutes abdominal breathing. Unisonal respiration or double breathing is characterized by the synchronous movements of the thorax and abdomen. This type of respiration has been observed in newborns (Miller and Behrle, 1952). Older infants' breathing patterns are predominantly of the abdominal type for both males and females (Gregor, 1902). Feldman (1920) attributes the predominance of abdominal breathing in an infant's early life to the conical shaped thorax, anterior–posterior diameter equal to or greater than lateral diameter, and the extension of the ribs at almost right angles to the spinal vertebra. Halvorson (1941) describes the exclusively costal, predominantly costal, unisonal, predominantly abdominal, exclusively abdominal, and paradoxical or dysynchronization between thoracic and abdominal movements as occurring in young infants. The thoracic type of breathing was reported by Clausen (1951) to occur most typically in adult women, while adult men predominantly use the abdominal type of breathing.

Normal breathing patterns have been described for adults and infants. According to Hoff and Breckenridge (1952), these patterns include eupnea, panting, and sighing. The breathing patterns each have their characteristic rhythm and amplitude. Eupnea, or quiet breathing, is effortless breathing in which the rate and amplitude of the cycles are approximately constant. A panting respiration pattern is distinguished by both increased rate and amplitude. Sighing, or gasping, is characterized by a markedly increased amplitude and reduced rate. Illustrations of these three types of breathing patterns are shown in Figure 1, where upward deflections represent the inspiratory and downward inflections the expiratory, phase of the respiration cycles.

Respiration rates appear to be variable among individuals when considering such differences as sex, age, and position of the body during recordings. Respiration rate decreases from birth to adolescence; it again increases in advanced age. Newborn babies have the most rapid rate, and reach the adult level of 12 to 16 cycles per minute (cpm) by about

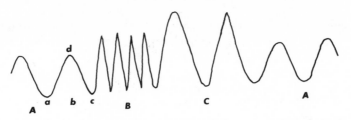

Figure 1 Eupnea (A), panting (B), and sighing (C) respiration patterns. The curves lead from left to right. A single respiration cycle (a–c) consists of inspiration (a–d), expiration (d–c), and amplitude (b–d).

16 years of age. Newborn respiration rates during sleep range from 24 to 76 cpm, with the average being 43 cpm for males and 36 cpm for females (Deming and Washburn, 1935). Halvorson (1941) recorded a mean rate of 32.3 cpm in sleeping infants. Adult respiration rates are slower in men than in women according to Clausen (1951). Several researchers have emphasized that rate is faster in an upright than in a recumbent position (Haladine and Priestly, 1935; Reed and Kleitmann, 1925). An individual's pulse rate, body temperature, height, weight, or the circumference of his thorax or abdomen does not appear to affect respiration rates or patterning (Clausen, 1951).

Deming and Washburn (1935) have studied the respiration of infants from birth through 13 weeks of age during sleep and found three principal normal breathing patterns, which they have termed "regular," "cogwheel," and "periodic" types of breathing. The regular pattern, or eupnea, is similar to that of adults, in which there are no pauses at the end of the expiration phase of the respiration cycle. The rate is generally uniform but more rapid than that of adults. A quick inspiration and prolonged jerky expiration with no pauses at the end of the expiration phase is the cogwheel type of breathing. In the periodic type of breathing, the amplitude of the respiration cycles waxes and wanes in recurring patterns. The periodic type of respiration is further delimited into a moderate periodic and an extreme periodic type. Cyclic variations without pauses at the end of the expiration phase occur in the moderate periodic type of breathing. When pauses, or breath-holding, of varying durations occur after a series of cycles at the end of the expiration phase, the pattern is termed an "extreme periodic" type of breathing. The extreme periodic breathing pattern of neonates is similar to the pathological breathing pattern in adults termed "Cheyne–Stokes respiration." However, in infancy, this type of breathing occurs during deep sleep (Czerny, 1892; Howard and Bauer, 1949). Figure 2 illustrates the cogwheel, moderate periodic, and extreme periodic respiration patterns.

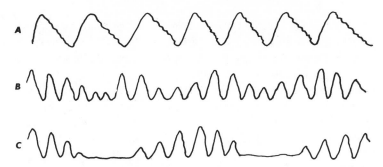

Figure 2 Cogwheel (A), moderate periodic (B), and extreme periodic (C) types of respiration patterns pneumographically recorded from normal newborn infants in our clinic. The curves lead from left to right. Inspiration carries the curve up, expiration down.

1. Respiration Patterns When Asleep. That hearing continues during sleep has been known for some time, and has been commented on by various writers. The physiologist Burdach (1838) wrote about this phenomenon as follows:

> In sleep the mind isolates itself from the external world and withdraws from its own periphery. . . . Nevertheless, connection is not broken off entirely. If we could not hear or feel while we were actually asleep, but only after we had woken up, it would be impossible to wake us at all [p. 482].

In his discussion of dreams, Freud (1958a) wrote that "we cannot keep stimuli completely away from our sense organs nor can we completely suspend the excitability of our sense organs. . . . Even in sleep the soul is in constant contact with the extra-corporeal world [p. 23]." According to Canestrini (1913), Mosso, in writing about the effects of respiration alterations during sleep, stated:

> These changes, occurring without our knowledge, represent one of the most marvelous arrangements which we may observe among the perfections of our organization. During interruption of consciousness our body is not helplessly exposed to the influences of the outer world, or to the danger to become a victim of its enemies [p. 54].

The effects of sleep on respiration patterns has been examined in a limited number of studies and is of interest to the understanding of respiration audiometry. There is no conclusive evidence that respiration patterns become deeper and more regular during sleep of adults, although there is some evidence that these changes do occur in sleeping infants.

Reed and Kleitmann (1925) were unable to differentiate sleeping from waking states by respiration patterns. Patterson (1934) found respiration to be deep and slow in drowsy states, and slow and shallow in sleeping states. Jenness and Wible (1937) report a definite tendency for respiration rate and amplitude to decrease in sleep. Reports that infants' respiration rates become slower and more regular during light sleep have been presented (Canestrini, 1913; Halvorson, 1941), and one study (Wagner, 1939) reported distinguishable respiration patterns between sleeping and waking states. In addition, determination of the depth of sleep on the basis of respiration patterns has also been reported (Reynard and Dockeray, 1939; Wagner, 1937). Halvorson (1941) concluded from his study of infants' breathing that the physiological state of the infant is reflected in his breathing. He noted respiration differences among profound sleep, early sleep, awake quiescence, restlessness, satiation-animated, pleasurable activity, fretting, and crying. He presented a quantitative scale to assess respiration variables into categories of the infant's physiological state. Although there appears to be no definitive answer to the effects of sleep on adult respiration patterns, there is some evidence that infant respiration patterns during sleep become more regular, and vary with the depth of sleep.

B. Theoretical Explanations of Respiration Alterations to Sound

Definitive explanations accounting for respiration alterations to threshold level sounds are not available with the present state of knowledge. However, there is research that does suggest possible explanations for this phenomena, and these are offered tentatively for the reader's consideration. Further research with man and animals, however, is greatly needed in order to understand better the neurological and psychological factors that produce respiration alterations to auditory stimuli.

1. Neurological Explanations. The cortical influence on respiration movements in man is demonstrated by voluntary breath-holding, hyperventilation, and alterations of respiratory rate, rhythm, and duration during speaking and singing. The slowing of respiration by electrical excitation of the cortex has been known since 1875, when Danilewisky reported on this phenomena from his research with the cat and dog. Similar observations have been reported with the cat (Preobraschensky, 1890), the dog (Bechterew, 1911), the monkey (Kaada *et al.*, 1949), and these three animals in combination (Bucy and Case, 1936). The latter researchers also observed that a slowing of respiration was "not influenced by section of the vagi, or of the phrenic nerves [p. 167]." From his research with animals, Smith (1938) concluded:

The presence in the cat, dog, and monkey of cortical areas possessing similar cytoarchitectual structure and yielding similar physiological responses, suggests the existence of a fundamental plan for the cortical evolution [p. 67].

And Bucy and Case (1936) observed in a 26-year-old man the arrest of respiration from electrical excitation of the cortex.

A comprehensive neurological discussion of respiration alterations from cortical centers is provided by Oberholzer and Tofani (1960). With reference to the particular area that controls respiration, they wrote:

Today, it is customary to separate a primary respiratory center in the reticular substance of the medulla and pons from the superimposed or secondary respiratory center in the mesencephalon and diencephalon, as also from the spinal effector centers in the spinal cord [p. 1111].

In their study of the cat, these investigators noted that a respiratory inhibition, with a decrease in the depth of inspiration and a prolongation of expiration, is most easily obtained by cortical stimulation. With reference to cortical and cerebellar influence on the respiratory activity of man they wrote: "For the most part, stimulation of the cortex results in an inhibition of respiration, for example, from the orbital face of the frontal lobe (30), from the anterior end of the island of Reil (150), and from the columna fornicis (176) [p. 1115]."[2] Respiration is a complex phenomenon, but research seems to indicate that it is influenced by cortical control. The arrest of respiration does occur in animals and man from electrical stimulation of different cortical areas.

2. *Psychological Explanations.* The psychophysiology of attention has interested early psychologists like William James (1950a) and Edward Titchener (1908) as well as modern psychologists (Berlyne, 1960; Rapaport, 1951; Woodworth and Schlosberg, 1954), and offers another possible explanation to account for respiration alterations. The exact relationship of attention to neurophysiology is not clear, but there are indications from research that attention to auditory stimuli, however explained, may account for alterations of respiration. Freud (1958b), in his "Two Principles of Mental Functioning," in 1911, wrote about auditory attention during sleep in this way:

A special function was instituted which had periodically to search the external world in order that its data might be familiar already if an ur-

---

[2] In the original article, (30) referred to Brookhart (1940); (150) to Penfield and Rasmussen (1950); and (176) to Segundo *et al.* (1955).

gent internal need should arise—the function of *attention.* This activity meets the sense-impressions halfway, instead of awaiting their appearance [p. 220].

Lehmann (1905) had written about the effects of attention on respiration in awake states as follows:

> It is a well-known experience of daily life that respiration becomes more hesitating, slower and shallower while listening to a weak sound. In my older experiment "About the Connection between Respiration and Attention" this appears clearly. Here sound, light, and electric stimuli were used near the stimulus threshold and the average of hundreds of measured respirations show that these are always the longest with sound stimuli [p. 55].

James (1950b) stated in 1890 that:

> *The effect upon respiration* of sudden sensory stimuli are also too well-known to need elaborate comment. We "catch our breath" at every sudden sound. We "hold our breath" whenever our attention and expectation are strongly engaged, and we sigh when the tension of the situation is relieved [p. 376].

The relationship of attention to breathing was also discussed by Woodworth and Schlosberg (1954):

> Another clear correlation is that between momentary attention and partial or complete inhibition of breathing. Sudden stimuli will make the subject "catch his breath." If he is listening to a faint sound, arrested breathing eliminates disturbing respiratory sounds [p. 171].

Canestrini's (1913) experience with presentations of acoustic stimuli to infants corresponded to his and other researchers' findings among adults. In general, respiration patterns were altered as a phenomena of catching the attention.

There has been some research directed to the auditory electrophysiology of attention. The influence of the efferent system on the cochlear nucleus is discussed by Worden (1966). Following the publication of a report by Hernandez–Peon *et al.* (1956), the influence of the cochlear nucleus on attention with cats received much interest. It was Worden who reviewed the research on modification of electrical activity in the cochlear nucleus during "attention" and concluded that, "at present, there is no solid evidence to support the hypothesis that attention is mediated by efferent gating of acoustic information processing in the cochlear nucleus [p. 107]." Rousey *et al.* (1971) observed elevated pure-tone thresholds in

15 of 17 subjects during a visual attention diversion task. There is some support by the research of Hubel *et al.* (1959) that there are attention units in the auditory cortex. Although the research with attention does not provide definitive explanations for alterations in respiration when auditory stimuli are presented, there are indications that this does occur and that attention may be a function of cortical control.

3. *Orienting Reflex.* The concept of the orienting reflex (OR), introduced by Pavlov (1947) and elaborated by Sokolov (1960a, 1963), offers another theoretical explanation for respiratory changes to threshold level auditory stimuli. The ability of the organism to distinguish external stimuli is necessary for the emergence of the orienting reaction. Pavlov (1947) stated that

> between the registering by the nervous system of a difference between external agents in general, and the differentiation of those very same agents with the aid of conditioned reflexes, there lies an essential difference. The former is revealed to be a stimulus process in the form of an orienting reaction, an investigatory reflex, only secondarily influencing conditioned reflexes either in inhibitory or disinhibitory fashion. The latter is expressed in the development of an inhibitory process appearing as a result, so to speak, of the struggle between stimulation and inhibition [p. 116].

The orienting reflex arises under any conditions of change in stimulation and is independent of strengthening, weakening, or qualitatively changing stimuli. The OR is differentiated from the adaptive reflex, which prepares the body for action, and the defense reflex (startle), which is the organism's response to high intensity stimuli. Sokolov (1963) differentiated the orienting from the defense reflex as follows:

> The defense and orientation reflexes are similar in that they bring into operation generalized reactions and are not limited to any given analyzer depending on the nature of the stimulus. On the other hand, they differ in their ultimate object, this being establishment of contact with the stimulus in the case of the former [p. 14].

The OR occurs when the nervous system detects a change in the stimulus or has distinguished one stimulus from another.

The OR is a response to all changes in the environment that mobilize receptors for the perception of new stimuli. The vascular components of the OR include changes in respiration, and the cortex plays the most important role in this process. Extinction of the OR is impossible in decorticate animals. Although above-threshold stimuli are extinguished in the OR, the hypothesized "neurodynamic model" prevents extinction of threshold or near-threshold stimuli. Sokolov (1960a) wrote that "the orienting reflex is greater to stimulations which are very close to threshold. The same reactions can be observed, in spite of hundreds of presentations [p. 230]." In another paper, Sokolov (1960b) stated: "If stimuli close to the threshold are administered, where formulation of a model is more difficult, then the orienting reaction is not extinguished, even if approximately 1000 stimuli are presented in a series of trials [p. 22]."

The theoretical position of the orienting reflex offers still another explanation for the cortical influence on respiration. In addition, it may explain the phenomenon of respiratory changes in threshold or near-threshold auditory stimuli.

III. STUDIES CONCERNING THE EFFECTS OF AUDITORY STIMULI ON RESPIRATION

Angelo Mosso, a physiologist in the late nineteenth century, investigated respiratory functioning of humans and animals by recording abdominal and thoracic movements with a Marey pneumograph. In 1878, he recorded his sleeping brother's respiration and pulse pressure changes to the sound of light taps on a table top. In his 1886 paper, "Periodische Athmung and Luxusathmung," he provides many pneumographic tracings of respiratory curve alterations to sounds in waking and sleeping humans and sedated dogs. His recording of "a short stopping of breathing" to slight noises is illustrated in Figures 18 and 19 of his paper. Canestrini (1913) quoted Mosso without citing the reference:

> We have seen that a voice, a noise, a touch, the influence of light, in short any outer sensory impression, can change the rhythm of respiration. . . . If in the moment when we perceive these functional changes, we observe a second impression which interrupts the sleep and when we question the testee immediately about the content of his consciousness, we receive in the majority of cases the answer that sleep has been very deep and that no memory remains of the outer impressions received during it [p. 54].

Other early research with respiration alterations to sensory stimuli has been reported by Mentz (1895) and Lehmann (1905). Although these researchers utilized auditory stimuli, Mosso appears to be the first person to record respiration alterations to sound by a pneumograph.

Silvio Canestrini (1913) assessed vision, hearing, taste, touch, and smell of newborn infants by noting changes in respiration patterns and fontanel pulse pressures as recorded by a Marey pneumograph. He recorded thoracic and abdominal respiration curves of 75 infants from 6 hours to 14 days of age, using uncalibrated sounds of a toy gun, tuning fork, mouth organ, bells, voices, whistles, and hand claps. Infants' responses to sounds were recorded when they were sleeping, awake and quiet, and awake and crying. Slight modifications of the respiration curves were noticed. He examined some of the sleeping infants' hearing 2 to 3 hours after feeding. Sounds loud enough to awaken the baby produced *increases* in respiration rate and amplitude; sounds soft enough not to awaken the baby produced *decreases* in respiration rate and amplitude. He observed amplitude reductions to soft sounds and amplitude increases to loud sounds in the awake and quiet infants. In the crying infant, the mother's speech, when loud enough to exceed the crying threshold, effected amplitude reductions.

Canestrini administered 279 auditory test stimuli to the infants and obtained positive respiratory responses to 228 (82%) of the stimulus presentations. He reported that 80% of the negative responses occurred when the babies were in deep sleep or angry and when the tuning fork, mouth organ, and the whispering of strangers were employed as stimuli. Although Canestrini was not attempting to measure auditory thresholds in the infants, his findings suggest that pneumographic tracings of respiration alterations to loud and soft stimuli could be recorded in the awake and sleeping infant.

In 1895, an Italian criminologist, Caesare Lombroso, reported measuring pulse rate and blood pressure alterations in individuals suspected of deception about criminal guilt.[3] Benussi (1914) recorded breathing and suggested that changes in the inspiration–expiration ratio could be used as another measure of deception. Respiration recordings have been an integral part of all lie-detection instruments since the appearance of the paper, "The Cardio-Pneumo-Psychogram in Deception," by Larson in 1923 (q.v., Trovillo 1939, 1940, for an excellent history on lie detection). According to Inbau (1942), the "occurrence of a suppression in respiration and an increase in blood pressure . . . is the most reliable and definite indication of deception [p. 13]." An Italian otolaryngologist, Mario Ponzo, hypothesized that modifications in respiration might be used to detect simulation of deafness (1915). In a later paper (1921), he presented the results of a study with 12 adults simulating a unilateral deafness. Respiration recordings were made with a Gutzman pneumograph. From a visual observation of the traces, he determined that uncalibrated "soft" and "loud" sounds produced a "breaking of the breath . . . a cav-

---

[3] In the first Italian edition, published in 1876, he did not mention using the sphygmomanometer or plethysmograph for interrogating criminals.

ing in of the respiratory apex (beginning of an inspiratory or expiratory act) and a prolongation of inspiration [p. 332]." Ponzo appears to be the first investigator to utilize respiration alterations specifically for assessing hearing. It was not until 40 years later that respiration alterations were systematically studied as a way to measure hearing sensitivity.

The first study combining pneumograph records and controlled auditory stimuli to assess hearing was conducted by Stubbs (1934). A total of 75 infants under 10 days of age were examined while asleep and in awake–inactive, silent–active, and crying–active states. She examined the effects of duration, intensity, and frequency of pure tones on respiration. A Western Electric 2A audiometer delivered tones through a speaker placed 10 inches above the level of the ears. The intensity of the pure tones was from 30 to 85 "sensation units," or units above the hearing threshold of two adults. Infants' gross body responses to the tones were observed by the examiner, while respiration was recorded by a pneumograph, and body movements by a stablimeter-polygraph. The most frequently observed respiration responses to the tones were an increase in rate and a decrease in amplitude. A higher percentage of these responses occurred with an increase of duration (1–15 sec), and a smaller percentage with an increase of intensity. Changes in frequency (128, 256, 1024, and 4096 cps) did not affect the percentage of infants' respiratory responses, except that sleeping infants responded more frequently to the lowest frequency than to the highest frequency. Responses to the duration, intensity, and frequency of the stimuli were not greatly influenced by the four physical states of the infant. Sex and age of the infants were not found to affect the percentage of respiration responses.

Rosenau (1961, 1962a,b) published results of his sleep-hearing test, "Die Schlafbeschallung." Respiration movements were recorded by a pneumograph connected to a kymograph. He used pure-tone and noise stimuli in these studies, and concluded that noise was the more effective stimulus for producing respiratory changes (1961). In his most comprehensive study (1962a), he tested children's hearing with 43 to 97 dB pure-tone stimuli delivered through a loudspeaker placed 50 cm above the ears. The duration of the stimulus was 250 and 500 msec. He stated that medium sound intensities (levels not specified) altered respiration patterns: "Depending on the time of the stimulation, it is a matter of forming 'steps' on inspiration, of a plateau-shaped spreading of the peak in the alternation between inspiration and expiration or of extending the intervals between two respirations [p. 198]."

In the same paper, Rosenau discussed his study with normal-hearing children, normal-hearing children with artificially induced deafness (ears plugged with paraffin-saturated gelatin), children with audiometrically verified organic hearing impairments, and children with verified absence of hearing. The normal-hearing children had a "mean reaction threshold" measured by respiration from 50 to 60 dB at 125, 400, 1250, and 4000 Hz. The difference between the audiometric threshold and the "mean reaction threshold" measured by respiration was from 40 to 55 dB for those with induced deafness, and 34 to 39 dB for the organically deaf group at the first three test frequencies. Mean reaction thresholds were less at 4000 Hz. Respiration alterations were obtained in the group without hearing only at 97 dB at 125 Hz, which was interpreted as a tactile response. Rosenau (1962b) made known his observation of respiration changes in children during sleep, that the deepness of the sleep had almost no effect on the change in respiration (when stimulated with sound intensities from 50 to 60 dB). He concluded from his studies that the sleep-hearing test could be used with children from 5 months to 6 years of age.

Some modifications of Rosenau's sleep-hearing test have been suggested by his associates to improve the recordings and to allow utilization of the test with awake children. Wagner (1963) employed a modified psycho-galvanometer and constructed a different "pneumobelt" to improve respiration recordings. Lehnhardt (1963) introduced a cadmium-sulfide-photo pneumograph to record more accurately thoracic movements for air- and bone-conduction assessments. He wrote:

> When the stimulus, after the proposal of Rosenau, begins in the first third of the inspiration, then during the last third of inspiration a shallowing typically occurs. It can show itself as a slight, perhaps only suggested, bend in the rising curve up to a distinct lessening of the depth of breath [p. 626].

He confirmed that the "reaction threshold," as found by Rosenau, was between 50 and 60 dB when the child is falling asleep. In addition, he found that thresholds were elevated by about 30 dB in deep sleep and 30 to 40 dB when the child was sedated with Luminal or rectal chloral hydrate.

Other research in Germany was conducted to reduce the time required for testing during sleep. Mahler and Wagner (1967) obtained respiration alterations in the waking state with a 20-impulse pure-tone stimulus. In order to save time, only the frequencies of 500 and 2000 Hz were tested. They said that "the certainty of the audiometric result appears considerably higher than the sleep sounding because the reactions are very obvious and therefore uncertainties of evaluation are very much absent [p. 515]." The investigators concluded that both the sleep and waking tests could be used with infants 6 months of age and older. Gerhardt *et al.* (1967) used rhythmic white-noise impulses synchronized with the subject's respiration rate as another way to test hearing sensitivity in the waking state. Changes in respiration rate and amplitude occurred with the first noise impulse: Irregular respiration was regularized; increasing the rate of the stimuli accelerated respiration rate up to some maximum; decreasing the rate of the stimulus decelerated respiration rate; and termination of the stimuli resulted in a rate decrease of ongoing rapid rates, and increased rates of previously slow rates. These changes occurred when subjects were falling asleep, but they were more distinct when the subject was awake. They claimed that this demonstrated efferent cortical control of respiration, in contrast to Rosenau's hypothesis of afferent control of respiration from the reticular formation during sleep.

Research with respiration alterations to sound has been conducted with infants in Japan and South Africa. During two experiments with sounds delivered through a speaker placed 15 cm from one ear, Suzuki *et al.* (1964) recorded awake infants' respiration with a pneumograph connected to a kymograph. Their first experiment was conducted with 45 normal neonates, from 5 hours to 7 days old, using a 500-Hz pure tone and an artificial sound (cow mooing). The stimuli were presented for a duration of 4 to 5 sec in 10-dB increments from 30 to 80 dB. They observed three respiration alterations:

> 1. Changes in rate or deepness of respiration, that is, becoming faster or slower in its rate or becoming deeper or shallower in its amplitude.
> 2. Decrease in regularity of respiratory movements which last 20 to 30 seconds after auditory stimulation. 3. Appearance of sudden deep inspiration [pp. 918–919].

The first two responses appeared at all intensity levels, but the appearance of deep inspirations increased significantly at 70- and 80-dB intensity levels. A second experiment was conducted with 61 neonates from 1 to 33 days of age. With a speaker placed 15 cm from the right ear, the infants were tested by 500- and 1000-Hz pure tones of 3- to 5-sec duration and at 10-dB increments of intensity from 40 to 90 dB. The average of respiration responses for these infants was found to be 62.8 dB.

Heron and Jacobs recorded infants' respiration changes to low-, middle-, and high-frequency modulated pure tones delivered through earphones. Respiration was recorded on a kymograph from a thermistor taped to the infant's nose. In one study (1968), the hearing of 150 7-day-old infants was tested with 40-, 60-, and 90-dB "modulated tones." The most frequent response was "breath holding or prolongation of inspiration probably a gasp," occurring one to three cycles after the beginning of the 5-sec stimulus tone, but after the tone was turned off. In another paper (1969), the hearing of 200 normal and 43 "at risk" neonates was tested with a low-, middle-, and high-frequency variable tone produced by a specially constructed "Frequency Modulated Audiometer" at 40, 60, and 100 dB. The most frequent respiration alteration to these stimuli was a "change of rate or depth of respiration or a 'gasp' reflex." The gasp occurred more frequently at the louder tones.

A series of papers has appeared reporting the use of the sound of a person's breathing, white noise, filtered white noise, and warble tones as a test of hearing (Kumpf, 1966, 1968a,b, 1970, 1972; Kumpf and Landwehr, 1970). In one series of experiments, the subject's breathing was recorded from a neck microphone, stored, and delayed for playback through earphones. While the subject's breathing was being traced on a level recorder, the delayed breathing sounds were amplified in increasing 5-dB steps. This procedure produced the Lee effect on the subject's breathing. In other experiments, white noise, filtered white noise, and warble tones were recorded on the channel of the recorder, and the intensity was continuously increased through an earphone placed on the test ear at a rate of 1 dB per second while the subject's breathing was recorded on the second channel. The white noise, warble tones, and the sounds of respiration were played into a level recorder to obtain a synchronized write-out for visual scoring, which Kumpf termed a "Pegeldiagram." A "decrement" or an "increment" of the breathing sound was reported to occur depending on the intensity level of the stimulus. Decrements, or a decrease in the amplitude of the breathing sound, occurred near auditory threshold and consisted of either pauses between inspiration and expiration or a reduction in the amplitude of the breathing sound. It was hypothesized that this phenomenon occurred because "it is not absolute silence which is 'breathtaking' but a weak acoustic stimulus which interrupts the silence [1972, p. 76]." Kumpf obtained these responses at intensity levels which compare well with the subject's voluntary threshold level. Strengthening, or an increase in the amplitude of the breathing sound, occurred when the level was about 30 dB or more above the subject's voluntary threshold level. This phenomenon was described as the "Lombard experiment with sound of breathing." Respiration responses recorded by this method were reported to measure successfully air- and bone-conduction thresholds with children when awake (Kumpf and Landwehr, 1970) and when under sedation (1972); but the procedure is not successful when the subject is sleeping deeply.

IV. RESPIRATION AUDIOMETRY

A. Recording and Scoring of Respiration Traces

1. Respiration Recording Instruments. In 1847, Karl Ludwig added a float to the mercury hemodynamometer developed in 1823 by Jean–Leonard–Marie Poiseulle to measure blood pressure. A stylus was attached to the float and connected to a recording cylinder. Thus, he introduced a graphic recording instrument, the kymograph (wave writer), to physiology. Respiration patterns were first recorded in 1855 by Vierordt and Ludwig, using a sphymograph connected to a kymograph. The "pneumographe" designed by Etienne–Jules Marey (1865, 1876) became the standard instrument for obtaining graphic writeouts of thoracic cage and abdominal movements during breathing. Respiration rate and patterning variations were obtained by placing the pneumograph around the thorax, or the abdomen, and connecting it to the stylus for recording on Ludwig's kymograph or on a polygraph developed by Marey. Mechanical–electrical systems using wire or rubber-filled tubing strain gauges (Hesse, 1959; Montague, 1957; Wade, 1954) and thermistors, which record temperature variations between inspired and expired air at the nares (Heron and Jacobs, 1969; Lipton *et al.*, 1964) permitted the measuring of small respiratory movement satisfactory for respiration audiometry. A completely electrical system of transthoracic impedance pneumography, employed by Atzler (1935) for cardiac measurements, has been used successfully for measuring breathing of humans (Geddes *et al.*, 1962; McCollum *et al.*, 1969) and of animals (Fenning, 1936; Fenning and Bonar, 1936). Other recording devices reported in the literature include the inspiration–expiration recorder (Burtt, 1918; Nixon, 1923), multiple capsule pneumography (Baglioni, 1929), body plethysmograph (Golla and Antonovitch, 1929), ordinate time recorder (Fleisch, 1935), pneumotachograph (Lee and Silverman, 1943), and the acoustic respirograph (Margolin and Kubie, 1943).

The initial research and clinical work with respiration audiometry at The Menninger Foundation employed a mechanical–electrical recording system with a mercury-in-rubber strain gauge. The present system consists of a bellows-actuated photoelectric cell strain gauge, stimulus timer, and a two-channel polygraph recorder with heat sensitive paper. A schematic drawing of the components connected to a patient is shown in Figure 3. An illustration of the recording unit and strain gauge designed by Rex Hartzell of the Bio-Medical Laboratory at The Menninger Foun-

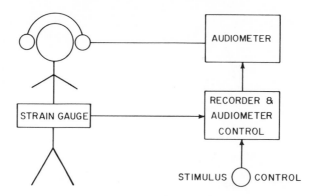

Figure 3 Schematic drawing of the respiration audiometry equipment on a patient.

dation is shown in Figure 4. The strain gauge is fitted snugly, but not tightly, around the chest of the person being tested. The movements of the chest during respiration lengthen or contract the bellows. The bellows' changes are recorded on the polygraph as upward deflections for inspiration and as downward deflections for expiration. One channel of the polygraph serves as the event marker to record precisely the point and duration of the 250 msec stimulus tone, and the second channel records the respiration cycle traces. The paper speed of the prototype polygraph can be set to run at 5 and 10 mm per sec. The slower speed is used for making recording stylus adjustments, and the faster speed is used during testing. The respiration trace is adjusted on the strip chart by a position control knob to permit free swings within the width of the paper chart. The amount of stylus deflection, or amplitude of the respiration cycles, is adjusted by a balance control knob. The amplitude of the respiration cycle recordings can vary between 25 and 60 mm in width. The position and balance controls can be readjusted during testing to compensate for body movements and respiration fluctuations.

These units are adaptable to single- or two-room arrangements, and, when connected to an audiometer, permit the testing of hearing sensitivity with pure tones delivered through earphones or a bone vibrator. The strain gauge and earphone placements on an infant are shown in Figure 5 and on an adult in Figure 6.

The hearing sensitivity of patients is tested while they remain relatively still, in a sitting or reclining position. They may be tested either when awake, when relaxed by medication, or when sleeping naturally. Infants may be tested while sitting or reclining on a parent's lap or in an infant's seat. For young children who may be frightened by the test environment, a parent remains with the child in the test room. The patient

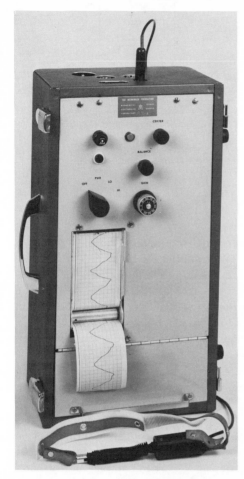

Figure 4 Prototype of the respiration recording unit and strain gauge.

is told that he will not feel anything from the "belt" that is placed around his chest, that he is to relax and remain as quiet as possible, that he does not have to say or do anything when he hears a tone, and that he may go to sleep if he wishes. An adjustment period is needed for some patients to relax sufficiently to regularize their breathing rate and pattern.

Resting respiration cycles are somewhat regular in amplitude and duration, and irregular during distraction and states of tension and anxiety. Extraneous body movements reduce the smoothness and regularity of the trace patterns and impair the differentiation of tone responses from body movements. For those who are unable to remain relatively quiet while awake, the testing is delayed until they become more relaxed or

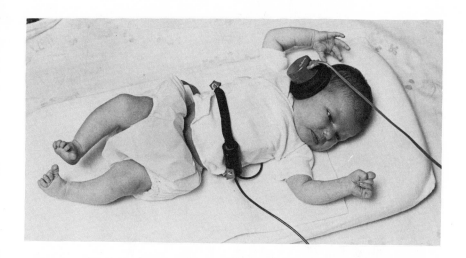

Figure 5 Strain gauge and earphone on a neonate. (Reproduced with permission of The Menninger Foundation.)

fall asleep. Infants usually fall asleep after feeding, which permits easy testing. Natural sleep can be produced for the testing of older children if parents keep them up later than usual the night before the test, get them up earlier than usual on the test day, or prevent napping during the day of the hearing examination. For those persons who are unable to relax or to fall asleep in the test room, sedation prescribed by a physician and administered by a nurse may be used. Liquid chloral hydrate for younger children and Sparine for older children have been used successfully in our clinic. The medication can be administered 15 to 20 min before testing begins, and provides about 1 hour of relaxation. When the respiration cycles have regularized, the testing can begin.

2. *Scoring Respiration Responses.* The search for valid respiration alterations following pure-tone presentations has examined automation, measuring, and visual methods of scoring. Although all three scoring procedures can be used successfully to infer auditory thresholds, the visual inspection procedure has been found to be the most practical method for clinical use (Rousey, 1969).

The three respiration cycle patterns to consider when presenting the tones and scoring the responses are the *resting, response,* and *recovery* cycles shown in Figure 7. The resting respiration cycles are the regular breathing cycles immediately preceding a tone presentation. The single cycle in which the pure tone is delivered is the response cycle. The re-

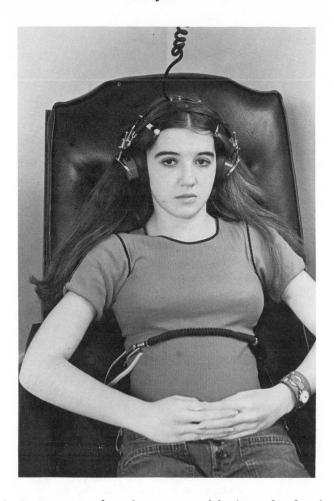

Figure 6 Strain gauge and earphones on an adult. (Reproduced with permission of The Menninger Foundation.)

covery respiration cycle is that cycle immediately following the response cycle.

When at least two resting cycles of approximately the same amplitude have been traced, the pure tone is presented at the *beginning of the inspiration phase* of the next cycle. This response cycle is examined for an alteration in the respiratory pattern by visually comparing it with the resting and recovery cycles. A valid cycle alteration will appear only in the response cycle—the cycle in which the tone is presented.

Research of hearing sensitivity by respiration audiometry has revealed

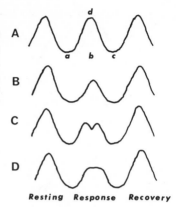

Figure 7 The resting, response, and recovery cycles used in respiration audiometry. A single respiration cycle (a–c) of a trace pattern recorded during eupnea (A) consists of inhalation (a–d), exhalation (d–c), and amplitude (b–d). The respiration alterations used for determining auditory thresholds include an amplitude reduction (B), a jamming or an M-shaped pattern (C), and a flattening (D) of the response cycle. The traces are recorded from left to right. Inspiration carries the curves up, expiration down.

three response cycle alterations related to hearing thresholds (Rousey, 1969). Figure 7 also illustrates respiration traces of eupnea and the three respiration alterations—a *reduction* of amplitude, a *jamming* of two cycles together or an *M-shaped* pattern, and a *flattening* of the positive peak. Clinical illustrations of amplitude reductions are shown in Figure 8,

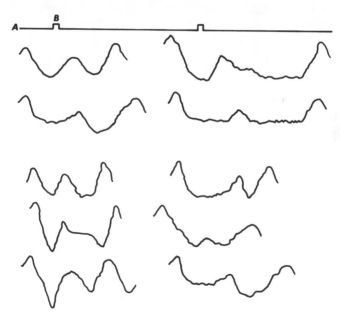

Figure 8 Clinical examples of amplitude reductions in the response cycle following presentation of a 250-msec pure tone at the beginning of inhalation. The second pen on the polygraph (A) deflects (B) to show the location and duration of the stimulus.

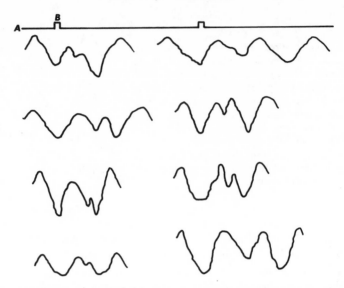

Figure 9 Clinical examples of jammed or M-shaped patterns in the response cycle following presentation of a 250-msec pure tone at the beginning of inhalation. The second pen on the polygraph (A) deflects (B) to show the location and duration of the stimulus.

jammed cycles in Figure 9, and positive-peak flattenings in Figure 10. From our experience, a reduction of amplitude occurs most frequently with presentations of pure-tone stimuli.

There are visual criteria used for determining a valid response cycle alteration. Attention must be given to the amplitudes of the resting, response, and recovery cycles when determining the existence of a reduced amplitude in the response cycle. If the amplitude of the recovery cycle exceeds the amplitude of the resting cycles, or if the amplitude of the resting cycles exceeds the amplitude of the recovery cycle, the cycle with the lesser amplitude is used for comparing a response-cycle reduction. If the amplitude of the recovery cycle is less than the amplitude of the response cycle, or if the recovery cycle is disturbed by some body movement, it is necessary to reestablish the resting cycles and to introduce the tone again at the same intensity level. A tone is presented no more than three times at one intensity level. The jamming of two cycles together or a flattened response cycle is not determined by the amplitude of the resting and recovery cycles. These two alterations need not be reduced in amplitude, although a reduction may occur. Any one or all of these three alterations—reduction, jamming, or flattening—may appear during the testing of a single patient.

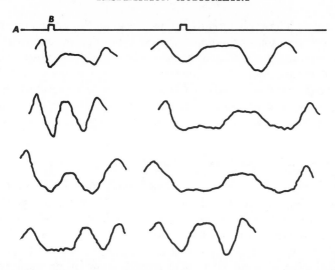

Figure 10 Clinical examples of flattenings in the response cycle following presentation of a 250-msec pure tone at the beginning of inhalation. The second pen on the polygraph (A) deflects (B) to show the location and duration of the stimulus.

The pure tones are delivered by the ascending method of standard audiometry in 5-dB steps, starting at 0 dB. An ascending presentation of the test tones is continued until two, and preferably three, scorable responses are recorded at successive 5-dB levels, or until the limits of the audiometer are reached. The ascending series is repeated, starting at 0 dB or at the intensity level 10 dB below the lowest response of the first ascending series. If three successive responses are recorded at this lower level, another ascending series should be made, starting at an intensity level 10 dB below the lowest response level in the second series. This procedure can be continued until the same three successive responses are recorded in two consecutive ascending series. The threshold for the test frequency is inferred to be the lowest intensity level of the two ascending series. This procedure is employed with each ear and test frequency. The frequencies typically tested in both ears at our clinic are 500, 1000, and 2000 Hz, with other frequencies and bone conduction being examined as indicated. Appropriate contralateral ear masking is used when there are significant air-conduction threshold differences between ears and when needed for bone-conduction testing.

In summary, the following criteria must be maintained when scoring respiratory alterations for valid auditory threshold determinations: (*1*) Only three respiratory alterations—a reduction of amplitude, a jammed or M-shaped pattern, and a flattening—are used for determining a response. (2) The cycle alteration must occur in the cycle immediately following presentation of the tone. (3) Two, and preferably three, of the described alterations must occur at consecutive 5-dB intensity levels before the cycle alteration at the lowest intensity level can be considered the threshold. Failure to observe this criterion may result in a false threshold, since it is conceivable that one of the three described breathing alterations might occur by chance with a presentation of the stimulus.

B. Research with Respiration Audiometry

1. Respiration Thresholds Compared with Standard Audiometric Thresholds. Research in the United States with indirect assessments of hearing sensitivity by recorded changes in breathing was initiated at The Menninger Foundation in 1964 by Clyde L. Rousey. Five studies were published in the next 5 years, testing the hypothesis that significant lengthening of the respiration cycle would occur at or near auditory thresholds for pure-tone stimuli produced by a clinical audiometer. The tones were delivered through earphones worn by the subjects while reclining on a couch in a supine position. The respiration cycle following introduction of a pure tone was hand-measured and compared with the length of the preceding cycles. The thresholds inferred from this measurement were compared with voluntary thresholds obtained by standard audiometry. Rousey *et al.* (1964) compared thresholds obtained by both test methods with 10 normal-hearing persons, 14 to 17 years of age. Only one ear was tested at 1000 Hz in 5-dB steps from 100 to −20 dB. They reported that 5 of 10 subjects slowed their breathing, i.e., lengthened the respiration cycle, at intensity levels that were within ±10 dB of voluntary thresholds. In another study (Poole *et al.*, 1966), respiration thresholds measured from cycle lengthenings were within ±15 dB; and retest thresholds were within ±10 dB of voluntary thresholds at 1000 Hz among 35 of 36 college-age subjects without ear pathology. Rousey and Reitz (1967) examined respiration cycle lengthenings in response to visual and auditory stimuli in two separate groups of subjects with normal hearing. In the visual study, the respiration alterations of four females and seven males, ages 17 to 25, were recorded while various intensities of a green-colored circle of light were presented. In the auditory study, the respiration alterations of 11 females, ages 21 to 50, were recorded. The 1000-Hz tone was presented five times to one ear of each subject in 5-dB steps from 50 through −15 dB. Although a consistent relationship between respiratory cycle lengthenings and predetermined visual thresholds was not found, respiration cycle lengthenings from the auditory stimulus were found to be within ±10 dB of voluntary thresholds in 10 of the 11 subjects. Respiration thresholds at 250 and 500 Hz were obtained by cycle measurements of 94 students attending the Kansas School for the Deaf, who had bilateral sensorineural hearing losses (Teel *et al.*, 1967). Of the respiration thresholds, 94% were within ±10 dB of these students' voluntary thresholds. Brooks and Gieschen (1968) examined 30 adults with voluntary thresholds between 10 and 55 dB at 4000 Hz and found that all respiration thresholds were within ±10 dB of voluntary thresholds ($r = .91$). These five studies demonstrated that the respiration thresholds determined from respiration cycle lengthenings were within ±10 dB of voluntary thresholds in 168 of the 181 ears tested (93%), and that the test–retest reliability examined in the one study was high.

A series of experiments was conducted next to investigate various parameters which influenced respiratory patterns at or near the threshold of hearing (Rousey, 1969). To circumvent the limitations of the hand-measuring of cycles employed in the first five studies, the initial experiments in this series of experiments utilized a semiautomated system to measure the cycles. The experiments with the semiautomated system were undertaken to ascertain the best estimate for comparing respiration thresholds to standard thresholds. These investigations compared: (*1*) the measurement of half-cycle duration with half-cycle amplitude; (*2*) the presentation of tones at the beginning of the inspiration phase with tones presented at the beginning of the expiration phase of respiration; (*3*) the presentation of the stimuli in ascending order with the descending order; and (*4*) the stimulus durations of 250, 500, 750, 1000, 1500, and 2000 msec. The more accurate estimates of the voluntary thresholds were obtained by automation from duration, or cycle lengthening measures, rather than from measures of amplitude changes. With the semiautomated system, it was found that accurate estimates of voluntary thresholds could be obtained with a 250-msec pure tone presented at the beginning of the inspiration phase of respiration, and by using the ascending method of tone presentation.

In another experiment in Rousey's series, respiration thresholds were obtained for 35 children with moderate to profound hearing losses, who attended the Kansas School for the Deaf. The relationship between their voluntary and respiration thresholds was not as high as had been found among the normal-hearing subjects in previous studies. Furthermore, the respiration thresholds of the hearing-impaired children determined from the semiautomated system and their voluntary thresholds did not compare as closely as did the hand-measured and voluntary thresholds of the deaf children tested by Teel and associates in 1967. This finding was attributed to the irregularity of the children's breathing patterns; the semiautomated system appeared to work effectively only when smooth sine-wave curves were traced.

Because the automated system approach was not sufficiently accurate for all clinical assessments, the trace records of selected subjects from previous experiments were reexamined for possible visual criteria that would accurately indicate thresholds. It was concluded that valid inferences could be made from "eyeballing" the entire trace record and noting any one, or combination, of three respiration alterations—reduction of amplitude, jamming of two cycles together, and flattening of the curve at either the positive or the negative peak. In addition, the lowest intensity level of two or three alterations at successive 5-dB increases of intensity was an indicator of threshold.

Two additional experiments using the newly established visual criteria were conducted to examine the effects of visual distraction and the effects of natural and sedated sleep on auditory thresholds determined by respiration cycle alterations. In the visual distraction study, 17 subjects, age 20 to 55 years, were tested while sitting instead of reclining. Voluntary auditory thresholds were obtained. Respiration thresholds were obtained (1) when subjects were distracted by matching random numbers flashed onto the wall every 2 sec, with instructions to push a button each time an odd number appeared, and (2) when subjects were not distracted by a visual stimulus. The voluntary thresholds were then compared to the "distracted" and "nondistracted" thresholds. The distracted thresholds were elevated from 10 to 85 dB in 15 of the 17 subjects. The nondistracted thresholds were within ±10 dB of the voluntary thresholds for all 17 subjects. The inference was made that the respiratory changes at elevated intensity levels during visual distraction are likely to be a cortical phenomenon. The final experiment in Rousey's 1969 series investigated the effects of sleep on respiration alterations in two groups of subjects. One group was composed of mild to severely retarded children residing at the Kansas Neurological Institute, who were tested during sleep induced by Sparine. The other group included normal adults tested during natural sleep. Sleep depth was monitored by EEG, and the respiration thresholds were noted during the second stage of sleep. Respiration thresholds of the retarded children were within ±15 dB of their known behavioral thresholds in 61% of the tone presentations. The influence of Sparine on some of these children often elevated their respiration thresholds by approximately 30 dB. Respiration thresholds for five of the six normal adults while sleeping naturally were within 5 dB of their voluntary thresholds. It was concluded that thresholds obtained during the second stage of natural sleep produced thresholds essentially similar to those found during the waking state.

In 1971, Rousey and Bradford compared the respiration thresholds during natural sleep to both voluntary and awake respiration thresholds of 20 brain-damaged orthopedically handicapped and 30 normal-appearing children. The sleep stages were monitored by EEG. Comparison of the voluntary thresholds with awake respiration thresholds was within ±15 dB for 49 of the 50 subjects. Of the children, 94% had respiration thresholds that were within ±10 dB of their voluntary thresholds. Although the mean thresholds inferred from respiration changes progressively decreased during stages 2, 3, and 4 of sleep as compared to awake thresholds, the use of the mean obscured the idiosyncrasy of respiration responses. A pronounced hearing loss was noted for some children in stages 3 and 4 of sleep, while essentially normal thresholds were found in other children during these deeper stages of sleep. For some children, the thresholds obtained during stage 2, the lightest stage of sleep, were not necessarily better than those obtained in deeper stages of sleep. This study suggested that when normal or near-normal thresholds are obtained during sleep, the estimate is probably close to the true threshold. However, decreased hearing sensitivity inferred during natural sleep may not be valid, and the hearing should be either reevaluated at another time or obtained during a waking state.

Bradford *et al.* (1972) compared the voluntary and respiration thresholds of preschool children. One experiment examined hearing sensitivity in one ear of each of 13 4-year-old children at 1000 Hz. Hearing thresholds were found to be within ±10 dB of voluntary thresholds in 11 of the 13 ears tested. Another experiment examined both ears of each of 16 children (2–7 to 4–10 years of age) at 500 and 4000 Hz. Of the 32 ears tested in this experiment, 81% of the respiration thresholds were within ±10 dB of the voluntary thresholds at 500 Hz. Differences of 10 dB or less were obtained in 91% of the ears tested at 4000 Hz.

2. *Respiration Audiometry with Neonates and Infants.* Previous research with respiration audiometry had been systematically studied only with children as young as 2–7 years of age. Pilot research with two young infants revealed that pure tones produced respiration cycle alterations in these infants similar to those alterations obtained with older children and adults. These findings motivated the testing of additional infants during the first year of life—shortly after birth, at 4 months, and at 12 months of age.[4]

---

[4] This study was supported by the Frank J. Phillips Foundation and the Research Section of the Children's Division of the Menninger Clinic. The use of facilities for some of the neonatal testing at Stormont–Vail and St. Francis Hospitals in Topeka, Kansas, are acknowledged.

Hearing sensitivity was tested during the three examination periods at 1000 and 3000 Hz and immediately retested at 1000 Hz, with pure tones produced by an audiometer calibrated to ANSI 1969 standards and delivered through an earphone. The audiometric testing was completed in non-sound-treated rooms when the noise levels were below those permitted for testing under earphones. With one ear toward the mattress, only the exposed ear was examined while the infants were sleeping naturally or lying quietly in a prone or supine position. An illustration of the strain gauge and earphone placement on an infant is shown in Figure 5.

Twenty-five full-term Caucasian newborns (14 boys and 11 girls) were tested from 2 to 24 days after their birth. The babies had no physical defects and the mothers no illnesses during pregnancy, and there was no known congenital hearing impairment in the families. The canals of the test ear were patent and free of vernix. Respiration thresholds at 1000 and 3000 Hz were 0 dB for 24 neonates and 5 dB for one neonate. All retest thresholds at 1000 Hz were 0 dB, except that one neonate with a test threshold of 0 dB had a retest threshold of 5 dB.

Of the original babies, 23 were available for testing at 4 months of age. Thresholds at 1000, 3000, and 1000 Hz were 0 dB for all of the infants. Hearing thresholds were obtained from 14 infants at 1 year of age. The hearing of four of the 1-year-olds could not be tested because they awakened when the strain gauge was placed on them, and they would not remain quiet or return to sleep. The families of the remaining children had moved from the city. Of the 14 infants examined at 12 months of age, thresholds of 0 dB were found at the test and retest frequencies for 13 infants. Figure 11 illustrates a typical respiration trace record obtained from the infants during the three examination periods. The fourteenth infant had an ear infection at the time of the scheduled 12-month examination. Her hearing was examined at 500, 1000, and 2000 Hz at that time, and again one month later after placement of pressure-equalization tubes in her ears. The trace records of this infant's responses during the four examinations are shown in Figure 12.

The findings of this study with normal infants during the first year of life demonstrated that pure tones alter newborn and infants' respiration patterns in a manner similar to that which had been observed with older children and adults. The test–retest reliability at 1000 Hz was excellent for all of the infants. This study suggested that respiration audiometry may be employed for determining neonatal and infant hearing sensitivity, and future research is planned to study the efficacy of respiration audiometry with high-risk infants.

3. *Respiration Audiometry with Deaf–Blind Children.* A diagnostic,

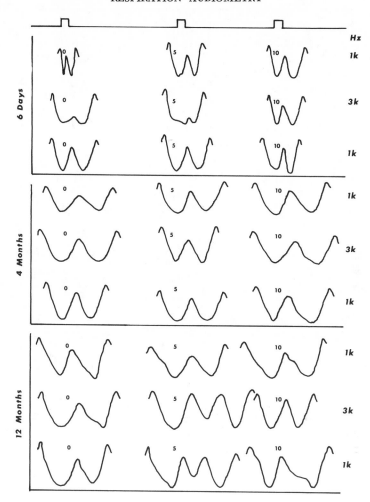

Figure 11 Test-retest respiration alterations from 1- and 3-kHz pure tones presented through an earphone to the right ear of an infant at 6 days, at 4 months, and at 12 months of age, while sleeping naturally. The decibel levels of the stimuli are shown by the numbers in the response cycle.

educational, and training program for deaf–blind children is maintained at the Kansas Neurological Institute in Topeka, Kansas. The severe neurological involvement of the children in this program prevented assessing their hearing by standard audiometric procedures, and their hearing sensitivity had never been determined. Therefore, an attempt was made to assess indirectly the hearing of the 14 children in this residential program

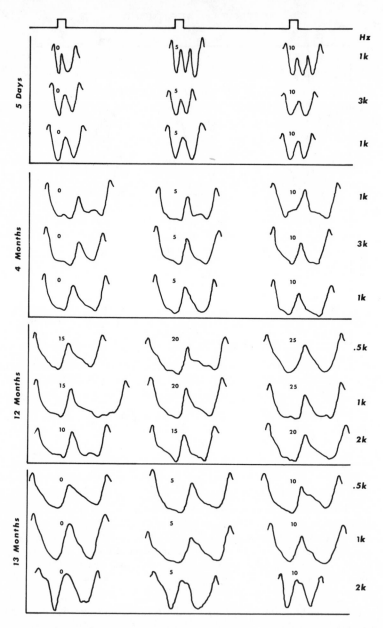

Figure 12 Test–retest respiration alterations from 1- and 3-kHz pure tones presented through an earphone to the left ear of an infant at 5 days and 4 months of age; from .5-, 1-, and 2-kHz pure tones when she had an ear infection at 12 months of age; and following placement of pressure-equalization tubes at 13 months of age. All thresholds were determined while she was sleeping naturally. The decibel level of the pure tones are shown by the numbers in the response cycle.

278

by respiration audiometry. The children, nine boys and five girls, ranged in age from 3 to 13 years. The intellectual development of all of them was classified as being at AAMD Level IV or V. Air-conduction thresholds at 500, 1000, and 2000 Hz were measured in both ears, using earphones and a commercial audiometer calibrated to ANSI 1969 standards. The hearing tests were conducted in a non-sound-treated room sufficiently quiet for determining thresholds under earphones. Hearing sensitivity was measured during natural sleep for two of the children. The remainder were tested after being sedated by Sodium Amytal, Sparine, or Seconal to reduce extraneous movements. Thresholds could not be obtained from two of the children because the medication was unsuccessful in calming them. Thresholds were obtained from both ears in one test session for 10 children, eight while sedated and two while sleeping naturally. Two of the sedated children required two testings because they either awakened or became so hyperactive after completion of the testing of one ear that further testing could not be done. During a second session, the activity was reduced sufficiently in these children to obtain threshold tracings in the untested ear and a retest of the previously tested ear. The test–retest thresholds for one ear of each of the two children were found to be the same, except that the retest thresholds were 5 dB better for one child at 1000 Hz and for the other child at 2000 Hz. The test-retest respiration trace records of one of the children are shown in Figure 13.

4. *Respiration Audiometry with Dogs.* Bradford *et al.* (1973) reported on the use of altered respiration responses as a procedure for assessing the hearing sensitivity of dogs. Hearing in the right ear only was tested with a normal-appearing Dachshund and a hearing-impaired Springer Spaniel, with pure tones produced by a commercial audiometer calibrated to ANSI 1969 standards. Placement of the strain gauge and earphone on the Dachshund is shown in Figure 14. The Dachshund's hearing was tested, while she lay quietly beside her owner, at 500, 1000, and 8000 Hz and retested 15 min later at the same three frequencies. This dog's hearing sensitivity was found to be 0 dB at the three frequencies during the test and retest examinations. The respiration trace records from which these thresholds were determined are shown in Figure 15. The Springer Spaniel had a bilateral absence of the tympanic membranes and auditory ossicles, presumed to have been congenital. Sedation with Acepromazine Maleate was required to reduce her respiration rate so that the trace records could be read. Hearing sensitivity was tested at 500, 1000, and 2000 Hz by air conduction and at 1000 and 4000 Hz by bone conduction. The air-conduction thresholds were depressed at all three frequencies, while the bone-conduction thresholds were 0 dB. These thresholds suggested a conductive type hearing loss compatible

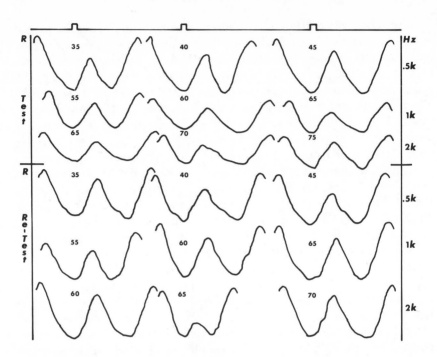

Figure 13 Test–retest respiration alterations from .5-, 1-, and 2-kHz pure tones presented through an earphone to the right ear of a 9-year-old deaf-blind girl when sedated by Sparine.

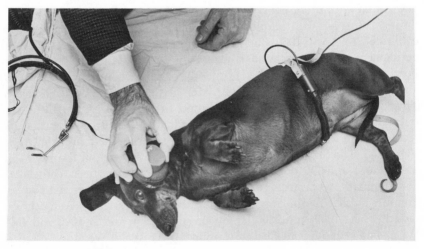

Figure 14 Strain gauge and earphone on a Dachshund. (Reproduced, with permission, from Bradford et al., 1973.)

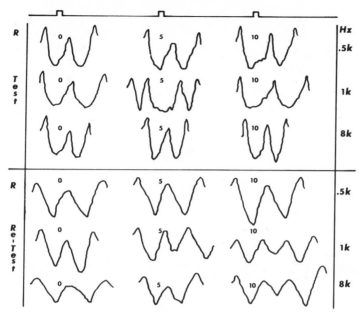

Figure 15 Test–retest respiration alterations from .5-, 1-, and 8-kHz pure tones presented through an earphone to the right ear of a Dachshund. The recordings were made while the dog was awake. The decibel levels of the stimuli are shown by the numbers in the response cycle. (Rproduced, with permission, from Bradford *et al.,* 1973.)

with the condition of her middle ear. The respiration trace records for the Springer Spaniel are shown in Figure 16.

The polygraph trace records of the two dogs revealed similarities to, and one difference from those observed with humans. The trace records with the Dachshund looked similar to records obtained from older infants and adults. The breathing rate of the Springer Spaniel was even more rapid with sedation than had been observed with sleeping newborns. The two double cycle reductions traced with this animal are probably related to her rapid respiration rate. The most frequent respiration alteration occurring in both animals was an amplitude reduction, although response-cycle flattening and M-shaped patterns did occur. This study suggested the practicability of using respiration audiometry for measuring hearing sensitivity by air and bone conduction with small and large dogs.

C. Summary

This section reviewed the research with respiration alterations as an indirect assessment of hearing sensitivity conducted at The Menninger

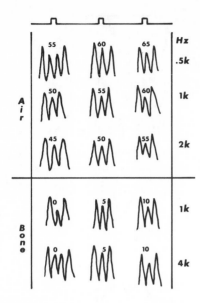

Figure 16 Respiration alterations from air-conduction (.5-, 1-, and 2-kHz) and bone-conduction (1- and 4-kHz) pure tones presented to the left ear of a Springer Spaniel. The recordings were made during induced sleep. The decibel levels of the stimuli are shown by the numbers in the response cycle. (Reproduced, with permission, from Bradford *et al.*, 1973.)

Foundation during the past 10 years. These studies have examined various parameters affecting respiration alterations and scoring methods in humans of varying ages, physical conditions, and hearing levels, and in humans and animals when awake and asleep. The studies, for the most part, compared voluntary thresholds with respiration thresholds to establish the validity between thresholds determined from the standard audiometric procedure and the indirect procedure. Studies of neonates' hearing during the first year of life, of deaf–blind children, and of dogs were reported, although threshold comparisons were not possible. This research has demonstrated the effectiveness of respiration audiometry for determining hearing thresholds with (1) humans and animals resting quietly, sleeping naturally, or in sedated sleep; (2) persons in a reclining or upright position; (3) 250 msec pure tones produced by a commercial audiometer and delivered through earphones; and (4) tones presented at the beginning of the inspiration phase of the respiration cycle. The respiration alterations at or near threshold were found to be an amplitude reduction, a jamming of two cycles together, or a flattening of the cycle immediately following presentation of the tone. These alterations can be readily noted by visual inspection of the trace records. The research has demonstrated that the respiration thresholds were within ±15 dB of voluntary thresholds in over 90% of the subjects among whom comparisons could be made.

V. CLINICAL USE OF RESPIRATION AUDIOMETRY

A. Difficult-to-Test Persons

A series of examples taken from our clinical files are presented to demonstrate the application of respiration audiometry with difficult-to-test infants and children, hearing-impaired children and adults, and an adult with expressive aphasia. Although corroborating voluntary data was available after respiration audiometry thresholds were obtained with some patients, other patients required a 2- or 3-year follow-up to substantiate the original inferences about hearing sensitivity.

CASE 1. Respiration thresholds were inferred from two normal-appearing infants during the pilot research with neonatal and infant testing. The trace records obtained during natural sleep from IR at 21 days of age are shown in Figure 17. Bilateral hearing sensitivity was found to be

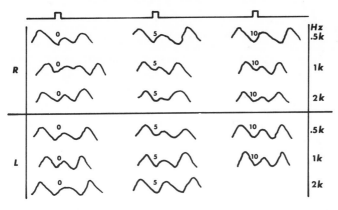

Figure 17 Respiration alterations from .5-, 1-, and 2-kHz pure tones presented through earphones to the left and right ears of 21-day-old IR. The recordings were made while she was awake.

0 dB at 500, 1000, and 2000 Hz. The hearing of AH was tested during natural sleep when she was 72 days of age. Her bilateral hearing sensitivity at 1000 and 2000 Hz was 0 dB. Retesting of her hearing at 83 days of age revealed identical bilateral thresholds except at 1000 Hz in the left ear, where her threshold was 5 dB. The test and retest respiration tracings of the left ear for AH are shown in Figure 18. Follow-up information from the parents indicated that IR, at 3 years of age, and AH,

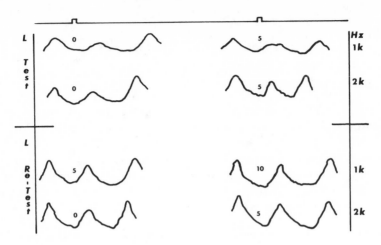

Figure 18 Respiration alterations from 1- and 2-kHz pure tones presented through an earphone to the left ear of AH, while sleeping naturally, at 72 (test) and 83 days of age (retest).

at 3½ years of age, had no hearing problems and had developed speech and language appropriate for their age.

CASE 2.   AS was referred to our clinic at 28 months of age because of unintelligible speech. His parents were concerned that he might be mentally retarded, since his wants and needs were communicated through gestures, pointing, and some guttural vocalizations. Because he sometimes ignored sounds and their speech, they also questioned his hearing. The pediatric evaluation indicated no medical problems to account for the delayed speech development. He localized to speech, noise, and warble tones at 20 dB in a sound field setting, suggesting that his hearing, at least in one ear, was not markedly impaired. Normal hearing sensitivity in both ears was found from respiration alterations obtained while he was awake. An illustration of the trace records for the right and left ears is shown in Figure 19. He was seen for individual speech therapy two times per week for the next 14 months at our clinic, and developed speech and language appropriate for his chronological age. Prior to termination of therapy, the original findings of normal hearing sensitivity as made from respiration alterations were substantiated from the voluntary thresholds obtained for the frequencies of 250 through 6000 Hz.

CASE 3.   DS was first fitted with a hearing aid in the right ear at 6½ years of age. The audiological data leading to the recommendation and fitting of the hearing aid was not available to us. The original hearing aid had to be replaced soon after fitting because he had lost it. Six months

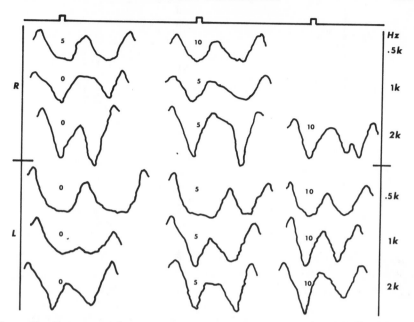

Figure 19 Respiration alterations from .5-, 1-, and 2-kHz pure tones presented through earphones to left and right ears of 28-month-old AS. The recordings were made while he was awake.

after being fitted with a hearing aid and prior to his being placed in a hard-of-hearing class, voluntary hearing thresholds were obtained at another clinic. These thresholds are shown in Figure 20. This hearing evaluation also revealed that word discrimination was impaired in the right ear; discrimination scores could not be obtained in the left ear. After attending the class for the hearing impaired for 2 months, he was transferred to a class for the mentally retarded because he seemed to hear but had difficulty understanding what he heard. He remained for the rest of the school year in the class for the mentally retarded. He was referred to our clinic that summer for a hearing evaluation because of poor academic achievement. Hearing sensitivity was found to be 0 dB through the speech frequencies in both ears; the respiration traces, which were recorded when he was awake, are shown in Figure 21. His word discrimination, as measured by the W-22 recorded test under earphones, was 6% in the right ear and 0% in the left ear. Following a complete medical, psychological, and psychiatric evaluation, he was diagnosed as being brain damaged, and transferred to a class for the neurologically impaired. After one year in this class, his hearing was evaluated again in our clinic. Voluntary air-conduction thresholds were found to be 0 dB for the fre-

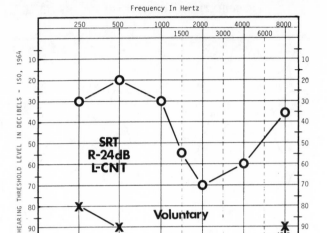

Figure 20 Voluntary pure-tone and speech reception thresholds of 6½-year-old DS.

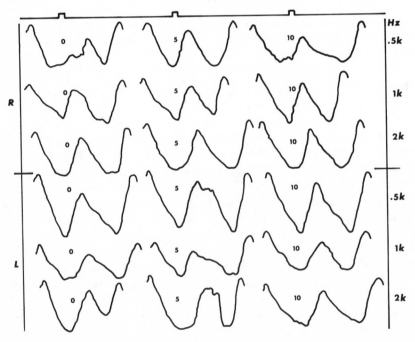

Figure 21 Respiration alterations from .5-, 1-, and 2-kHz pure tones presented through earphones to the right and left ears of DS. The recordings were made while he was awake.

quencies of 250 through 4000 Hz, and 10 dB at 8000 Hz in both ears; bilateral speech reception thresholds were 0 dB. These results corroborated the findings of normal hearing sensitivity made from the respiration alterations obtained the previous year. His word discrimination scores were again found to be as depressed as those obtained during the previous evaluations.

CASE 4. JH had a history of spinal meningitis in early infancy. A bilateral hearing impairment was suggested by respiration alterations obtained when he was 19 months of age. After being fitted with a hearing aid, the child and his parents attended a parent–home program for one year. From the age of 3 years, he attended a preschool program for hearing-impaired children. Respiration trace records, obtained when he was 5 years and 7 months of age, are shown in Figure 22. Respiration thresholds, shown in Figure 23, were found to be within ±15 dB for the frequencies of 500 through 2000 Hz.

CASE 5. SS, a 10-year-old boy, was evaluated at our clinic upon the referral from his special school. The case history revealed that the boy

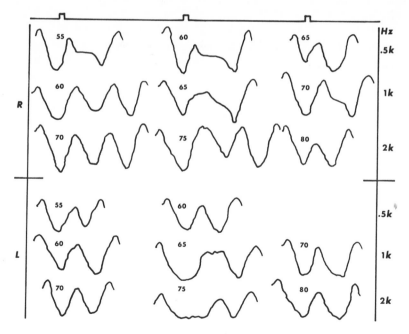

Figure 22 Respiration alterations from .5-, 1-, and 2-kHz pure tones presented through earphones to the right and left ears of JH. The recordings, made at 5 years and 7 months of age in June, 1972 were traced while he was awake.

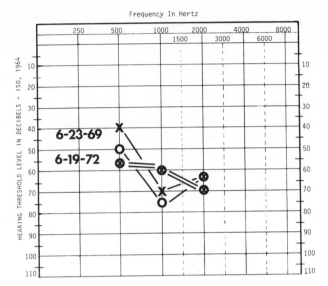

Figure 23 Thresholds determined from respiration alterations of JH at 19 months compared to thresholds determined from the respiration alterations shown in Figure 22.

was born by Caesarian section following five maternal miscarriages, had difficulty breathing for about 30 min after delivery, and within his first 24 hours had begun to have grand mal convulsions. He was later diagnosed by a neurologist as having a diffuse, congenital encephalopathy with the precise cause unknown but suspected to be anoxia. His delayed motor, language, and speech development had necessitated his enrollment in various special programs for children. At 7 years of age, a bilateral slight to severe hearing loss was detected at another clinic, and a body hearing aid was fitted in his right ear. The voluntary thresholds obtained at that clinic and the ones from which the recommendation for amplification was made are shown in Figure 24. Although he was fitted with a hearing aid, he had not worn the aid consistently. Because of his history of "brain damage" and inconsistent responses to speech with and without the hearing aid, the evaluation in our clinic was requested.

During an initial evaluation, hearing thresholds were determined from respiration alterations. As shown in Figure 25, bilateral sensitivity for the speech frequencies was within normal limits. During a second evaluation, these findings were substantiated by his voluntary responses for the frequencies of 250 to 6000 Hz. Speech reception thresholds were also 0 dB. Valid word discrimination scores could not be obtained because of his articulation deviations. However, the marked difficulty with word

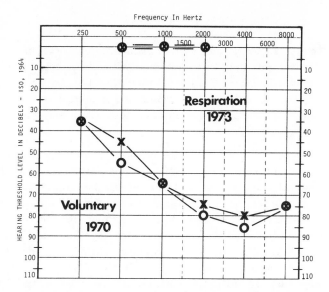

Figure 24 Voluntary pure-tone thresholds obtained at another clinic in 1970 compared to thresholds determined from the respiration alterations of SS shown in Figure 25, obtained in 1973.

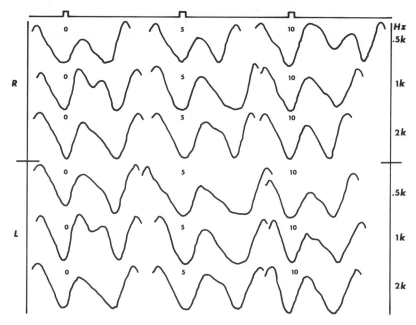

Figure 25 Respiration alterations from .5-, 1-, and 2-kHz pure tones delivered through earphones to the right and left ears of 10-year-old SS. The recordings were made while he was awake.

discrimination was not incompatible with his neurological diagnosis. This impairment in discrimination, in conjunction with his normal peripheral hearing, contraindicated the need for amplification. On the basis of this evaluation, the hearing aid was removed and his educational program was directed toward the central rather than the peripheral hearing impairment.

CASE 6. HD was a 57-year-old male whose hearing was assessed as part of an evaluation for physical disability compensation. He reportedly acquired a bilateral hearing loss at 6 months of age from measles. He entered a state school for the deaf when he was 7 years old and remained there until he was 21 years of age. While attending the school for the deaf, he became skilled in sign language, finger spelling, and a trade. After graduation from the school, he was successfully employed for the next 34 years, until he retired because of arthritis. Although he had attempted to use a hearing aid in the past, he had received no training in its use and had not proceeded beyond a few disappointing trials. His hearing sensitivity was measured by respiration audiometry when he was awake and sitting quietly in a chair. As shown in Figure 26, it was determined that he had some low-frequency residual hearing in both ears.

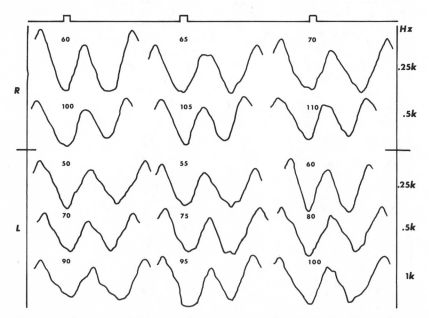

Figure 26 Respiration alterations from pure tones delivered through earphones to the right and left ears of 57-year-old profoundly deaf HD. The recordings were made while he was awake.

There were no scorable respiration alterations at the maximum intensity of the audiometer above 500 Hz in his right ear and 1000 Hz in his left ear. These thresholds were later confirmed by voluntary threshold testing, after instructions were conveyed to him by finger spelling and he responded with head nods.

CASE 7. RO was a 65-year-old male who had sustained a right hemiparesis and aphasia secondary to a left cerebral infarction 9 months prior to an evaluation in our clinic for language therapy. He arrived at our clinic with a neurological diagnosis of expressive aphasia, which was corroborated by our language assessment. Hearing sensitivity is routinely attempted with older aphasic patients evaluated in our clinic because of possible presbycusis. Voluntary thresholds were obtainable with this man by head-nodding responses. Figure 27 shows his respiration traces for both ears at the frequencies of 1000, 2000, and 4000 Hz. When compared to his voluntary thresholds, these thresholds noted from respiration alterations were the same at four frequencies and within 5 dB at two frequencies.

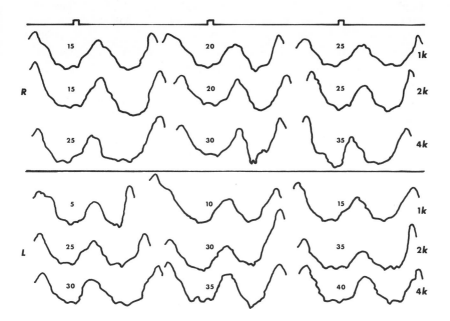

Figure 27 Respiration alterations recorded when awake from 1-, 2-, and 4-kHz pure tones delivered through earphones to the right and left ears of 65-year-old RO, obtained 9 months after a left cerebral infarction. The recordings were made while he was awake.

B. Psychogenic Hearing Losses[5]

1. Introduction. It is a common experience for all of us, as it was for Falstaff in Shakespeare's play, *Henry IV*, not to hear things that are spoken to us. When we "do not listen" or when we are "inattentive," our hearing can be restored by conscious efforts to "pay attention." However, some persons claim to have difficulty hearing when neither their past history nor their otologic examination reveals a reasonable cause for this claim. Matthew Henry (no date) exemplifies this by his comment that there are "none so deaf as those that will not hear." Patients who claim to have poor hearing but whose behavior or audiometric test findings may not substantiate a hearing deficit, all too often are considered to be neurotic and are classified as malingerers or hysterics (Grinker and Spiegel, 1945; Ingalls, 1946; Johnson *et al.*, 1956; Truex, 1946). In the first century A.D., the Greek physician, Galen of Pergamum, wrote about feigned illnesses in his treatise, "How to Detect Malingerers" (Veith, 1955). Malingering is commonly defined as the willful, deliberate, and fraudulent feigning or exaggeration of an illness or injury for the purpose of a consciously desired end. However, Brosin (1967) wrote that "most psychiatrists agree that genuine, conscious simulation of symptoms is uncommon. Such actions are difficult to plan and even more difficult to maintain [p. 750]." It is noteworthy that the prevalence of malingering, or at least confirmation from the person that he has been simulating an impairment, is very low with auditory impairments. Hopkinson (1967) reported only four or five such voluntary admissions in 17 years of clinical practice with a civilian population, and Grinker and Spiegel (1945) found only one or two cases among World War II veterans. Hysteria, as a clinical entity in an adult civilian population occurs quite rarely, and childhood hysteria is even less frequently encountered (Proctor, 1958; Robins and O'Neal, 1953). A review of the literature revealed only two psychiatrically confirmed cases of hysterical deafness in children (Berk and Feldman, 1958; Rank, 1942). It would appear that the feigning of a hearing loss and hysterical deafness do occur, but not frequently enough in a civilian population for understanding the severity of the patient's problem or for making a proper referral. The diagnostic task of the audiologist is made difficult by a predisposition toward the assumption of organic disorders, and by a frequent lack of knowledge of psychiatric etiologies. Audiometric test discrepancies have been accounted for by the use of such euphemistic terms as "nonorganic" (Martin, 1972),

[5] My appreciation is given to J. Tarlton Morrow, Jr., M.D., and Clyde L. Rousey, Ph.D., for their critical reading and constructive suggestions.

"exaggerated hearing level" (Engelberg, 1970), "pseudohypacusis" (Goldstein, 1966), and "functional" (Ventry and Chaiklin, 1962). Although physicians for many years have considered psychogenic etiologies in understanding their patients, audiologists do not routinely consider psychic factors when evaluating a patient's hearing.

2. *Psychogenesis.* A person's claim of hearing difficulty is a statement that is tested every day in an audiological clinic. The patient's assertion is assumed to be true, and the goal of the audiologist is to determine the amount of the loss and the site of the lesion (Martin, 1972). However, Hopkinson (1967) wrote that "the question of whether the patient with nonorganic hearing loss is malingering or is psychogenic is an academic one to the audiologist [p. 293]." This position, shared by many other audiologists, seems to indicate that audiologists are more interested in organic pathology than in psychic pathology, or are unaware of the potential impact of emotional factors on hearing sensitivity. The question is raised as to why this would be outside their realm of interest, since the ear is an audiopsychic organ, and hearing is a psychoacoustic phenomenon. Lipkin (1969) provides one answer in writing about functional disorders in medicine:

> It is often assumed that, first, "functional" means that the illness is not very important; second, that the suffering is not real ("it's all in the head" or "supratentorial"), though this tendency is dying out; third, that functional means difficult or impossible, or very time-consuming to treat; and fourth, that the patient whose illness is called functional is "a crock," and dull (as if it were the patient's obligation to interest the physician) [p. 1013].

Audiological training programs appear to put a great deal of emphasis on the organic, while providing minimal training in the "psychology of hearing." As a matter of fact, publications on the psychology of hearing have been restricted to studying persons' reactions to deafness (Levine, 1960; Mindel and Vernon, 1971; Ranier and Altshuler, 1967a,b; Ranier *et al.*, 1963; Rousey, 1971a; Schlesinger and Meadow, 1972; Solomon, 1943; Zeckel, 1950). Many professionals working with hearing impairments seem to ignore or overlook psychic factors related to hearing. Coleman's admonishment to otolaryngologists in 1949 could be heeded by audiologists today:

> The interrelationship between emotional experiences and physiological processes is no longer a speculative one. . . . The alteration of clinical symptomatology by psychic factors has been repeatedly witnessed by us as otolaryngologists. To underestimate the importance of these psychosomatic factors in otolaryngology is a disservice to our patients [p. 709].

The vast literature on psychogenic deafness and psychogenic factors related to otitis media, mastoiditis, otalgia, vestibular disturbances, and
otosclerosis summarized by Dunbar (1954) should not be ignored.

If the audiologist's role is to determine a patient's true hearing level,
this will not be possible without taking cognizance of psychogenic factors
in the hearing loss of some patients. Twenty-five years ago, Canfield
(1949) commented succinctly about this, as follows:

> Baffling diagnostic problems in audiometry have recently yielded to a
> more profound realization that hearing is not just a function of the ana-
> tomical structure known as the ear. When the brain and psyche are nor-
> mal, the usual audiometric procedures denote the hearing acuity with
> practical accuracy. But when the mental process is deranged, or func-
> tions abnormally, the signals sent to it by the ear may be grossly dis-
> torted. When these conditions are present, standard audiometry does
> not accurately measure the organic as contrasted with the psychogenic
> hearing loss [p. 12].

To understand any patient requires looking at the whole person—his
soma as well as his psyche. It was Hippocrates who commented, "In
order to cure the human body it is necessary to have knowledge of the
whole of things" (Dunbar, 1954). This counsel can be used with benefit
by audiologists.

The "lesion" in all patients is either organic, psychic, or a combination
of both. The term "psychogenic," as defined by Kaplan (1967), "is used
to signify that the eitology of a disease, sign or symptom, or its progress
or exacerbation, is, at least in part, psychologically determined [p 1120]."
The otolaryngologist Coleman (1949) found from his experience that one-
third of his patients had no "definite bodily disease to account for their
symptoms, illness or incapacitation," one-third were those "whose symptoms are part of or dependent on emotional factors," and the remaining
third were patients with organic disease for which "psychic disturbances
are a significant etiological factor [p. 713]." Hunter and Cawthorne
(1963) described two categories of patients seen by them, as follows:

> first, those in whom deafness is the chief symptom and who are for that
> reason likely to have been considered organically afflicted for the long-
> est time; and second, a group in which deafness, an exaggeration of
> deafness, or a merely apparent deafness is part of a more widespread
> psychological disturbance or indeed a major psychiatric syndrome [p.
> 205].

And it was Rosen (1953) who postulated that "symptoms and even syndromes . . . may mask schizophrenic reactions or hold suicidal depres-
sions in check [p. 424]." That restoration of hearing following surgery for

otosclerosis has been reported to result in either suicide or psychosis (Lester, 1971; Linn, 1953) suggests one of the defensive functions of not hearing and the tragedy of mechanically removing that defense without psychiatric support.

(a) *Psychogenic deafness as a symptom.* A person's claim of a hearing deficit is a symptom of organic and/or psychological impairment. Among audiologists, there is a clear understanding of organic symptomatology, since most audiological tests address themselves to finding the answer to organicity. However, there exists less understanding of psychological symptoms. Rousey (1971b) defines psychological symptoms in this way:

> A symptom (1) contains elements around hidden libidinal needs, (2) serves as an aggressive discharge in an external sense, (3) also has elements of self-directed aggression, (4) is a compromise between the aforementioned items and reality, (5) serves as a salvaging device to maintain one's equilibrium, and (6) is a distress signal to individuals in the environment [p. 820].

It is clear that symptoms reflect both the pathology and the maladaptive behaviors that give some integration and unity to the person. Psychiatric disorders are expressions of failure of the adaptive process (Mack and Semrad, 1967). Perkins (1938) defined a normal, healthy person "as one who can retain all his organs and tissues in a state of efficient function and physical organization against those external and internal forces that are constantly tending to disturb him." Menninger (1963), in his discussion of malingering, indicated that "no healthy person, no healthy-'minded' person would go to such extremes and take such devious and painful routes for minor gains that the invalid status brings to the malingerer [p. 208]." This observation is applicable to persons with psychogenic hearing losses. According to Prazic (1963), "we must consider the arising of the psychogenic deafness as a symptom of a certain psychic disturbance, or of a psychic alteration, or of a real psychic illness [p. 133]." Therefore, psychogenic deafness is best considered a significant symptom of psychopathology, a condition in which the audiologist can play a major role in diagnosis and psychiatric referral.

(b) *Not hearing as a defense against psychosis.* Defense mechanisms are psychological devices used to protect oneself against anxiety-provoking thoughts and experiences. They are used in everyday life to some extent but become pathological when used so extensively that interaction with one's environment becomes seriously distorted. Denial is a common defense mechanism that, with overuse, prevents a healthy interaction with the environment. Linn (1953) wrote that

in denial the ego reacts to some external reality as if it did not exist. . . .
A fact in the outer world may be denied, for example, because it represents a danger related to inner instinctual demands, rather than to any
danger inherent in that fact in contemporary reality [p. 700].

Denial, as a defense, is maintained at a high cost to one's efficiency and
relationship to reality. Excessive use of denial may be a precipitating
factor of psychosis (Mack and Semrad, 1967) or a protective device to
prevent psychosis (Davis and Fowler, 1960).

Dissociation can result from attempts to escape tension and anxiety by
separating one part of psychic life from the rest. Dissociation, according
to West (1967), is "a psychophysiological process whereby information
—incoming, stored, and outgoing—is actively deflected from integration
with its usual or expected associations [p. 890]." Cameron (1963) further
explains this psychic phenomenon by saying:

Dissociation becomes abnormal when the once mild and transient expe-
dient becomes too intense, lasts too long or escapes from the person's
control. It becomes abnormal whenever it leads to separation from the
surroundings which seriously disturbs object relations [p. 340].

It was Isakower (1939) who emphasized the role of hearing in maintaining contact with reality. It is postulated by this writer that denial of
hearing and dissociation from the environment occurs with some persons
to prevent psychic decompensation or psychosis itself. It seems naive to
"counsel" such persons to relinquish their "deafness" since such counsel
is usually unsuccessful (Ventry and Chaiklin, 1965) and very dangerous
to the well-being of the person.

  (c) Childhood psychosis. With many children, a differential diagnosis
requires a team effort because of the complexity of factors and behaviors
presenting themselves. Young children with delayed speech development
and those who appear nonresponsive to speech are frequently referred
to the audiological clinic because they are suspected of being hearing
impaired. The problem of differentiating mental retardation from deafness was reported as early as 1821 by Itard. Recognition of severe emotional disturbance or psychosis in young children has been made only
since the 1940s. Kanner (1944) described 11 children whose symptoms
constituted what he termed "early infantile autism." Among other symptoms, these children lacked auditory responses to people. Myklebust
(1954) considered autism to be a form of "psychic deafness." Most professionals now consider autism to be but one form of childhood psychosis.
Bender (1947) described "schizophrenia in childhood" and considered
it to be an organic abnormality. Mahler (1952) described a "symbiotic

psychosis" and considered it to be different from infantile autism. Autistic and schizophrenic children reportedly have been misdiagnosed as deaf or mentally retarded (Gelinier–Ortigues, 1955; Hefferman, 1955; Klein, 1956).

3. *Clinical Examples.*[6] Numerous tests have been developed for the detection of hearing "deception." Krugelstein, in his 1828 book, *Malingering and Disease,* tells about getting a response from a patient suspected of having normal hearing by informing him that his "fly is open" (Jacobson, 1898). Other procedures include the Stenger test (1900), the Lombard voice test (1911), and the more recent, sophisticated test made possible with electronics. Hanley and Tiffany (1954) found from their review of the literature that over 40 tests have been developed to detect deception. They reported that almost all of these tests were limited by "lack of reliability, dependence upon patient naiveté, and necessity for 'expert' interpretation [p. 197]." The utilization of respiration alterations, as described in Section IV of this chapter, is offered as a practical clinical procedure for testing persons suspected of having a psychogenic hearing impairment. Clinical material taken from our files is presented to illustrate the efficacy of respiration audiometry for testing such patients in any clinic setting. Although these patients had their hearing tested as part of psychiatric evaluation, the patients had been seen previously in numerous audiological clinics and must be considered as typical potential patients who are seen by any audiologist.

CASE 8. JL was evaluated in our clinic when he was 46 months of age. The limited vocalizations that he used were unintelligible. The neurological examination revealed poor motor coordination and soft neurological signs. Because he seemed to ignore people who spoke to him, there was also the concern that he might be either mentally retarded, autistic, or deaf. He localized to warble tones at 60 dB in a sound-field setting. Evaluation of his hearing sensitivity was made by respiration audiometry. From the awake respiration tracings, shown in Figure 28, it was determined that he had normal hearing sensitivity in both ears for the frequencies of 500 through 2000 Hz. Following the hearing evaluation and enrollment in a nursery school for emotionally disturbed children, his normal hearing sensitivity was substantiated by his psychotherapist and nursery school teacher. He was diagnosed as being autistic, rather than mentally retarded, on the basis of psychological evaluations. Two years after the hearing evaluation, he was talking, although his speech con-

---

[6] My thanks are extended to Estela Beale, M.D., and Cotter Hirschberg, M.D., for permission to use material about one of their patients.

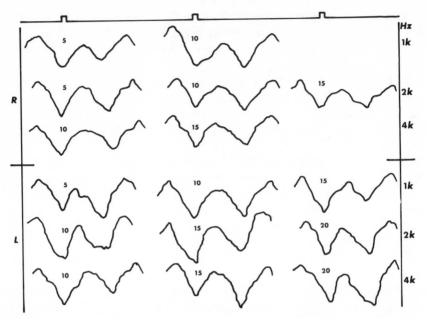

Figure 28 Respiration alterations from .5-, 1-, and 2-kHz pure tones presented through earphones to the left and right ears of 46-month-old JL. The recordings were made while he was awake.

tained numerous articulation errors. The therapists have observed that his speech became completely intelligible when he wanted his desires made known.

CASE 9. As an infant, MN was slow in developing speech and was suspected by his mother of being hearing impaired. His hearing was first tested by standard audiometric procedures when he was 4 years old. This and other evaluations during the next 2 years revealed a bilateral hearing impairment. He was fitted with a hearing aid just before his sixth birthday, enrolled in a state school for the deaf, and discharged 5 months later because the school officials observed that "he acted as if he had too much hearing to remain in the school." A similar opinion was expressed by his teacher after he was placed in a public school classroom for hearing-impaired children. An evaluation at our clinic was requested to assess further his hearing and assist the school in educational planning.

A review of the available records revealed no hearing impairments in his immediate family or medical problems known to cause a hearing deficit. He was born into a family that experienced much marital strife, separations, and finally a divorce when he was 5 years old. Because of the inadequate early care given to him by the family, he was first placed

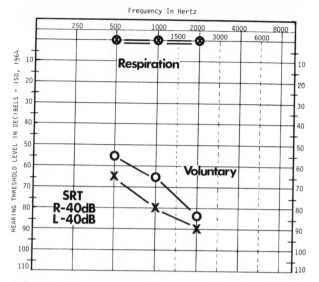

Figure 29 Voluntary pure-tone and speech reception thresholds compared to thresholds inferred from respiration alterations of MN shown in Figure 30.

in a foster home at 3½ years of age. He was living with his sixth foster family at the time of our evaluation. His speech and language development was not age appropriate, but his speech was better than expected for a child with a hearing loss comparable to his voluntary thresholds. Voluntary thresholds, as obtained in our clinic and shown in Figure 29, were not inconsistent with previous voluntary thresholds obtained at other clinics. His bilateral speech reception thresholds of 40 dB suggested that the voluntary thresholds were not valid. The air-conduction thresholds of 0 dB through the speech frequencies were noted from the respiration alterations shown in Figure 30. Because of these findings, it was recommended that he not wear the hearing aid. Following the evaluation, the boy was placed in a regular classroom for the remainder of the school year. His teachers and foster mother reported that he was functioning well without the hearing aid. Further follow-up on this boy was not possible because he was taken out of the state by his mother at the end of that school year.

CASE 10. RS was the fourth of five children born in a family that had no known hearing disorders. He had no medical problems known to cause a hearing impairment. His developmental milestones were normal except for speech. Although he was saying single words at 1 year of age, his

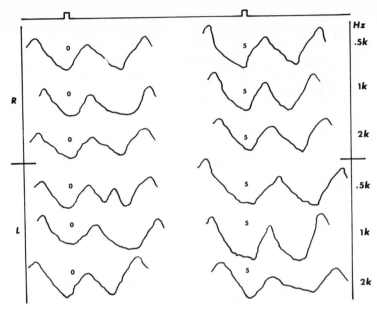

Figure 30 Respiration alterations from .5-, 1-, and 2-kHz pure tones presented through earphones to the right and left ears of 7-year-old MN. The recordings were made while he was awake.

later language did not develop beyond single words and short phrases. By the age of 3 years, he was fascinated by light bulbs and manifested rocking, withdrawal, and behavior management problems, all of which the parents tried to ignore. They had some question about a possible hearing impairment because of his inconsistent responses to speech. A diagnosis of "untreatable nerve deafness" was given to the family by different physicians, but standard audiological data indicating a bilateral hearing loss was not obtained until he was 7 years of age. After that hearing evaluation, the boy remained in the home without benefit of a hearing aid or education for another year. Because the parents were unable to manage him, another audiological test was requested. A profound hearing impairment, as shown in Figure 31, was again determined by voluntary responses. He was fitted with a hearing aid and enrolled in a state school for the deaf just before his eighth birthday. The parents did not believe that the school for the deaf was the correct place for him, for they thought he heard "better than he shows." They did consent to the placement because of his poor speech, bizarre behavior, and unmanageability in the home. A review of the records from the school for the deaf contained many references to this boy's normal hearing. One

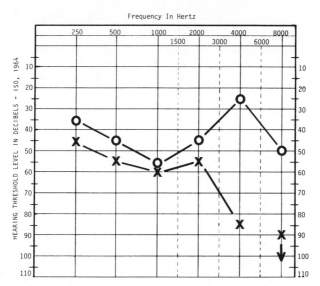

Figure 31 Voluntary thresholds given by RS at another clinic at 8 years of age.

teacher reported, "I've seen him react to speech, and the question asked was not in a loud voice. But he generally shows no reaction to the spoken word." Another teacher reported that "he gets much of his speaking vocabulary through hearing. He does not wear a hearing aid or earphones." Still another teacher reported that "he can talk if he wants to. He understands much if not all a person says to him." His academic achievement was slow, and he was a constant discipline problem to the staff by his provoking, kicking, and hitting other students and teachers, breaking windows, and destroying furniture at the school. He was discharged from the school 3 years after admission, with the recommendation that he receive psychiatric help because of his aggressive and unmanageable behavior. The parents were unwilling to accept this recommendation and he was again taken home, where he remained without attending school until that fall. Because of the family's inability to cope with his strangeness, they did consent to an evaluation for admission to a state mental hospital. As space limitations did not permit immediate admission to the hospital after the evaluation, he was again taken home, where he remained for another 8 months without treatment. He was finally admitted to the state hospital at 11 years, 8 months of age.

This boy's hearing was evaluated by respiration audiometry during the preadmission evaluation for placement, and again after his admission to the hospital. He would not cooperate for voluntary threshold testing during either evaluation. His bilateral hearing sensitivity was determined by the initial respiratory evaluation to be 0 dB through the speech frequencies. The hearing test by the respiration method during the second evaluation required administering 30 mg of Sparine to reduce extraneous body movements. From that evaluation, his hearing sensitivity, as determined from the respiration alterations shown in Figure 32, was again considered to be within normal limits in both ears.

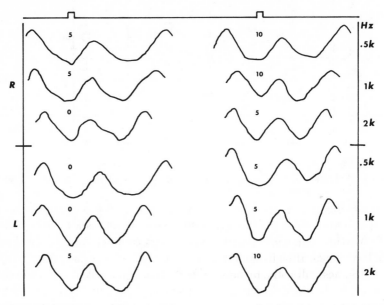

Figure 32 Respiration alterations from .5-, 1-, and 2-kHz pure tones presented through earphones to the right and left ears of RS at 11 years and 8 months of age following administration of Sparine.

The examining psychiatrist reported that his language was simple, personalized, and concrete; he spoke in single words, nouns, and verbs to convey ideas. His communication, play, and drawings consisted of compulsive, repetitive dealing with light bulbs, tornadoes, and destruction of people by heat from fire and the sun. The boy was seen for 30 hours of individual play therapy over a 5-month period. It was found that his hearing and speech functioning would fluctuate, but that he was able to articulate all speech phonemes, including the high-frequency sibilants. Other examiners reported that "when upset, R. is unable to understand others and others are unable to understand him. However, when he is angry, he uses a voice that sounds like a hearing child." During the 5-month therapy period, he had been observed to verbalize clearly four- and five-word sentences, and to respond to softly spoken speech, to unseen birds chirping outside, and to bushes brushing against the window when his back was turned toward it. About 14 months after admission to the hospital, his hearing was retested at another center, where test results substantiated the original findings of normal hearing sensitivity obtained by respiration audiometry. His bilateral voluntary thresholds were found to be normal for the frequencies of 250 through 8000 Hz (pure tone average, or PTA, 8 dB), and evoked cortical responses obtained from pure tones were as low as 15 dB through the speech frequencies in both ears. This boy's latter diagnosis of a schizophrenic reaction of childhood with symbiotic features could account for his "hearing loss." The hospital treatment team has recommended long-term institutionalization for this boy.

CASE 11. RR, a 13-year-old female, was admitted to a state mental hospital for evaluation because of her suspiciousness of others, impulsive behavior, poor concentration, mood swings, and hallucinations. She had a lifelong history of headaches, tinnitus, and vertigo, although previous medical and neurological examinations revealed no organic impairment. This girl was born to a nomadic and highly unstable couple who were divorced before she was 3 years of age. The father obtained custody of the girl, but the mother maintained a periodic but continuing battle to regain custody. During the next 7 years, she experienced 12 separations from the family while living with various parents, stepparents, and relatives. She was often moved from the home of one rejecting parent or relative to another, and had been witness to the parents' physical battles, sexual promiscuity, and alcoholism. She reportedly had been threatened with bodily harm (such as having her tongue cut out if she didn't stop talking so much) and had been battered by her mother and stepmother. She had scars on her lower legs from boiling water, and on her chin from physical beatings. Her father himself had said that he "bounced her off the wall a couple of times." There were also reports of incestuous relations with her brother, cousin, and an older uncle. Her father divorced his second wife and remarried again when the patient was 10 years old. This marriage was chaotic, with the new stepmother attempting suicide several times.

Since entering school, her adjustment had been poor and her educational achievement limited. She was considered at one time to be mentally retarded. However, for the 3 years preceding her admission to the hospital, she was described by her teachers as being an "insecure dependent loner" who seemed to "live in a world of her own." A bilateral hearing loss was detected during a public school hearing screening test and was later confirmed by audiological testing at another clinic. Voluntary air-conduction and speech reception thresholds obtained at that

304 LARRY J. BRADFORD

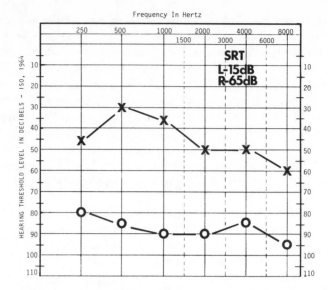

Figure 33 Voluntary pure-tone and speech reception thresholds obtained from RR at another clinic.

center are shown in Figure 33. Shortly after admission to the hospital, the patient said that she was "deaf in her right ear and could not hear very well in her left ear." She denied experiencing either tinnitus or vertigo at that time. The discrepancy between her previously obtained pure-tone averages and speech reception thresholds, as well as our observation of no articulation or voice quality deviations, suggested that her hearing sensitivity was better than her voluntary thresholds. Voluntary thresholds obtained in our clinic approximated those previously obtained, but the bilateral respiration thresholds were 0 dB at 1000 Hz. Her hearing sensitivity was measured 1 month later by both respiration and voluntary methods. Auditory thresholds of 0 dB were determined from respiration alterations at the frequencies of 500, 1000, and 2000 Hz. These are shown in Figure 34. These thresholds were corroborated when voluntary thresholds for the same three frequencies and speech reception thresholds were obtained at 0 dB in both ears.

After admission to the hospital, she told the examining psychiatrist of her visual hallucinations of predatory animals and ferocious monsters. However, she stated that, "I can make them disappear if I want, and people too, by just closing my eyes." She also reported being able to "close up" her ears so as not to hear ugly and frightening things. With her ears closed up, she was able to "know what will happen in the future," which included fantasies of life without conflict and a reunion with her

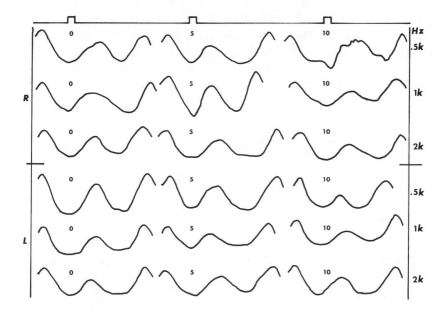

Figure 34 Respiration alterations from .5-, 1-, and 2-kHz pure tones presented through earphones to the right and left ears of RR. The recordings were made while she was awake.

idealized natural mother. The respiration data indicating normal hearing sensitivity permitted the psychiatric treatment team to understand her defenses relating to the hearing impairment. She was diagnosed as having childhood schizophrenia with predominantly presymbiotic features, which will require long-term residential treatment.

CASE 12.   LM was almost 18 years old when she was admitted to our hospital because of depression, withdrawal, and isolation from her family and peers. This girl had a long history of feeling that life was hopeless and futile, and considered herself to be defective and isolated from others because of a hearing impairment. She was born 6 weeks prematurely, weighing 4 lbs and 10 oz. Because of her slow speech development, immature behavior, and poor motor coordination, there was concern that she might be aphasic, brain damaged, or mentally retarded. A clinging, dependent, and negativistic relationship had developed between the girl and her mother at an early age. As she moved into childhood, she became passively dependent upon her father, since he was the only one who supposedly understood her.

A series of voluntary audiological thresholds, obtained when she was between 3 and 4 years old, indicated a bilateral hearing impairment.

She had been fitted with a hearing aid at about 3 years of age, and was wearing an aid in her left ear at the time of admission. Although auditory testing had indicated a hearing impairment at the time she was given the hearing aid, there were also observations indicating that she was not hearing impaired. When she was 4 years of age, one examiner reported that

> the absence of the hearing aid did not seem to lessen her ability to perceive and react to conversational speech. The effect of the hearing aid was rather the reverse—it tended to create increased withdrawal and anxiousness in the child instead of aiding her. With the hearing aid she was less verbally communicative and more unsure of herself. At times, she also uses the speech difficulty as a way to demand attention from others, to cling dependently to them, and to exert control over them.

During the third year of life, she was saying single words and responded to her name when it was said outside of her range of vision. When looking at a book, she was able to repeat names of the objects that were said by her mother, without seeing her face. Around 4 years of age, her intelligence was found to be within a normal range on the Merrill Palmer Scale. She had been enrolled in a private school for the deaf at 5 years of age and had made "great strides in communication." She had remained at this school for 3 years and then entered public school, where she remained until the tenth grade. Because of emotional and scholastic problems, she entered an "open school." Her academic and social adjustment did not improve, and her depression progressively worsened. A suicide attempt precipitated the hospital admission.

The voluntary audiograms from different clinics consistently revealed a bilateral hearing impairment. The air-conduction and speech reception thresholds obtained voluntarily in our clinic shortly after her entrance to the hospital are similar to previously obtained voluntary thresholds. These are shown in Figure 35. Hearing sensitivity, as determined by respiration alterations for the frequencies of 500 through 8000 Hz, was found to be within normal limits in both ears. The trace records for the right and left ear at 500, 1000, and 2000 Hz are shown in Figure 36.

After entering the hospital, her psychiatrist observed that her hearing difficulty fluctuated "in response to the subject at hand." About 3 months after admission, she "confessed" that she did not need the hearing aid to hear. However, she was only able to tolerate going without her hearing aid for a short period of time. Without her hearing aid, she reported feeling "depressed, empty and like all of my defenses are gone." On one occasion, she threw her hearing aid against the wall, stating that all of this was a "lie." She started to wear the hearing aid again and has been

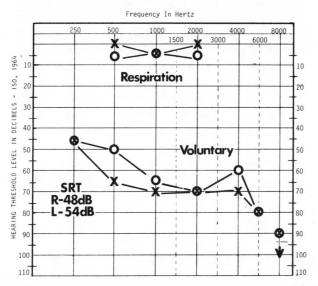

Figure 35 Voluntary pure-tone and speech reception thresholds of LM obtained at our clinic compared to the thresholds determined from the respiration alterations shown in Figure 36.

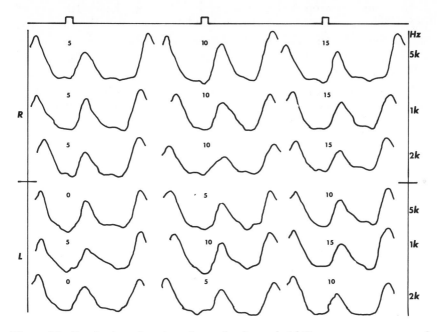

Figure 36 Respiration alterations from .5-, 1-, and 2-kHz pure tones presented through earphones to the right and left ears of LM. The recordings were made while she was awake.

unable to give it up. The audiological information obtained from respiration audiometry will permit her psychiatrist to focus on the reasons she has been using a hearing loss all of these years.

CASE 13. CM was a 19-year-old male who was admitted to our hospital following three separate psychotic breaks associated with separation from his mother. The psychotic episodes were accompanied by delusions and auditory hallucinations. The first episode occurred on the day he received news of his acceptance at an out-of-state university. He was hospitalized at another hospital for 6 weeks because of ideas ranging from being the world's most popular boy, destined to become the President of the United States, to having been killed in an automobile accident and living on as a spirit. In the fall, he entered the university that had originally accepted him for admission. Shortly after enrollment, he was hospitalized for the second time because of an exacerbation of paranoid and delusional thinking and the discontinuation of his university studies. The third psychotic episode began about 8 months later, when he began to express exaggerated ideas about his importance in the world. He considered himself to be the real embodiment of Christ in the second coming, and Newton feeling the apple fall on his head. He also experienced auditory hallucinations in which trucks and the devil were saying things to him. Following the third psychotic episode, he entered our hospital and was diagnosed as manifesting paranoid schizophrenia.

This patient had been a full-term baby weighing 9 lbs. and had been delivered following an easy labor. Five days after birth, he was transfused because of an Rh blood incompatibility. His development was normal in all areas except speech and language. His history reported the development of a very close relationship between mother and son, there being much marital strife between CM's parents, and the mother feeling that her son needed to be protected. The mother had previously had a miscarriage and had mourned the loss of that baby. The mother advised us that her son had been diagnosed as having a "high frequency hearing loss" and had been fitted with a hearing aid in his right ear at 3 years of age. He had worn a hearing aid since that time and was wearing a glasses-type hearing aid when admitted to the hospital. There were no audiological or medical reports available to us to substantiate the mother's report. After the initial diagnosis of a bilateral hearing loss, the mother had begun preparing herself to teach her "deaf" son to speak and read. He had never received any professional help because his mother had insisted on being his special teacher. She reported, "As a result of my intensive care, he was able to speak by the time he was 4 years old." With her encouragement, he did excel in school and was a superior student throughout high school. His intelligence was in the superior range, as measured on the Wechsler–Bellevue Scale after admission to the hospital.

An audiological evaluation was completed shortly after CM's admission to the hospital. Because of significant discrepancies between his speech reception thresholds and voluntary pure-tone threshold averages, his hearing sensitivity was evaluated by respiration audiometry and was found to be within normal limits. His voluntary thresholds and thresholds from respiration alterations are shown in Figure 37.

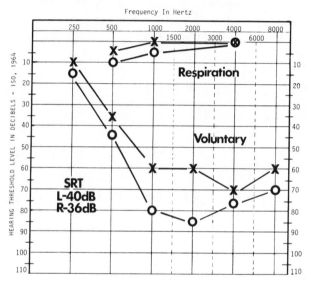

Figure 37 Voluntary pure-tone and speech reception thresholds compared to the thresholds determined from respiration alterations of CM, recorded while awake.

The information about his normal hearing was utilized during his hospitalization and psychiatric treatment. Although he never admitted to being able to hear normally, he gradually used his hearing aid less during psychotherapy sessions and on the hospital ward. One year after admission, he was discharged from the hospital to live independently in an apartment while attending a local university. He eventually was able to discontinue wearing his hearing aid, obtain a bachelor's degree in 3 years, and enter graduate school at an eastern university.

CASE 14. GR was the only child born to a 15-year-old mother and 29-year-old father. Shortly after GR's birth, his father deserted the family, and the boy had little or no later contact with him. After the separation, the boy lived with and was cared for by various maternal relatives while his mother worked away from home. During the first 6 years of his life, he experienced many moves, rejections, and a lack of care until he became a ward of the court at 6 years of age, following the divorce of his parents. His early development appeared normal except that at 2 years of age his only words were "mamma" and "dadda." At 2½ years of age, he was hospitalized for 6 weeks because of pneumococcic meningitis, and his mother was advised that he could have a residual hearing impairment. When he was 3 years old, a pediatrician found his speech to be unclear, but observed that "at times he can't hear but at other times he acts like he can hear." However, an otologist diagnosed the boy as having a "postmeningitis nerve deafness." At the age of 8 years, one physician estimated that his hearing appeared to be adequate in his left ear but impaired in his right ear. Another physician diagnosed him at 12 years of age as having a bilateral "typical profound postmeningitic sensorineural deafness." A hearing aid was recommended for him at that time, although the physician speculated that the boy would not get "any speech amplification at all with the hearing aid." Our records indicate that he was taken to a faith healer and that he underwent brain surgery to correct his hearing loss. He was also taken in a small airplane by his mother, in the hope that the high altitude would improve his hearing. Information about actual hearing-aid usage at any time was not available to us.

He was enrolled at a state school for the deaf at 6 years of age. Records from the school indicated that he "was so emotionally upset most of the time that his teacher did not accomplish very much with him." He was placed in a private school for the deaf at 8 years of age and remained there until completing the ninth grade at 19 years of age. The boy had limited contact with his mother after enrollment in school because she had remarried and moved to another part of the country.

His adjustment and achievement in the private school appeared to be marginal, as he vacillated from passive compliance to violent outbursts. Just before his graduation from school, it was recommended that he be seen by a psychiatrist. The parents did not follow this recommendation until the occurrence of a psychotic episode after he left the protective environment of the private school. Since he had acquired some skill in electronics while attending school, he entered a trade school, which enrolled deaf students, for further training in this specialty. He was unable to adjust academically and socially, and dropped out after attending for only a year. He returned to the city in which his mother and stepfather lived. He did not live in the home, for his stepfather was tired of supporting him and insisted that he was old enough to live on his own. During the next year, GR became increasingly suspicious of people, expressed the fear that something had happened to his brain, threatened to kill his mother, lost several menial jobs, and finally refused to get out of bed to go to work. He was committed to a state mental hospital, where he remained for 3 months and was diagnosed as being schizophrenic. Following his discharge, he again began to verbalize ideas of persecution and to manifest violent behavior. When he was 22 years of age, he was admitted to our hospital with a diagnosis of paranoid schizophrenia. While a patient at our hospital, he neither had nor wore a hearing aid.

During voluntary auditory testing, thresholds were obtained in his left ear which suggested a mild to profound sloping impairment, as shown in Figure 38. He denied hearing any of the tones presented to his right

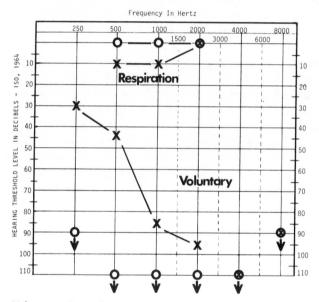

Figure 38 Voluntary thresholds compared to thresholds determined from respiration alterations of GR recorded while awake.

ear. However, he said, "I do not hear a tone," as the tones were presented to his right ear at intensity levels within the normal hearing range. He also responded to tones in his right ear when a tone was quickly switched to that ear while his left ear was being tested. From the bilateral respiration traces obtained for the frequencies of 500, 1000, and 2000 Hz, his hearing sensitivity was found to be within normal limits, as shown in Figure 38. These results were substantiated 9 months later when normal sensitivity was again inferred from respiration alterations. During his hospitalization, he learned to play a guitar, which he probably would not have been able to do if his true hearing loss was at the level to which he voluntarily admitted. Clinical observations repeatedly demonstrated that he responded appropriately to normal conversation-level speech and even to softly spoken speech when his back was turned to the speaker. On one occasion, he told his psychiatrist that he was "not as interested in listening as he was in talking." His speech had a deaf-like quality, but he was quite intelligible when he elected to talk. On another occasion, he told a story suggesting the fear he experienced if he were consciously to admit to hearing normally, and indicating his unconscious need to deny hearing in order to prevent his own symbolic death. He told of a boy with a hearing loss who jumped out of an airplane with a parachute, and, on the way down, had his hearing restored. The boy was unable to believe his good fortune, and according to the patient, went up the next day and jumped again. This time his parachute did not open and he was killed.

After a year's hospitalization, the patient was withdrawn by his mother and sent to another private psychiatric facility. There is no follow-up information on this patient after his discharge from our hospital.

In each of these clinical cases, the patient had used a hearing loss as a coping device for adapting to his environment. In some cases, the voluntary thresholds obtained early in life had resulted in patients being placed in educational programs for the deaf. The utilization of an indirect hearing test, such as respiration audiometry, could have prevented these misdiagnoses and suggested the need for a psychiatric referral. These cases illustrate the usefulness of respiration audiometry for determining the hearing sensitivity of persons with a psychogenic hearing loss.

VI. SUMMARY

This chapter has reviewed the literature on respiration alterations in response to sound. Although this phenomenon has been known for almost 100 years, it has been only during the past 10 years that the alterations have been employed for measuring hearing. The respiration audiometric procedure developed at The Menninger Foundation was presented as an innocuous way to measure hearing sensitivity. Research comparing voluntary thresholds and respiration thresholds of normal-hearing and hearing-impaired children and adults was presented to demonstrate the validity of the technique. On the basis of this research, the respiration thresholds obtained with difficult-to-test humans and with animals on whom voluntary thresholds could not be obtained are considered to be valid. Psychogenic factors were discussed to provide an understanding of how a "hearing impairment" can be a symptom of a maladjustive behavior used to prevent further psychic decompensation. Clinical examples illustrating the efficacy of respiration audiometry in our clinic were offered to encourage use of, and further research on, respiration audiometry by others.

REFERENCES

Atzler, E. (1935). *Handb. Biol. Arbmeth.* **5,** 1073.
Baglioni, S. (1929). *Arch. Fisiol.* **27,** 132.
Bechterew, W. von (1911). "Die Funktionen der Nervencentra." Gustav Fisher, Jena.
Bender, L. (1947). *Amer. J. Orthopsychiat.* **17,** 40.
Benussi, V. (1914). *Arch. Psychol.* **31,** 244.
Berk, R. L., and Feldman, A. S. (1958). *New England J. Med.* **259,** 214.
Berlyne, D. E. (1960). "Conflict, Arousal, and Curiosity." McGraw-Hill, New York.
Braatoy, T. (1947). "De Nervose Sinn." Cappelen, Oslo.
Bradford, L., and Rousey, C. (1972). *Maico Aud. Lib. Ser.* **10** Rep. 6.
Bradford, L., Rousey, C., and Bradford, M. (1972). *Laryngoscope* **82,** 28.
Bradford, L., McKinley, J., Rousey, C., and Klein, D. (1973). *Amer. J. Vet. Res.* **34,** 1183.
Brookhart, J. M. (1940). *Amer. J. Physiol.* **129,** 709.
Brooks, R., and Gieschen, E. (1968). *J. Kansas Speech Hear. Ass.* **9,** 1.
Brosin, H. W. (1967). *In* "Comprehensive Textbook of Psychiatry" (A. M. Freedman and H. I. Kaplan, eds.), pp. 748–759. Williams and Wilkins, Baltimore, Maryland.
Bucy, P. C., and Case, T. J. (1936). *J. Nerv. Ment. Dis.* **84,** 156.
Burdach, C. F. (1838). "Die Physiologie als Erfahrungswissenschaft," Vol. 3. Voss, Leipzig.
Burtt, H. E. (1918). *Psychol. Bull.* **15,** 325.
Cameron, N. (1963). "Personality Development and Psychopathology." Houghton Mifflin, Boston, Massachusetts.
Canestrini, S. (1913). *Monogr. Gesamtgeb. Psychiat.* (*Berlin*) **5,** 1.
Canfield, N. (1949). "Audiology: The Science of Hearing." Thomas, Springfield, Illinois.
Clausen, J. (1951). *Acta Psychiat. Scand. Suppl.* **68,** 1.
Coleman, L. D. (1949). *Laryngoscope* **59,** 709.
Czerny, A. (1892). *Jahrb. Kinderheilkd.* **33,** 1.
Danilewsky, B. von (1875). *Pfluegers Arch.* **11,** 128.
Davis, H., and Fowler, E. P., Jr. (1960). *In* "Hearing and Deafness" (H. Davis and S. R. Silverman, eds.) (rev. ed.), pp. 80–124. Holt, New York.
Deming, J., and Washburn, A. H. (1935). *Amer. J. Dis. Child.* **49,** 108.
Dunbar, F. (1954). "Emotions and Bodily Changes," 4th ed. Columbia Univ. Press, New York.
Engelberg, M. W. (1970). "Audiological Evaluation for Exaggerated Hearing Level." Thomas, Springfield, Illinois.
Feldman, W. (1920). "The Principles of Ante-Natal and Post-Natal Child Physiology." Longmans, Green, New York.
Fenning, C. (1936). *J. Lab. Clin. Med.* **22,** 1279.
Fenning, C., and Bonar, B. E. (1936). *J. Lab. Clin. Med.* **22,** 1280.

Fleisch, A. (1935). *Handb. Biol. Arbmeth.* 5, 905.

Freud, S. (1958a). In "Standard Edition of the Complete Psychological Works of Sigmund Freud," Vol. 4, pp. 1–95. Hogarth Press, London.

Freud, S. (1958b). In "Standard Edition of the Complete Psychological Works of Sigmund Freud," Vol. 12, pp. 218–226. Hogarth Press, London.

Geddes, L. A., Hoff, H. E., Hickman, D. M., and Moore, A. G. (1962). *Aerosp. Med.* 33, 28.

Gelinier-Ortigues, M-C. (1955). In "Emotional Problems of Early Childhood" (G. Caplan, ed.), pp. 231–247. Basic Books, New York.

Gerhardt, H. J., Wagner, H., Thomschke, I., and Pasch, B. (1967). *Z. Laryngol. Rhinol. Otol.* 46, 235.

Goldstein, R. (1966). *J. Speech Hear. Disord.* 31, 341.

Golla, F. L., and Antonovitch, S. (1929). *Brain* 52, 491.

Gregor, K. (1902). *Arch. Kinderheilkd.* 35, 272.

Grinker, R. R., and Spiegel, J. P. (1945). "War Neuroses." McGraw-Hill (Blakiston), New York.

Haladine, J. S., and Priestly, J. G. (1935). "Respiration." Oxford Univ. Press, London and New York.

Halvorson, H. M. (1941). *J. Genet. Psychol.* 59, 259.

Hanley, C. N., and Tiffany, W. R. (1954). *Arch. Otolaryngol.* 60, 197.

Hefferman, A. (1955). In "Emotional Problems of Early Childhood" (G. Caplan, ed.), pp. 269–292. Basic Books, New York.

Henry, M. (no date). "Commentaries on the Whole Bible." Revell, New York.

Hernandez-Peon, R., Scherrer, H., and Jouvet, M. (1956). *Science* 123, 331.

Heron, T. G., and Jacobs, R. (1968). *Int. Aud.* 7, 41.

Heron, T. G., and Jacobs, R. (1969). *Int. Aud.* 8, 77.

Hesse, G. E. (1959). *Brit. J. Anaesth.* 31, 229.

Hoff, H. E., and Breckenridge, C. G. (1952). *J. Neurophysiol.* 15, 47.

Hopkinson, N. T. (1967). *J. Speech Hear. Disord.* 32, 293.

Howard, P. J., and Bauer, A. R. (1949). *Amer. J. Dis. Child.* 77, 592.

Howell, W. H. (1928). "A Textbook of Physiology," 10th ed. rev. Saunders, Philadelphia, Pennsylvania.

Hubel, D. H., Hensen, C. O., Rupert, A., and Galambos, R (1959). *Science* 129, 1279.

Hunter, R., and Cawthorne, T. (1963). *Int. Aud.* 2, 250.

Inbau, F. E. (1942). "Lie Detection and Criminal Interrogation." Williams and Wilkins, Baltimore, Maryland.

Ingalls, G. S. (1946). *Occup. Ther. Rehabil.* 25, 62.

Isakower, O. (1939). *Int. J. Psychonal.* 20, 340.

Itard, J.-M.-G. (1821). "Traité des Maladies de l'Oreille et de l'Audition." Mequignon-Marvis, Paris.

Jacobson, L. (1898). "Lehrbuch der Ohrenheilkunde für Aerzte und Studirende," 2nd ed. Thieme, Leipzig.

James, W. (1950a). "The Principles of Psychology," Vol. 1, pp. 402–458. Dover, New York.

James, W. (1950b). "The Principles of Psychology," Vol. 2. Dover, New York.

Jenness, A., and Wible, C. L. (1937). *J. Gen. Psychol.* 16, 197.

Johnson, K. O., Work, W. P., and McCoy, G. (1956). *Ann. Otol. Rhinol. Laryngol.* 65, 154.

Kaada, B. R., Pribram, K. H., and Epstein, J. A. (1949). *J. Neurophysiol.* 12, 347.

Kanner, L. (1944). *J. Pediatr.* **25**, 211.

Kaplan, H. S. (1967). In "Comprehensive Textbook of Psychiatry" (A. F. Freedman and H. I. Kaplan, eds.), pp. 1120–1124. Williams and Wilkins, Baltimore, Maryland.

Klein, I. J. (1956). *Nerv. Child* **10**, 135.

Kumpf, W. (1966). *Arch. Klin. Exp. Ohren Nasen Kehlkopfheilkd.* **186**, 80.

Kumpf, W. (1968a). *Arch. Klin. Exp. Ohren Nasen Kehlkopfheilkd.* **191**, 593.

Kumpf, W. (1968b). *HNO* **16**, 52.

Kumpf, W. (1970). *Deutsch. Med. Wochenschr.* **95**, 1416.

Kumpf, W. (1972). *Fortschr. Med.* **90**, 74.

Kumpf, W., and Landwehr, F. J. (1970). *Monatsschr. Ohrenheilkd. Laryngorhinol.* **104**, 535.

Larson, J. A. (1923). *J. Exp. Psychol.* **6**, 420.

Lee, R. C., and Silverman, L. (1943). *Rev. Sci. Instrum.* **14**, 174.

Lehmann, A. (1905). "Die Körperlichen Äusserungen Psychischer Zustände." Reisland, Leipzig.

Lehnhardt, E. (1963). *Arch. Klin. Exp. Ohren Nasen Kehlkopfheilkd.* **182**, 623.

Lester, D. (1971). *Amer. Med. Ass.* **216**, 678.

Levine, E. S. (1960). "The Psychology of Deafness." Columbia Univ. Press, New York.

Linn, L. (1953). *J. Amer. Psychoanal. Ass.* **1**, 690.

Lipkin, M. (1969). *Ann. Intern. Med.* **71**, 1013.

Lipton, E. L., Sleinschneider, A., and Richmond, J. B. (1964). *Pediatrics* **33**, 212.

Lombard, E. (1911). *Ann. Mal. Oreil. Larynx* **37**, 101.

Lombroso, C. (1895). "L'Homme Criminel." Alcan, Paris.

Ludwig, K. W. F. von (1847). *Arch. Physiol. Wissensch. Med.* (*Berlin/Leipzig*) **14**, 241.

Mack, J. E., and Semrad, E. V. (1967). In "Comprehensive Textbook of Psychiatry" (A. F. Freedman and H. I. Kaplan, eds.), pp. 269–319. William and Wilkins, Baltimore, Maryland.

Mahler, K. F., and Wagner, F. (1967). *Monatsschr. Ohrenheilkd. Laryngorhinol.* **101**, 512.

Mahler, M. S. (1952). In "Psychoanalytic Study of the Child," Vol. VII, pp. 286–305. Int. Univ. Press, New York.

Marey, E.-J.-M. (1865). *J. Anat. Physiol. Norm. et Pathol. Homme Animaux* (*Paris*) **2**, 428.

Marey, E.-J.-M. (1876). "Physiologie Experimentale," Vol. 2. Libraire de L'Acad. de Med., Paris.

Margolin, S., and Kubie, L. S. (1943). *J. Clin. Invest.* **22**, 221.

Martin, F. N. (1972). In "Handbook of Clinical Audiology" (J. Katz, ed.), pp. 357–373. Williams and Wilkins, Baltimore, Maryland.

McCollum, M., Burch, N. R., and Roessler, R. (1969). *Psychophysiology* **6**, 291.

Menninger, K. (1963). "The Vital Balance." Viking Press, New York.

Mentz, P. von (1895). In "Philosophische Studien" (W. Wundt, ed.), pp. 371–393, 563–602. Engelmann, Leipzig.

Miller, H. C., and Behrle, F. C. (1952). *Pediatrics* **10**, 272.

Mindel, E. D., and Vernon, M. (1971). "They Grow in Silence." Nat. Ass. for the Deaf, Silver Springs, Maryland.

Montague, J. D. (1957). *Lancet* **2**, 126.

Mosso, A. (1878). *Arch. Anat. Physiol.* (Leipzig) **44**, 441.

Mosso, A. (1886). *Arch. Anat. Physiol.* (Leipzig) **52**, 37.

Myklebust, H. R. (1954). "Auditory Disorders in Children." Grune and Stratton, New York.

Nixon, H. K. (1923). *J. Exp. Psychol.* **6**, 383.

Oberholzer, R. J. H., and Tofani, W. O. (1960). In "Handbook of Physiology" (J. Fields, ed.-in-chief), Vol. II, pp. 1111–1129. Amer. Physiol. Soc., Washington, D.C.

Patterson, A. S. (1934). *J. Neurol. Psychopath.* **14**, 323.

Pavlov, I. P. (1947). "Complete Works" (Poln. sobr. trud.), Vol. IV. U.S.S.R. Acad. Sci. Press, Moscow.

Penfield, W., and Rasmussen, T. (1950). "The Cerebral Cortex of Man." Macmillan, New York.

Perkins, W. H. (1938). "Cause and Prevention of Disease." Lea and Febiger, Philadelphia, Pennsylvania.

Pitts, R. F. (1946). *Physiol. Rev.* **26**, 609.

Ponzo, M. (1915). *Arch. Ital. Otol.* **26**, 42.

Ponzo, M. (1921). *Arch. Ital. Otol.* **32**, 321.

Poole, R., Goetzinger, C., and Rousey, C. (1966). *Acta Oto–Laryngol.* **61**, 143.

Prazic, M. (1963). *Int. Aud.* **2**, 133.

Preobraschensky, S. S. (1890). *Wien. Klin. Wochenschr.* **3**, 793, 832.

Proctor, J. T. (1958). *Amer. J. Orthopsychiat.* **28**, 394.

Ranier, J. D., and Altshuler, K. Z. (1967a). "Comprehensive Mental Health Services for the Deaf." Columbia Univ. Press, New York.

Ranier, J. D., and Altshuler, K. Z. (eds.) (1967b). "Psychiatry and the Deaf." U.S. Dept. Health, Education, and Welfare, Social and Rehabilitation Serv., Washington, D.C.

Ranier, J. D., Altshuler, K. Z., and Kallman, F. J. (eds.) (1963). "Family and Mental Health Problems in a Deaf Population." New York Psychiatric Inst., Columbia Univ., New York.

Rank, B. (1942). *Amer. Imago* **3**, 41.

Rapaport, D. (1951). "Organization and Pathology of Thought." Columbia Univ. Press, New York.

Reed, C. I., and Kleitmann, N. (1925). *Amer. J. Physiol.* **75**, 600.

Reynard, M. C., and Dockeray, F. C. (1939). *J. Genet. Psychol.* **55**, 103.

Robins, E., and O'Neal, P. (1953). *Nerv. Child* **10**, 246.

Rosen, H. (1953). *Psychosom. Med.* **15**, 403.

Rosenau, H. (1961). *Arch. Klin. Exp. Ohren Nasen Kehlkopfheilkd.* **178**, 476.

Rosenau, H. (1962a). *Z. Laryngol. Rhinol. Otol.* **41**, 194.

Rosenau, H. (1962b). *Paediat. Grenzgeb.* **1**, 27.

Rousey, C. (1969). "Indirect Assessment of Hearing Sensitivity by Changes in Respiration." Final rep., Project No. 6-1572. Dept. Health, Education and Welfare, U.S. Office of Education, Bur. of Education for the Handicapped, Washington, D.C.

Rousey, C. L. (1971a). *J. Speech Hear. Disord.* **36**, 382.

Rousey, C. L. (1971b). In "Handbook of Speech Pathology and Audiology" (L. E. Travis, ed.), pp. 819–836. Appleton, New York.

Rousey, C. L., and Bradford, L. J. (1971). "An Indirect Hearing Sensitivity Assessment by Respiration in Brain Damaged and Orthopedically Handicapped Children as Compared to Normal Appearing Children During Varying States of Waking and Sleeping." Easter Seal Grant N-7010.

Rousey, C., and Reitz, W. (1967). *Psychophysiology* **3**, 258.

Rousey, C. L., Snyder, C., and Rousey, C. G. (1964). *J. Aud. Res.* **4**, 107.

Rousey, C. L., Engle, M., and Houchins, R. (1971). *J. Aud. Res.* **11**, 322.

Schlesinger, H. S., and Meadow, K. P. (1972). "Sound and Sign: Childhood Deafness and Mental Health." Univ. California Press, Berkeley, California.

Segundo, J. P., Arana, R., Migliaro, E., Villar, J. E., Garcia Guelfi, A., and Garcia Austif, E. (1955). *J. Neurophysiol.* **18**, 96.

Severinghaus, J. W. (1962). *Ann. Rev. Physiol.* **24**, 421.

Smith, W. K. (1938). *J. Physiol.* **1**, 55.

Sokolov, E. N. (1960a). *In* "The Central Nervous System and Behavior" (M. A. B. Brazier, ed.), pp. 187–276. Josiah Macy, Jr. Foundation, New York.

Sokolov, E. N. (1960b). *Vopr. Psikhol.* **4**, 61–72.

Sokolov, E. N. (1963). "Perception and the Conditioned Reflex." Macmillan, New York.

Solomon, J. C. (1943). *Ment. Hyg.* **27**, 439.

Stenger, P. (1900). *Arch. Ohrenheilk.* **50**, 197.

Stubbs, E. M. (1934). *In* "Studies of Infant Behavior" (G. B. Stoddard, ed.), Vol. 9, pp. 75–135. Univ. Iowa Stud. in Child Welfare.

Suzuki, T., Kamijo, Y., and Kiuchi, S. (1964). *Ann. Otol. Rhinol. Laryngol.* **73**, 914.

Teel, J., Winston, M., Aspinall, K., Rousey, C., and Goetzinger, C. (1967). *Arch. Otolaryngol.* **86**, 172.

Titchener, E. B. (1908). "Lectures on the Elementary Psychology of Feeling and Attention." Macmillan, New York.

Trovillo, P. V. (1939). *J. Crim. Law, Criminol. Police Sci.* **29**, 848.

Trovillo, P. V. (1940). *J. Crim. Law Criminol. Police Sci.* **30**, 104.

Truex, E. H., Jr. (1946). *Conn. St. J. Med.* **10**, 907.

Veith, I. (1955). *Bull. Cleveland Med. Lib.* **2**, 67.

Ventry, I. M., and Chailkin. J. B. (1962). *Asha* **4**, 251.

Ventry, I. M., and Chailkin, J. B. (1965). *J. Aud. Res.* **5**, 179.

Vierordt, K. von, and Ludwig, G. (1855). *Arch. Physiolog. Heilk.* **14**, 253.

Wade, O. L. (1954). *J. Physiol.* **124**, 193.

Wagner, H. (1963). *Z. Laryngol. Rhinol. Otol.* **42**, 139.

Wagner, I. F. (1937). *J. Genet. Psychol.* **51**, 17.

Wagner, I. F. (1939). *J. Genet. Psychol.* **55**, 121.

West, L. J. (1967). *In* "Comprehensive Textbook of Psychiatry" (A. F. Freedman and H. I. Kaplan, eds.), pp. 885–899. Williams and Wilkins, Baltimore, Maryland.

Woodworth, R. S., and Schlosberg, H. (1954). "Experimental Psychology" (rev. ed.). Holt, New York.

Worden, F. G. (1966). *Progr. Physiolog. Psychol.* **1**, 45–116.

Wyss, O. A. M. (1963). *Ann. Rev. Physiol.* **25**, 143.

Zeckel, A. (1950). *J. Nerv. Ment. Dis.* **112**, 322.

Chapter Nine

Cardiotachometry[1]

Rita B. Eisenberg[2]

I. INTRODUCTION

The use of cranial blood pressure and related cardiac measures as indicators of sensory or other functions dates back some 60 years (Kessen
et al., 1970), and cardiac measures in particular have acquired wide
currency within the past decade. For instance, investigators in psychology, obstetrics, pediatrics, and a number of other disciplines now
employ heart rate (HR) quite regularly to disclose the effects of sensory stimuli, to monitor foetal status, and to study the organization of
behavior (Graham and Jackson, 1970; Lewis, 1974; Steinschneider,
1971). Audiologists, however, have shown little interest in cardiac measures; Few have explored them, and even fewer have persisted beyond
preliminary inquiries. Beadle (1962), working under David Crowell
at the University of Hawaii, was the first to report work in this area,
but the initial report remains her sole contribution to the literature.
Bench (1969, 1970), using the electrocardiogram, studied intensity and
frequency discrimination by neonates as well as the relations between
HR and arousal, but apparently did not consider the application of
cardiac measures to auditory testing. Lassman, at the University of
Minnesota, attempted to measure auditory thresholds by HR, but found

[1] This work was supported in part by an institutional grant from the National
Institutes of Health, R01 HD 00732, and a personal grant from the Grant Foundation.

[2] Bioacoustic Laboratory Research Institute, St. Joseph Hospital, Lancaster, Pennsylvania.

the experience frustrating (personal communication). Jerger, at Baylor University, explored the possibility of transmitting cardiac data by telemetry but, despite some success, shelved this work for more rewarding activities (personal communication). Schulman (1970a,b), who has done a great deal of work on cardiac measures of auditory sensitivity during early life and has developed an automatic device for computing threshold responses to pure tones, recently qualified earlier statements on the validity of such responses during the neonatal period (1973).

Despite this discouraging catalog, work at the Bioacoustic Laboratory suggests that cardiac measures of audition not only are feasible, but are potentially important (Eisenberg, 1974). In our opinion, the significance they someday may attain depends partly on the context in which they are approached and partly on whether or not an adequate research and development effort can be mounted by audiologists.[3]

In laboratory work with HR measures, we have been concerned mainly with suprathreshold responses to speech-like sounds. There are specific reasons for this. First, we are convinced that traditional measures of threshold cannot cast light upon the dysfunction underlying developmental disorders of communication and related clinical entities (Eisenberg, 1970a, 1971, 1972). Second, it has become increasingly clear that speech-like sounds are prepotent during early life, whereas pure tones and other "constant" signals (Eisenberg, 1970b) are ineffective (Eimas et al., 1971; Hutt et al., 1968; Lenard et al., 1969; Turkewitz et al., 1972a,b). This chapter, therefore, has the dual purpose of introducing audiologists (or other interested specialists) to HR measures, and relating procedures to the directions we believe a bona fide pediatric audiology eventually must take. First, methods of measuring HR are discussed, with particular reference to the use of a cardiotachometer. Next, the nature of Bioacoustic Laboratory research is described and our experimental conditions are detailed. Then, preliminary results of current laboratory studies are reviewed and related to other investigations of sensory-evoked cardiac activity. Finally, the present status of research in this area is summarized, and suggestions are made for further study.

Before proceeding to factual material and current thinking on cardiac measures, a caveat seems in order. This chapter represents the first

---

[3] It is worth noting that audiologists, with the exception of Jerger and Lassman, have initiated no research with HR. Beadle's study was directed by the Department of Psychology, and all of the other investigators cited in the introduction are psychologists who, for one reason or another, have focused on audition.

general airing of laboratory efforts to study stimulus-bound cardiac behavior in infancy (Eisenberg, 1974), and it covers an area in which no standardized methodology exists. The reader, therefore, is urged to consider the contents of the chapter as a report of work in progress. Procedures for the measurement and treatment of HR data, though adaptable to other situations, were designed specifically for the Bioacoustic Laboratory situation. The preliminary findings to be reviewed here remain to be confirmed by large-sample results and by other investigators. The opinions to be offered inevitably are biased.

II. HEART RATE MEASURES

A. The Electrocardiogram

The electrocardiogram, or EKG, which reflects action potentials in cardiac muscle cells, yields a pattern of strip-chart deflections referable to intervals of the cardiac cycle. These deflections, which conventionally are characterized at P, Q, R, S, and T waves, afford a great deal of important diagnostic information respecting mechanisms of heart action. However, numerous investigations have shown little of this information to be pertinent when the purpose of cardiac measures is to study perception or some other selected aspect of human behavior. Under these conditions, HR has emerged as the least troublesome and, consequently, most widely applied indicator of function (Eichorn, 1970).

The salient deflection in the EKG record is the "R wave," which appears as a prominent spike (see Figure 2), and the HR measure accordingly can be extrapolated from the full EKG complex by counting the number of R waves per unit of time. However, this is a tedious, time-consuming task that tends to be short on accuracy, hard on the eyes, and seemingly endless on arithmetic computations. Fortunately, cardiotachometers are available now, and experimental chores have been reduced appreciably.

B. The Cardiotachometer

The cardiotachometer is essentially a beat-to-beat metering device that is triggered by the R wave of a subject under test. Electronic circuits built into the instrument continuously measure the time intervals (tau, or t) between successive R waves, convert them to instantaneous rates, determine the reciprocals of those rates ($1/t$), and display and/or record the resulting values on a calibrated scale as "Nixie" read-outs of instantaneous heart rates and/or as strip-chart deflections convertible to such rates. Reciprocals must be determined because the period between successive R waves, measured in milliseconds (msec), is not identical with HR in beats per minute (bpm) (Khachaturian *et al.*, 1972). This means, then, that the formula

$$HR = \frac{60}{tau(t)}$$

must be applied for conversion. For example, a tau, or R–R interval, of 0.3 sec (300 msec) would yield an instantaneous HR of 200 bpm.

This example is a clue to the massive amounts of data generated by HR studies. A half-hour recording on an average adult, whose HR usually varies between 60 and 70 bpm, would generate something on the order of 2000 data bits; a like recording on an average 1-month-old infant, whose HR may span a 100-beat range, would generate something in the neighborhood of 6000 data bits. Thus, cardiac measurement presents serious problems with respect to data reduction and retrieval, and how one resolves them depends partly upon the resources available. Under most conditions, however, computer treatment of the data is mandatory.

III. BIOACOUSTIC LABORATORY RESEARCH INVOLVING HEART RATE MEASURES

A. Introduction

Our group at the Bioacoustic Laboratory first became interested in cardiac measures of auditory behavior in 1962 or thereabouts, during a period when a number of electrophysiological indicators were under investigation (Eisenberg, 1965). We became involved in cardiotachometry somewhat later, when reports from the Department of Pediatrics at the New York Upstate Medical Center in Syracuse came to our attention (Lipton *et al.*, 1961; Richmond *et al.*, 1962; Steinschneider, 1971).[4] All of the HR findings to be considered in this chapter were collected in conjunction with behavioral and electroencephalographic (EEG)

---

[4] We learned the tools of the HR trade by visiting at Syracuse, and some of the technical procedures, e.g., electrode placements, are based on Steinschneider's recommendations.

data and, inasmuch as the experimental situation from which they derive is complex, it may be well to spell out both the questions being asked and the conditions under which they were approached.

B. Research Questions

Our long-term objectives, though perhaps overly ambitious, are specific. The first objective is to develop *clinically viable* techniques for measuring auditory processes in early life. This means that study methods must neither require nor assume subject cooperation, and that they must apply under any condition of arousal. The second objective is to acquire normative information on auditory processing as a function of age and stimulus variables. This means that study methods must be applicable to control subjects at any stage of development, and valid under a wide range of stimulus conditions. The third objective is to determine what kinds of perceptual and central specializations may underlie the ontogeny of verbal communication. This means that study methods must be addressed to both coding and integrating functions, and that "probe" stimuli must have some direct bearing on verbal communication. The fourth objective is to apply all of this information to the design of predictive auditory tests for the pediatric-aged. This means that study methods eventually must prove applicable in average clinical situations as well as in research-oriented facilities.

At this point, we are concerned mainly with the third objective, and our procedures are designed to attack it in complementary ways. On the one hand, we approach the perception of speech-like sounds by studying stimulus-bound activity per se—seeking to characterize behavioral, HR, and EEG responses to a synthetic speech signal in terms of such conventional parameters as latency and magnitude. On the other hand, we approach integrating functions, or "listening" behavior, by studying the cumulative effects of repeated stimulation on individual indices—plotting a dynamic curve referable to changes in physiologic equilibrium over time.

C. Subjects

The bulk of our data pertains to infants under 2 months of age. However, the population studied thus far spans a range between 13 hours and 27 years, and it includes a few high-risk newborns as well as older male subjects with known or suspected central nervous system (CNS) dysfunction.

D. Stimulus Conditions

The stimulus to which all of the cardiac data to be considered here refer was the synthetic vowel, "ah," which is a prominent constituent of the young infant's vocal repertoire. This 1.16-sec signal,[5] with a fixed rise and decay of 25 msec, was recorded on magnetic tape at 90-sec intervals (onset to onset)[6] for sound-field presentation at the conversationally loud level of 60 dB (re 0.0002 μbar).

E. Apparatus for Data Acquisition and Storage

A condensed diagram of Bioacoustic Laboratory circuitry is shown in Figure 1. The acoustic signals, recorded on magnetic tape and controlled

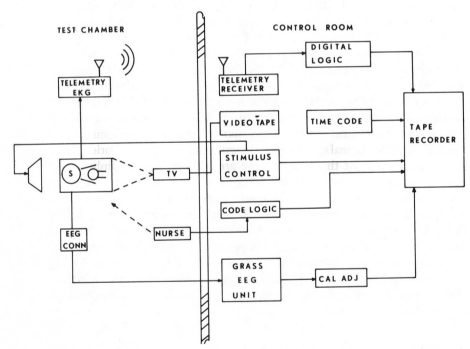

Figure 1 Schematic of Bioacoustic Laboratory system for data acquisition and storage.

---

[5] Generated at Haskins Laboratories, New Haven, Conn.

[6] An unconventionally long interstimulus interval was employed because we were concerned mainly with statistical means of characterizing the cardiac response, and earlier studies with patterned signals of several kinds had shown delays of this order to be required for attainment of stable poststimulus patterns.

through digital logic modules, are fed to amplifier and attenuator networks by way of an electronic switch that gates speakers only when a signal is presented.[7] Behavioral, cardiac, and EEG outputs from a subject in the test chamber are routed to appropriate display and monitor units in the control room and also to specified channels of an Ampex FR-1800-L tape recorder. An eight-track recording format on the tape recorder permits storage of (1) all acoustic events occurring in the test chamber; (2) two channels of HR information (the EKG complex and the heart beat); (3) coded stimulus and artifact markers; (4) three channels of EEG information and (5) real-time, in the form of the IRIG B standardized electrical time code.

F. Circuitry for Obtaining Heart Rate Data

The Bioacoustic Laboratory system for heart rate measurement is shown in Figure 2. We have chosen to employ telemetry for two reasons. From a practical standpoint, it precludes the possibility of electrical hazards arising from simultaneous use of EEG and cardiac indicators. From a long-range planning standpoint, it affords hope for the development of pediatric study procedures permitting reasonable freedom of movement in a test environment.

As can be seen from the block diagram, the EKG from a subject in the test chamber is routed to a Lexington Neurological Amplifier (Model A-103 B). The amplified cardiac complex thus obtained then goes to a special FM transmitter[8] operating at 108 MHZ—a frequency that is relatively free both of commercial transmission in the Lancaster area and of hospital equipment interference. This transmitted signal is received in the control room by a commercial FM tuner (Sony, Model 150). The output of the tuner, amplified in its turn and conditioned by digital logic circuitry,[9] provides a uniform square pulse for each heart beat. The uniform pulses, representing the successive R waves, are fed into a standard cardiotachometer (Gilford, Model 122) for conversion to instantaneous rates. The output of the cardiotachometer, in the form of a DC level proportional to HR, finally is routed to a number of on-line devices: An indicator button on the Gilford, together with its Nixie read-out, permits visual monitoring of each heart beat; a speaker permits

---

[7] This precludes the possibility of electrical noise during interstimulus intervals.

[8] This device, like the signal conditioner elsewhere in the circuit, was designed by Dr. Anthony Marmarou of the Bioacoustic Laboratory staff.

[9] Amplitude thresholds are incorporated into the logic to exclude extraneous noise sources.

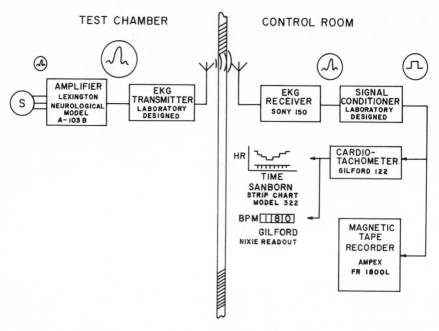

Figure 2 Schematic of Bioacoustic Laboratory system for telemetric transmission of heart rate data.

auditory monitoring; the Ampex FR-1800-L permits storage of the continuously recorded data; and a two-channel strip-chart recorder (Sanborn, Model 322) permits visual inspection of the cardiotachometer output.

G. Placement of EKG Electrodes

Careful placement of electrodes is crucial to obtaining artifact-free HR data, and an investigator is well advised to work out his own reasonably foolproof physical procedures before any large-scale studies are attempted. It is emphasized, therefore, that the laboratory methods outlined here, which have proved satisfactory with very young babies and adult males, are not necessarily applicable to other kinds of subjects.[10]

We employ the same electrodes (Beckman, No. 650944, .062 inches)

---

[10] Infants older than 6 months of age, for instance, tend to be frightened of the test situation and, unlike relatively passive younger babies, many of them will

with subjects in all age groups, and follow strict pretest and test protocols designed to guard against technical problems that conceivably might arise during experimental procedures.

The pretest, or "prep," routine begins on the afternoon or evening before any scheduled study session, when two sets of electrodes are left to soak overnight in a solution of normal (physiological) saline. On the following morning, well before a subject arrives on the scene, these units are thoroughly rinsed and dried, after which preliminary procedures for their placement are instituted. Specifically, the electrodes required for immediate test use, as well as others to serve as spares, are coated with an electrolytic gel (Burton Parsons EKG Sol) and laid on a work table, ready for attachment.

The test routine per se begins with the arrival of the subject in the test chamber. As soon as the subject's chest is bared (and prior to feeding, in the case of infants), the skin area to which electrodes subsequently will be attached is cleaned, dried, and coated lightly with the EKG gel (to promote absorption). About half an hour later[11] (or, for infants, when feeding and associated care have been completed), the cardiac electrodes are applied. Only three of these, attached with clear plastic tape, are required for cardiotachometer work. Two electrodes are placed on the anterior chest wall, one in the third interspace just to the left of the sternum and the second (ground) adjacent to the left nipple; the third is attached at the midline over the vertebral column, at the same level.[12]

---

struggle actively during the placement process. Female subjects, however "liberated" and cooperative, take a dim view of having their chests exposed for prolonged periods of time. There are expedients, though: For older infants, the best technique is to try to establish rapport, get the placement procedures over with as quickly as possible, and allow for prolonged adaptation time; for adult subjects of either sex, excellent cardiac data can be obtained when electrodes are attached to the extremities.

[11] In the case of adults, this half hour or so is utilized for obtaining identifying data, briefing subjects, and so forth. Briefing statements routinely are variations on the following themes: (1) we are interested in how HR (and/or brain wave) patterns change over time; (2) you will be hearing some sounds from time to time, but they are not important, and you don't have to listen for them or do anything when you happen to hear them; (3) if you feel like it, you can take a nap but, in any case, try not to move about while the experiment is going on.

[12] In our experience, the back electrode never comes loose, even when there is an enormous amount of gross movement: The two spares, therefore, constitute ready replacements for the chest electrodes.

H. General Procedures for Data Collection

Each experimental session routinely is preceded by a strict "monitor" protocol assuring (1) "optimal" physical conditions for auditory study (Eisenberg, 1965), (2) electrical safety, and (3) efficient communication between the test chamber and the control room.

Infant subjects are fed immediately upon arrival at the Bioacoustic Laboratory,[13] and whatever associated care is required for their comfort and well-being (burping, diaper changes, and the like) is provided. All subjects are stripped to the waist to permit easy placement of cardiac electrodes and observation of respiratory movements.[14] They remain lying down throughout the experimental period and, depending on age, the bed in which they rest is an infant crib, an infant recliner, or a standard hospital mattress.

When all physical preparations (electrode placements, subject-in-circuit calibrations, and so on) are completed, all personnel other than the subject and an attending nurse–observer leave the test chamber. The nurse is responsible for seeing that all subjects are settled comfortably in a supine position such that an overhead speaker, which constitutes the source of all test signals, is at the midline between both ears.

When it is assured that data acquisition can proceed satisfactorily, an adaptation period begins. The duration of this period is variable, depending upon a subject's age, activity level, and pertinent individual factors (Eisenberg, 1965).

The experiment proper, consisting of 30 trials, is preceded and followed by a basal run providing information on behavioral, HR, and EEG patterns under "no sound" conditions.

Behavioral data, recorded by the nurse–observer in the test chamber, are coded on IBM cards for comparison with similarly treated filmed data. EEG data recorded on a strip chart are scored on a single-trial basis by a trained technician; those stored on the tape recorder eventually are subjected to off-line analysis.[15] In the same way, on-line cardio-

---

[13] Feeding is done by the parent or usual caretaker who, when appointments are scheduled, is instructed that infants must be (1) healthy, (2) hungry, and (3) sleepy when they arrive at the Bioacoustic Laboratory.

[14] Respiration rates (counted by the nurse–observer) are noted, at specified intervals, throughout the study session.

[15] For the present, only a Computer of Average Transients (CAT 400 B) is used.

tachometer tracings are inspected visually while the continuous data, stored on tape, are available for computer treatments of various kinds.

I. Analysis of Heart Rate Data

As previously noted, methods of dealing with HR measures have not been standardized. It is hardly surprising, then, that the literature abounds with alternative suggestions for data analysis. These alternatives are discussed in detail in recent review papers (Graham and Jackson, 1970; Khachaturian *et al.*, 1972; Lewis, 1974; Steinschneider, 1971), and there is no need to consider their specific merits and demerits here.

By and large, the critical problems in analyzing HR data relate to the nature of mechanisms controlling cardiac function and the inherent instability of stimulus-bound events. That is to say, since cardiac output reflects activity in interrelated physiological systems, we cannot reasonably expect HR responses to assume some fixed pattern that is independent of changing relations among those systems. Indeed, it seems clear that an organism's prestimulus level of arousal determines, to greater or lesser extent, the mode and magnitude of cardiac and other responses to sensory stimuli (Eisenberg 1965; Eisenberg *et al.*, 1964; Graham and Jackson, 1970; Steinschneider, 1971). Moreover, centers controlling HR and respiration are coupled in the brain stem (Campbell, 1965; Evans and Mulholland, 1969; Lipton *et al.*, 1965, 1966; Parmalee *et al.*, 1972), and such variables as the depth and regularity of breathing or a subject's smoking habits will exert profound effects on the cardiac wave form under stimulus and nonstimulus conditions alike. Certainly, in work at the Bioacoustic Laboratory, we have found no stage of development during which stimulus-bound activity is invariant. Particularly during the earliest months of life, when systems for cardiac control are immature and consequently very unstable, this variance must be dealt with realistically.

In our experience, statistical treatments based on assumptions that system or response characteristics can be predicted reliably (Jones *et al.*, 1969) simply do not prove out, and exploratory use of numerous parametric procedures, some of them complex and highly sophisticated, has resulted in ambiguous or even conflicting findings. Specific efforts at analysis in the time domain have tested the use of ensemble averaging, time-shifted correlation matrices, polynomial regression, and analysis of variance. Not one of these commonly recommended techniques has permitted the extraction of adequate response criteria. Not one of them has proved potent statistically on a single-trial basis. At a descriptive level, they have yielded nothing more than confirmation of trends that were apparent during preliminary eyeballing.

The foregoing is by way of stressing that most of the statistical alternatives suggested in the literature have been tested at the Bioacoustic Laboratory, and none of them has been found satisfactory at all stages of development or under all stimulus conditions. We have, of necessity, become pragmatists, fitting our methods to our objectives, our measures, and our stage of research development.

IV. SOUND-EVOKED CARDIAC CHANGES

A. The Statistical Questions to Be Answered

At this point, it is too early to be concerned with characterizing sound-evoked HR responses on a single-trial basis; and indeed, we are beginning to wonder whether such an approach is warranted. Whether or not this turns out to be the case, however, the first questions to be asked must deal with fundamentals. Can we prove the existence of response? Can we demonstrate that cardiac measures are valid under differing conditions of arousal? Can we derive general descriptors that, regardless of stimulus or subject variables, refer to operations in VIIIth nerve channels? Can we develop dynamic measures that refer to central mechanisms affecting operating efficiency in those channels?

Each of these questions carries with it a set of sub-questions, some of which are bound to vary with experimental design. In laboratory work, for instance, the use of a fixed interstimulus interval (ISI) creates a whole series of statistical problems relative to time-dependent phenomena, such as anticipation of and habituation to the stimulus.[16] Although these subsidiary problems remain unresolved, we have managed to bypass them in attacking the more immediate questions noted above. To do so, we have adopted a series of nonparametric treatments that, in addition to yielding some of the answers now needed, may afford baselines for resolution of the subsidiary problems. These treatments,

---

[16] Even the most cursory visual inspection of our data makes it clear that, for all age groups, including newborns, temporal conditioning to a synthetic vowel takes place within as few as five trials. This finding was totally unexpected. It was assumed, on the basis of considerable pilot work with tonal sequences and other kinds of "patterned" signals (Eisenberg, 1970b), that time-dependent phenomena of this sort would be precluded by the use of a 90-sec interstimulus interval.

which uniformly involve the use of interval histograms, will be considered later with reference to their applications; and inasmuch as the statistical manipulations to be covered in this section may be new to some readers, they will be discussed with reference to sample data on individual subjects.

B. When Is a Change in Heart Rate a Response?

To answer the question of whether or not a response exists, we can consider data on a typical 43-day-old control: A baby younger than 2 months or so is a particularly telling exemplar because, at early stages of development, instantaneous heart rates may change by as much as 20 or 30 beats in the absence of any external stimulation. The cardiac system, then, is very labile in infancy. If we seek unequivocal proof of response, we need to show (1) that the distribution of heart rates during some sample of time subsequent to stimulus onset (T_o) differs significantly from the distribution found during some like period of time immediately preceding stimulus onset; and (2) that the differences between these two samples differ significantly in degree and/or in kind from differences that characterize contiguous nonstimulus samples. The first set of time intervals clearly must be selected from either side of T_o; the second set can be selected from any portion of the data sufficiently remote from T_o to be assumed independent of stimulus effects.

The samples, or epochs, used at the Bioacoustic Laboratory were selected only after careful visual inspection of many HR records. They cover 40 sec of real time in each trial and permit comparison of matched samples as follows:

1. a 10-sec stimulus-bound epoch (T_o to $T_o + 10$ sec) with the like nonstimulus epoch immediately preceding it in time (T_o to $T_o - 10$ sec);
2. an alternate nonstimulus epoch of 10 sec ($T_o - 5$ to 15 sec) with the 10-sec epoch immediately preceding it ($T_o - 15$ to 25 sec).[17]

As a first step toward proving response, interval histograms are extracted from these 40 selected sec of each trial, and the distribution of taus, or interbeat intervals in seconds, during each of the epochs is

---

[17] Putting this another way, we are dealing with the 65–85 sec of time subsequent to stimulus onset. The 5-sec interval immediately prior to T_o was excluded from consideration when visual inspection of strip-chart data showed anticipatory HR changes to occur during this particular epoch.

obtained. These tau distributions then are converted to equivalent heart rates according to the formula

$$HR = \frac{60}{tau(t)}$$

Such conversion, though not essential, is useful because most data on stimulus-evoked cardiac changes are presented with reference to heart rates rather than to interbeat intervals.

As a next step, both sets of data, i.e., those describing the two 10-sec epochs around stimulus onset and those describing the two 10-sec epochs remote from stimulus onset, are accumulated sequentially, in three-trial blocks, over the entire 30-trial schedule.

Finally, in order to quantify the significance of differences among epochs, the cumulative distributions (trials 1–3, 1–6, 1–9, and so on) are subjected individually to the Kolmogorov–Smirnov (K–S) Two-Sample Two-Tail Test (Siegel, 1956).

The general approach is illustrated in Figures 3 and 4, which refer, respectively, to HR distributions in the vicinity of stimulus onset (Figure 3) and HR distributions remote from stimulus onset (Figure 4). Statistical (K–S) values for the accumulative groupings are shown in the pertinent graphs, A through J, in each figure. In both cases, taus and HR equivalents are shown on the abscissa and, to point up the effects of increasing sample size, graphs are arranged in descending order. For purposes of graphic treatment, the approximately equal number of observations in each of the sample sets[18] has been converted to percentage values.

From these figures, the two questions posed at the beginning of this section can be answered with some confidence. Statistically significant differences between HR distributions for the 10-sec period preceding stimulus onset and the like period beginning with stimulus onset are found consistently. Statistically significant differences between the contiguous epochs remote from stimulus onset are found only inconsistently. In the first set of comparisons (Figure 3), it is true that differences between distributions show the statistical values declining from .001 to .05, as more and more trials are accumulated; but the decline clearly is systematic, and the statistical values never reach a point of no significance. In the second set of comparisons (Figure 4), however, differences between the distributions, when they occur, are less significant, and the statistical values show no systematic relation to sample size.

---

[18] These range between 82 and 84 for trials 1 through 3, and between 796 and 801 for trials 1 through 30.

These illustrative findings, which are supported by similar data on a few other control subjects in selected age groups, have obvious implications for further study. From a clinical standpoint, it seems entirely likely that, as further data are accumulated, the approach outlined here will yield strict, objective (statistical) criteria for determining response. From a research standpoint, at least two useful avenues of inquiry are opened. First of all, since the significance of differences between pre- and poststimulus distributions decreases systematically with sample size, the relative potency of given acoustic signals should prove measurable with reference to the number of trials required before statistical significance is lost or, alternatively, reduced appreciably. Second, since significance levels are highest when the number of trials included is limited, it should prove possible to determine, on an operational basis, the optimal (minimal) number of trials that applies to any given stimulus condition or study purpose.

C. Arousal Level as a Determinant of Heart Rate Activity

As one examines the accumulative histograms in Figures 3 and 4, it can be seen that both stimulus-bound and nonstimulus HR distributions shift considerably over a 30-trial (45 min) schedule. Since our study procedures yield correlative indices of prestimulus state, *i.e.*, EEG and behavioral ratings in addition to the HR values, we can assume with good reason that these shifting distributions reflect changes in physiological equilibrium.[19] The question of what these changes may mean is discussed later in this chapter. For the present, the issue is whether or not they affect the validity of response measures. The answer is that they seem not to do so. Although infant heart rates tend to be similarly labile in the presence or absence of stimulation, evidence for the existence of response remains unaffected even when modes of response activity are altered. It is clear, for instance, that the nature of the differences between the pre- and poststimulus distributions in Figure 3 varies according to the dispersion of HR values along some dynamic continuum. Thus, when the prestimulus distribution is concentrated near the middle of this continuum (graphs A through C), the sole descriptor is deceleration. On the other hand, when the prestimulus heart rates are

---

[19] Correlations among the individual indices are far from perfect, but there is excellent general correspondence among behavioral, EEG, and cardiac measures of arousal level. For any given subject, lower cardiac rates are associated with sleep and doze states and slow brain-wave frequencies, while higher cardiac rates are associated with waking states and relatively faster brain-wave frequencies (see Table I).

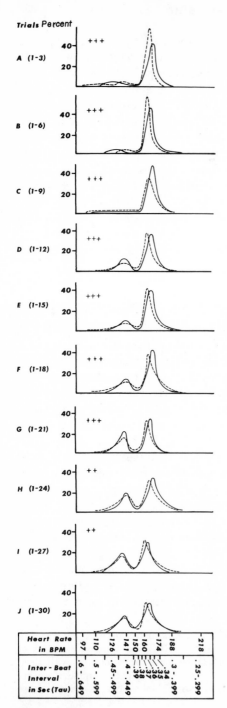

Figure 3 Distribution, by accumulative three-trial blocks, of infant heart rates before and after stimulus onset. Before (——) = T_o to T_o − 10 sec; after (– – –) = T_o to T_o + 10 sec. The significance of differences between each sample pair, according to the K–S Two-Sample Two-Tail Test, is shown as +++ (.001), ++ (.01), and + (.05)

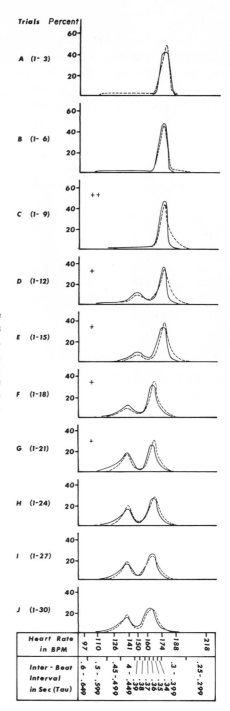

Figure 4 Distribution, by accumulative three-trial blocks, of infant heart rates during contiguous nonstimulus epochs. Solid line (——) $= T_0 - 15$ to 25 sec; broken line (– – –) $= T_0 - 5$ to 15 sec. Where differences between samples are significant by the K–S test, p values are shown in the pertinent graphs as ++ (.01) and + (.05).

distributed more or less in bimodal fashion (graphs G through J), there seem to be relatively fewer low heart rates during the stimulus period, suggesting the existence of accelerative changes during some trials. By the same token, it seems likely that the occasional findings of statistically significant differences between the contiguous nonstimulus samples, as shown in Figure 4, reflect nothing more than chance alterations in physiological states that occur within particular epochs.

The value of an interval histogram approach is that it provides a reliable and flexible method of treating cardiac data on either a single-trial or an accumulative-trial basis. On a single-trial basis, it holds great promise as an index of prestimulus state because the dispersion of HR values over relatively long epochs is more representative of internal equilibrium than is some arbitrarily selected reference point shortly before stimulus onset. On an accumulative-trial basis, the approach has a number of uses. It allows us to deal objectively with response activity that is complex, atypical, or "fragile." It tells us something about the inherent variability of our data. It suggests whether or not a typical response in fact exists.

D. Heart Rate as a Clue to Auditory Processes

Figure 3 suggests rather strongly that if there is not a typical response to the synthetic vowel used in our experiments, there certainly is a predominant response. In all the graphs shown in that figure, the heart rates most frequently represented during poststimulus epochs are shifted by an interval (five to eight beats) below those most frequently represented during prestimulus epochs. The same trend has been found for all subjects at whom we have managed to look thus far, regardless of age or state variables. This trend has not appeared in association with pure tones, noise bands, or any unmodulated signals of the kinds thus far explored (Eisenberg, 1965; Graham and Jackson, 1970; unpublished laboratory data). It seems possible, then, that cardiac deceleration may be one special functional property of complex sound patterns and speech-like stimuli. If indeed this is the case, as we believe it to be, the data reported here have important implications for our thinking about infant perception in general and auditory perception in particular. It has been argued, for instance, that the direction of HR responses reflects the nature of an organism's transactions with his external environment (Lacey and Lacey, 1970; Lacey et al., 1963; Lynn, 1966): Decelerative changes, which presumably are associated with an orienting system (Graham and Clifton, 1966; Sokolov, 1963), relate to acceptance of stimuli; accelerative changes, which presumably are associated with defense reflexes, relate to their rejection. The hypothesis, which has sparked a small amount of controversy (Obrist *et al.*, 1969, 1970) and a large amount of useful research (Graham and Jackson, 1970; Lewis, 1974; Porges *et al.*, 1973), gains scant support from our data: Correlative findings from a number of individual subjects show that decelerative HR changes to the signal used in our experiment cannot be associated easily with given patterns of overt or cortical activity.

Figure 5, which refers to the same 43-day-old control considered in Figures 3 and 4, is a case in point. Here we have selected six trials which, by visual inspection, were associated with marked and prolonged cardiac deceleration, we have graphed HR distributions for the two epochs encompassing stimulus onset, and we have tried to relate them to behavioral and EEG state ratings (see Table I) as well as to modes of response. From this analysis and from similar efforts with other subjects, it can be said that, whatever the prestimulus HR, purely decelerative responses are as likely to be found during sleep states as they are during wakeful ones. Although decelerative responses tend most frequently to be associated with cortical arousal, either localized or diffuse, they appear also in relation to EEG flattening, responsive

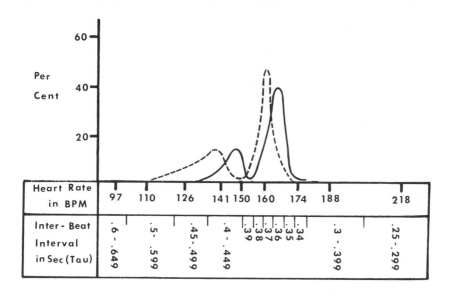

Figure 5 Distribution, for selected decelerative trials, of infant heart rates during 10 sec before (———) and 10 sec after (---) stimulus onset. N = 6; p (by K–S test) = <.0001. Correlative data on prestimulus state ratings (behavior and EEG) are shown in Table I.

TABLE I

PRESTIMULUS STATE RATINGS ASSOCIATED WITH SELECTED
DECELERATIVE RESPONSES (FIGURE 5)

Trial number	Prestimulus state ratings			
	Behavior		EEG	
1	Awake–Quiet	(IV)	Awake–Quiet	(IV)
2	Sleep	(II)	Doze	(III)
3	Doze	(III)	Doze	(III)
5	Doze	(III)	Doze	(III)
13	Awake–Quiet	(IV)	Awake–Quiet	(IV)
20	Sleep	(I)	Sleep	(II)

N.B.: Roman numerals bracketed with each descriptor refer to
Bioacoustic Laboratory codes; they are shown here merely to
indicate that correspondence among behavioral and EEG state
ratings is not as exact as verbal labels might suggest. State
classifications, whether verbal or numerical, are based upon
commonly accepted criteria.

motor activity, and even (though rarely) no response. There are suggestions, however, that decelerative HR changes bear on attentive
mechanisms, even in earliest life. In the infant under consideration here,
eight out of 13 trials associated with clearly detectable HR decrement,
whether of shorter or longer duration, were classified as orienting–quiet
behavior (Eisenberg, 1965) of one kind or another, while the remaining
five were scored under various categories of arousal.

Cardiac properties of the "probe" stimulus discussed in this chapter
obviously cannot be defined operationally with any real precision right
now. However, preliminary analysis of grouped and single-trial data
permits some general statements that bear upon the organization of
auditory mechanisms.

1. For all age groups, including newborns, reliable HR responses to
   a schedule of 30 trials with a prolonged, uninflected synthetic
   vowel of 60 dB can be found at least 70% of the time.
2. The predominant change in the HR pattern is a prolonged deceleration of considerable magnitude. In infants, single-trial changes
   may be well in excess of 20 beats and persist for periods in excess
   of 6 sec; in adults, single-trial changes may be in excess of 10 beats.
3. This decelerative response seems to be independent of a subject's
   level of arousal, a finding that assumes considerable theoretical importance since Newman and Symmes (1973) have reported the ex-

istence in monkey auditory cortex of selective "vocalization detector cells" having similar properties.

4. Although latency to peak magnitude of response varies greatly both within and among subjects, such latencies tend to be in excess of values reported in the literature for other kinds of signals. In infants under the age of about 2 months, peak magnitude most often is found 6 or more sec subsequent to stimulus onset.

All things considered, the HR data analyzed to date lend support to laboratory speculations that speech-like sounds may be processed at relatively high levels of the auditory system (Eisenberg, 1970b, 1973).

E. Repeated Stimulation as a Determinant of Dynamic Equilibrium

Up to this point, discussion has centered about what might be considered "static" measures of hearing, i.e., we mainly have been concerned with HR changes during selected periods of time associated with signal presentation. Now, however, let us consider an alternate line of inquiry and examine the long-term effects of a fixed presentation schedule on cardiac dynamics.

The approach toward defining a dynamic curve represents an adaptation of Bioacoustic Laboratory procedures that already have proved useful in studying behavioral responses to sound. Briefly, just as "state" is assumed to constitute a measure of equilibrium in interconnected systems governing overt behavior (Eisenberg, 1965, 1970b; Eisenberg et al., 1964), the distribution of heart rates over time is assumed to constitute a measure of equilibrium in systems governing cardiac behavior. This distribution derives from a series of histograms.

1. *Steady-state, or basal, equilibrium* is defined by HR distributions during the two rest periods preceding and following presentation of the acoustic battery (see Section III, H).
2. *Stimulus-bound, or dynamic, equilibrium* is defined on a trial-by-trial basis, according to individual histograms for 90 sec of time encompassing stimulus onset ($T_0 - 30$ sec through $T_0 + 60$ sec).

In analyzing these continuous data,[20] our basic questions have to do with whether or not dynamic measures can differentiate among subjects

---

[20] An initial sequence of 36 histograms per subject is involved in this analysis. Individual runs cover 90 sec of time and, together, the 36 histograms cover a period commencing 2.7 min prior to the first acoustic presentation (three histograms) and ending 2.7 min after the final presentation. In effect, we simply divide the continuous data into segments the computer can handle efficiently.

according to age, neurological status, or other factors. These are questions that computer programs could approach quite easily but, unfortunately, financial strictures have prevented us from implementing plans for automatic processing. To approach the questions on a preliminary basis, therefore, we selected two infants and two adults as experimental "prototypes" and subjected the individual histogram print-outs to manual treatments. The nature of such treatments and the results we have been able to glean from them are discussed below with reference to Figure 6.

In order to compress the mass of 120 stimulus-bound histograms for purposes of this chapter, each of the 30 90-sec print-outs for each of our four subjects was reduced to a set of five percentile points, referable to individual HR ranges. It was assumed, since the 90-sec histograms contain values that refer in unequal part to stimulus and nonstimulus conditions and since responses tend mainly to be decelerative, that the most representative region for looking at cardiac dynamics was that lying between the 25th and 87th percentiles. Thus, the lower boundary of the cardiac range was defined as that heart rate below which 25% of the HR values fell; the higher boundary as that above which 12.5% of the HR values fell; and the intervening points (50%, 62.5%, and 75%, respectively) were included to provide some slight degree of refinement. Then, to compress the data still further, the 30 trials per subject were segmented into six consecutive five-trial blocks, and the mean HR value for each block was plotted. Figure 6, then, is designed to yield information on whether and how sequential stimulation affects cardiac dynamics. It affords a number of provocative trends.

First, it is immediately apparent that cardiac boundaries change over trials and that, for three out of four subjects, in much the same way, HR levels tend to fall during middle trials (11–20) and then to return toward the initial range. It is difficult to evaluate the significance of this trend in terms of such time-dependent phenomena as anticipation or habituation until computer procedures for dealing separately with response and nonresponse epochs can be implemented, but we are convinced that the trend is real because analysis of our behavioral and EEG state ratings yields essentially the same results.

Second, the normal infant, despite differences in cardiac function that are reflected in higher HR levels and greater lability over time, behaves very similarly to the normal adult. It accordingly seems likely that similar control mechanisms in the nervous system, which presumably relate to attentive behavior, are operating in both age groups.

Third, since the high-risk infant is the only subject to show a systematic decline in HR over trials, it seems possible that measures of car-

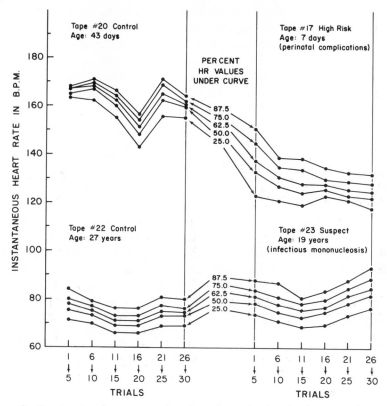

Figure 6 Heart rate change as a function of regular bombardment with a synthetic vowel sound.

diac dynamics under defined stimulus conditions may afford important diagnostic information. There is no reason to suppose that the trend seen here relates to age, since eyeballed data on control infants in the age range between 28 hours and 11 days shows them to behave much like the control infant shown in Figure 6.

The significance of differences between the control and suspect adults cannot be evaluated adequately at this time.[21] However, the tendency toward a wider dynamic range and increased HR lability is of some interest, because similar trends have been noted for the few "suspect" infants (Eisenberg *et al.*, 1964) on whom 90-sec interval histogram printouts are available.

---

[21] This particular suspect adult was included for study because of temporary nervous system dysfunction associated with severe infectious mononucleosis, and we are hoping to do a follow-up run now that his recovery seems complete.

Although basal data could not be analyzed in depth for purposes of this chapter, they were examined on a preliminary basis, and there is no evidence whatever for systematic changes in HR during either pre- or poststimulation runs. Both for infants and for adults, cardiac patterns appear to be stable during these "no sound" periods. Therefore, whether or not one accepts the notion that dynamic measures bear upon attentive mechanisms and/or the neurological integrity of subjects, the fact that heart rates and correlative indicators seem to change systematically under conditions of regular stimulation has important implications for the design of auditory study procedures that might prove useful with uncooperative subjects of any age. Unless we unreasonably are willing to assume that systematic changes over time can occur in the absence of sensation, we reasonably must assume that the dynamic curve associated with a train of signals constitutes an implicit measure of hearing. Such a measure conceivably could tell us as much about auditory function as threshold determinations, and it certainly could tell us something different. In any case, hearing sensitivity need not always be assessed solely on the basis of explicit yes-or-no responses to individual signal presentations, and normal auditory competence involves far more than normal hearing sensitivity.

V. A SUMMING UP

The research considered here is still in its developmental phase and, after more years than comfortably can be contemplated, it at least can be said that solutions to the problems of HR audiometry are in sight. Purely technical problems relative to data acquisition have been resolved and, short of circumstances beyond laboratory control, data attrition is negligible. A great many approaches recommended by other investigators have failed to fulfill their initial promise, but a few have evolved that seem to be holding up nicely. Tentative answers to some of the fundamental questions posed by HR and other autonomic measures may be available. Given the use of potent stimuli, for instance, it seems probable that the existence of response can be defined unequivocally, regardless of state or movement variables; and it seems possible that operational definitions of auditory processes and central influences can be established. The curve describing changes in state over a stimulus battery, whether measured by HR or by some alternative indicator, can tell us whether or not a subject hears suprathreshold signals; and there seems a good chance that it may be able to differentiate between normal subjects and those at risk of communicative disorders or other forms of subtle CNS dysfunction.

A. The Present Status of Heart Rate Measures

Once this is said, it must be emphasized that much remains to be done before HR audiometry can become a routine clinical procedure. The answers obtained at our laboratory may or may not be valid for all signals and for all intensities. Indeed, since the work considered here was undertaken with sounds of conversational loudness, it remains to be seen whether the statistical techniques developed will disclose response at or near threshold levels. We, of course, are hopeful that the procedures outlined will prove useful under many stimulus conditions and with large numbers of subjects. Even if by some miracle they should prove infallible, however, these procedures still would have to be simplified and standardized before they could acquire general clinical utility. In sum, then, cardiotachometers and related gear for measuring cardiac change at present must be viewed as research instruments with a rosy future. Exactly how rosy that future will be depends heavily upon whether *audiologists* are willing to do the spade work still required while deferring clinical applications until all of the validating data have become available. The history of GSR audiometry and electronic screening devices for newborns provides cautionary tales it would be well to heed (see Ventry, in this volume, and Eisenberg, 1971).

There is little reason to suppose that HR measures can be refined for clinical use within the immediate future, unless, of course, there is a dramatic surge in the number of audiologists exploring such measures. The work is urgently needed because differential diagnosis in the pediatric aged will remain an exercise in futility unless reliable objective objective techniques can be developed. Behavioral procedures, however carefully designed, cannot be freed from the element of examiner bias. Most of the electrophysiological procedures discussed in this volume can disclose hearing loss, but few of them are amenable to the disclosure of central problems. PGSR and EEG audiometry, which perhaps might serve in this regard, have specific drawbacks. The former has been discredited for use with the population it best might serve; the latter is extremely expensive and fraught with special difficulties relative to movement artifacts, changing maturational patterns, and the effects of arousal level. By comparison, then, cardiotachometry has some specific advantages. It has been found to yield valid data on newborns, infants, and even such difficult-to-test subjects as autistic teenagers (Eisenberg and Coleman). It is relatively inexpensive as compared with such alternatives as evoked-cortical response audiometry. It is almost totally free of movement artifact and, consequently, well-suited to telemetric procedures. It is past the stage of purely preliminary exploration.

B. An Approach toward the Definition of Individual Responses

Given traditional audiological concerns, future research undoubtedly will be directed toward methods of validating and characterizing HR responses on a single-trial basis. From a practical standpoint, of course, experiments employing variable rather than fixed interstimulus intervals (ISIs) will be needed. In this context, however, it may be worthwhile to outline some relevant pilot work at the Bioacoustic Laboratory.

Our approach toward data analysis involves a promising combination of nonparametric and parametric techniques. In essence, it is a method whereby the incidence and mode of cardiac responses can be defined according to the frequency and nature of statistically significant shifts in HR distributions during periods associated with stimulus presentation.

Treatment of the stimulus-bound data revolves around segmenting into smaller units each of the 30 sets of 90-sec histograms detailed in Section IV,E.

1. The histogram distribution for each initial 10-sec unit ($T_0 - 20$ to 30 sec), assumed to be uncontaminated by stimulus effects, is used as a "window," or comparator, to be shifted along the time axis in selected steps. The *existence of a response event* then is defined on the basis of statistically significant differences between the non-stimulus window and one or more 10-sec epochs in the immediate vicinity of T.

2. *Response-time boundaries* are defined by contiguous intervals of statistically significant shift, and *response peak(s)* by the period(s) of maximum shift within those boundaries.

3. *Mode of response*, defined by the direction of HR shift during peak periods, accordingly may be characterized broadly as accelerative, decelerative, or some combination of the two.

In effect, the purpose of nonparametric treatments is to provide a logical and orderly basis for parametric analysis. The 90-sec histograms for individual trials, sorted into homogeneous groups, can be ranked according to cardiac boundary conditions and equated with behavioral states or other correlative indices. A measure analogous to behavioral response pattern (Eisenberg, 1965; Eisenberg et al., 1964) can be obtained by sorting individual trials into homogeneous groups according to the direction of HR shift, and computing the relative frequency with which particular kinds of shifts occur. Further, since the magnitude and latency of responses can be defined with reference to *response onset* as well as stimulus onset, temporal conditioning, habituation, or other phenomena associated with repeated stimulation should become demonstrable. Finally, the time and magnitude characteristics of specific response modes can be determined by lining up homogeneous groups of trials with reference to response onset in order to obtain conventional measures of central tendency and variance.

No claims are made for the efficacy of the approach just outlined, and most of the procedures specified are unthinkable in the absence of computer facilities. Given such facilities, however, the techniques seem viable; and the rationale behind them has implications for the design of alternative procedures that are simpler and less expensive.

C. The Future of Heart Rate Measures

It seems to me that the future of HR measures and, indeed, of many electrophysiological techniques depends partly on whether or not we can begin to think about auditory function in new and more imaginative ways. The fact is that a substantial proportion of today's clinical population is made up of the very young and the very old, both of whom present hearing problems other than, or in addition to, deafness. Our management of these groups leaves much to be desired, mostly because we have no test procedures that define their problems in operational terms. One of our most pressing tasks is to devise and standardize such procedures.

What this means in terms of pursuing work on HR measures is that we have to make some hard decisions respecting the directions research most productively can take in the immediate future. As things now stand, we have a choice between addressing ourselves to one set of questions that may define hearing loss and another set of questions that may define some aspects of auditory competence. In my judgment, the definition of hearing loss can and should be deferred, if for no other reason than because alternatives are available. If we focus on it unthinkingly, the travail of dealing with single-trial data cannot be bypassed, and clinical applications for cardiotachometry lie far in the future. If we defer it and concentrate on the development of suprathreshold test procedures, we have a good chance of coming up with a great deal of very useful information, and clinical applications for cardiotachometry may not be very far away. Some of these potential applications have been considered in this chapter, and there doubtless are others we somehow may have overlooked. I would hope, therefore, that this chapter, whatever other purposes it may serve, will stimulate some critical thinking about audiological measures in general and cardiac measures in particular.

REFERENCES

Beadle, K. B., and Crowell, D. H. (1962). *J. Speech Hear. Res.* 5, 112.
Bench, J. (1969). *Int. Audiol.* 8, 615.
Bench, J. (1970). *Int. Audiol.* 9, 314.
Campbell, H. J. (1965). "Correlative Physiology of the Nervous System." Academic Press, New York.
Eichorn, D. (1970). *In* "Carmichael's Manual of Child Psychology" (P. H. Mussen, ed.), Vol. I, pp. 157–287. Wiley, New York.
Eimas, P. D., Siqueland, E. R., Jusczyk, P., and Vigorito, J. (1971). *Science* 171, 303.
Eisenberg, R. B. (1965). *J. Aud. Res.* 5, 159.
Eisenberg, R. B. (1970a). *Asha* 12, 119.
Eisenberg, R. B. (1970b). *J. Speech Hear. Res.* 13, 454.
Eisenberg, R. B. (1971). *J. Aud. Res.* 11, 148.
Eisenberg, R. B. (1972). *Develop. Psychobiol.* 5, 97.
Eisenberg, R. B. (1973). *Proc. Symp. Neuroontogeneticum, Prague,* Charles Univ., Prague (in press).
Eisenberg, R. B. (1974). *In* "Sensory Capabilities of Hearing-Impaired Children" (R. E. Stark, ed.), pp. 23–30. University Park Press, Baltimore, Maryland.
Eisenberg, R. B., and Coleman, M. P. Electrophysiological Correlates and Serotonin Metabolism in Normal and Autistic Children (unpublished laboratory study).
Eisenberg, R. B., Griffin, E. J., Coursin, D. B., and Hunter, M. A. (1964). *J. Speech Hear. Res.* 7, 245.
Evans, C. R., and Mulholland, T. B. (eds.) (1969). "Attention in Neurophysiology." Appleton, New York.
Graham, F. K., and Clifton, R. K. (1966). *Psychol. Bull.* 65, 305.
Graham, F. K., and Jackson, J. C. (1970). *Advanc. Child Develop. Behav.* 5, 69–117.
Hutt, W. J., Hutt, C., Lenard, H. G., Bernuth, H. v., and Muntjewerff, W. F. (1968). *Nature* (London) 218, 888.
Jones, R. H., Crowell, D. H., and Kapuniai, L. E. (1969). *Psychol. Bull.* 71, 352.
Kessen, W., Haith, M. M., and Salapatek, P. H. (1970). *In* "Carmichael's Manual of Child Psychology" (P. H. Mussen, ed.), Vol. I, pp. 287–447. Wiley, New York.
Khachaturian, Z. S., Kerr, J., Kruger, R., and Schachter, J. (1972). *Psychophysiology* 9, 539.
Lacey, J. I., and Lacey, B. C. (1970). *In* "Physiological Correlates of Emotion" (P. Black, ed.), pp. 205–228. Academic Press, New York.
Lacey, J. I., Kagan, J., Lacey, B. C. and Moss, H. A. (1963). *In* "Expressions of the Emotions in Man" (P. H. Knapp, ed.), pp. 161–196. Int. Univ. Press, New York.
Lenard, H. G., Bernuth, H. v., and Hutt, S. J. (1969). *Electroencephalogr. Clin. Neurophysiol.* 27, 121.

Lewis, M. (1974). *In* "Methods in Physiological Psychology" (R. F. Thompson and M. M. Patterson, eds.). Academic Press, New York.

Lipton, E. L., Steinschneider, A., and Richmond, J. B. (1961). *Psychosom. Med.* **23**, 461.

Lipton, E. L., Steinschneider, A., and Richmond, J. B. (1965). *New England J. Med.* **273**, 201.

Lipton, E. L., Steinschneider, A., and Richmond, J. B. (1966). *Child Develop.* **37**, 1.

Lynn, R. (1966). "Attention, Arousal, and the Orienting Reaction." Pergamon, Oxford.

Newman, J. D., and Symmes, D. (1973). Paper given before the Society for Neuroscience, San Diego, California.

Obrist, P. A., Webb, R. A., and Sutterer, J. R. (1969). *Psychophysiology* **5**, 696.

Obrist, P. A., Webb, R. A., Sutterer, J. R., and Howard, J. C. (1970). *Psychophysiology* **6**, 569.

Parmalee, A. H. Jr., Stern, E., and Harris, M. A. (1972). *Neuro-paediatrie* **3**, 294.

Porges, S. W., Arnold, W. R., and Forbes, E. J. (1973). *Develop. Psychol.* **8**, 85.

Richmond, J. B., Lipton, E. L., and Steinschneider, A. (1962). *Psychosom. Med.* **24**, 66.

Schulman, C. A. (1970a). *Psychophysiology* **6**, 690.

Schulman, C. A. (1970b). *Develop. Psychobiol.* **2**, 172.

Schulman, C. A. (1973). Paper given before the American Speech and Hearing Ass. Detroit, Michigan.

Siegel, S. (1956). "Nonparametric Statistics." McGraw-Hill, New York.

Sokolov, E. N. (1963). "Perception and the Conditioned Reflex." Macmillan, New York.

Steinschneider, A. (1971). *In* "Early Childhood: The Development of Self-regulated Mechanisms" (D. N. Walcher and D. L. Peters, eds.), pp. 73–105. Academic Press, New York.

Turkewitz, G., Birch, H. G., and Cooper, K. K. (1972a). *Develop. Psychobiol.* **5**, 7.

Turkewitz, G., Birch, H. G., and Cooper, K. K. (1972b). *Develop. Med. Child Neurol.* **14**, 487.

Chapter Ten

Evoked Cortical Response Audiometry

Donald C. Hood [1]

I. INTRODUCTION

We have learned much about human brain potentials since Berger's first report in 1929 (Berger, 1929). It was not until 10 years later that we first learned of the effects of auditory stimulation on human brain-wave activity or electroencephalogram (EEG) by Davis (1939). Interest generally waned in studying the effects of auditory stimulation on the EEG until 1954, when Dawson reported on a photographic superimposition technique for looking at low voltage potentials evoked by auditory stimulation. Determination of hearing sensitivity by the use of auditory evoked cortical potentials became the subject of much research in the mid-1950s and early 1960s (Dawson, 1954; Derbyshire *et al.*, 1956; Walter, 1961), and continues to be a major concern of persons involved in obtaining this type of response. As electronic and computer technology grew, so did the ability to detect and analyze lower voltage cortical evoked responses to auditory stimulation, such as the fast or middle cortical evoked response (Goldstein, 1965) and the brainstem or early evoked response (Jewett and Williston, 1971; Jewett *et al.*, 1970).

For many years, evoked cortical response audiometry (ECRA) was considered the panacea for testing hearing sensitivity in uncooperative persons, children, the mentally retarded, and adults giving unreliable responses during standard audiometric testing. Not all research has focused on using the evoked cortical response to obtain estimates of hearing sensi-

---

[1] Department of Otolaryngology, The Hospital for Sick Children, Toronto, Ontario, Canada.

tivity. Walter (1964) was able to demonstrate a very late component of the evoked cortical response, sometimes referred to as "very slow" (300 msec to several seconds), whose presence was contingent on some foregoing event or stimulus. Much research is currently being conducted regarding the effects of patient state and stimulus parameters on the so-called late or slow response (50 to 300 msec). This work will be described later in the chapter.

What this chapter will attempt to do is bring together a body of knowledge about four known components of the auditory evoked cortical response: brainstem or early response, fast or middle response, late or slow response, and contingent negative variation or very late response. Earlier texts dealing with these responses forced the reader to search through a chapter in an attempt to glean all information about the component of a particular response. This chapter will present a discussion of each component separately, so that information about a given component will be all together.

The four components of the evoked cortical response will be discussed in "chronological" order, i.e., the brainstem component or early response, which occurs between about 1 and 8 msec after presentation of an auditory stimulus, will be discussed first; the fast or middle component, which occurs between about 8 and 60 msec after onset of the stimulus, will be discussed second; the late or slow evoked cortical response component, occurring between 50 and 300 msec after stimulus onset is third; and contingent negative variation or very late response, occurring later than 300 msec after onset of the stimulus, will be considered last. There may be other components of the auditory evoked cortical response present in brain-wave activity, but presently we are not aware of them.

The following areas will be considered for each of the first three components mentioned above: (1) nature of the response, (2) types of response measurement and analysis, (3) effect of stimulus parameters, (4) effect of subject state, (5) purpose of testing for this response, (6) discussion, and (7) suggestions for further research. The contingent negative variation will not be discussed in the above format, since we do not have as much knowledge of the characteristics of this response component. Rather, a more general discussion will focus on the contingent negative variation.

II. BRAINSTEM OR EARLY RESPONSE

A. Nature of the Response

The brainstem component or early response, which was first reported by Jewett and his associates in 1970, is a moderately large (1 to 10 μvolt) polyphasic wave occurring from 1 to 8 msec after the onset of an auditory stimulus (Hood, 1971; Jewett and Williston, 1971; Jewett *et al.*, 1970). These researchers hypothesized that this very early component was neural in origin, since the earliest known myogenic potentials associated with auditory stimulation have been recorded at approximately 14 msec (Bickford *et al.*, 1964). Jewett and Williston (1971) have identified seven peaks of the brainstem or early response and proposed that each of the peaks is generated in a particular region of the brainstem, but there has not yet been full verification of this (see Figure 1). Peak I is thought to be N_1 of the cochlear response seen with electrocochleography (Chapter 3). Peak II arises from the cochlear nucleus or from double firings of the VIIIth nerve. Efferent axons from the cochlear nuclei, both crossed and uncrossed, may, as well, contribute to peak II. The researchers describe peaks III through VII as arising from multiple generators in the subcortical auditory regions. In humans, peak V is the most prominent, and was always present in their subjects who were awake and quiet.

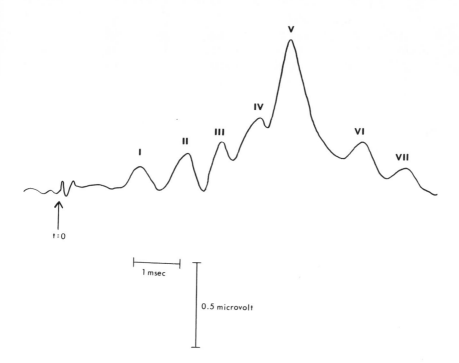

Figure 1   Early or brainstem response illustrating the seven peaks described by Jewett and Williston (1971). Note that peak V is the most prominent; $t = 0$ indicates the onset of the stimulus.

B. Types of Response Measurement and Analysis

The early response is best described by labeling the observed peaks and noting their latencies with respect to the onset of the stimulus. Amplitudes may be expressed as the voltage measured from the baseline observed before a stimulus is presented to each of the peaks rather than from a peak to a trough, as will be mentioned for the middle and late response.

This component may be measured using surface electrodes on the scalp (vertex) and on the earlobe or mastoid. Jewett and Williston (1971) suggested avoiding the use of polarity in describing this response, since they found that the polarity of the response is peculiar to the recording site. They found that, when the vertex electrode was referred to the earlobe, the seven major peaks were positive. The latency of peak V with this recording arrangement was between 4.6 and 5.1 msec.

Electrode pickup is differentially preamplified, filtered, amplified, and fed into an averaging computer. The averaged early response is then either displayed on a cathode ray oscilloscope (CRO) and photographed, or printed on an X–Y plotter for later visual analysis. An analysis bandpass of 1.6 to 2500 Hertz (Hz) proved to give the clearest early response (Jewett and Williston, 1971). They noted that, as the upper bandpass limiting frequency was lowered to 100 Hz, the response became much less distinct. This finding is supported by other reports (Lane *et al.*, 1974; Mendel and Goldstein, 1969a) that use of different bandpasses in analysis of evoked responses yields greatly different-looking evoked responses.

C. Effect of Stimulus Parameters

There is little data regarding the effect of change in stimulus parameters on the brainstem or early response. Jewett and Williston (1971) and Hood (1971) found good responses when click sensation levels were between 60 and 75 dB. The former writers tested for this response using stimulus rates from 2 to 50 per sec, and found the best rate to be 2 per sec. At rates faster than this, the response waveform became less distinct, and at a rate any slower than 2 per sec, the test took too long because several hundred stimuli had to be presented before a good response was averaged. Hood (1971) had to present 512 clicks at a rate of 3 per sec in order to obtain a good brainstem response.

D. Effect of Subject State

There are no reported studies of changes in response among awake, natural sleep, and sedated sleep states. One might think that, since this is a response generated peripheral to the cerebral cortex, sedations might have less effect on this component.

E. Purpose of Testing for This Response

The main reason for looking at the brainstem response may be to investigate lower levels of the auditory system. It may prove to be particularly helpful in investigation of hearing impairments found in persons with suspected brainstem lesions. For example, in such patients we might expect to see portions, or perhaps all, of the brainstem response missing or altered in some way.

F. Discussion

It seems odd that a response component as large as the brainstem response was not reported before 1970 by persons doing electrocochleography. Perhaps researchers believed that such early components were myogenic, particularly after the many reports on early myogenic responses to auditory stimulation (Bickford *et al.*, 1964; Mast, 1963, 1965).

Electrocochleography is the measurement of both cochlear electrical potentials and neural cochlear potentials in humans (see Chapter 3). Recording of these potentials involves looking at the first several milliseconds after the onset of the auditory stimulus. As discussed previously, both clinicians and researchers neglected events occurring after about 2 msec and before 8 msec, until Jewett and associates decided to investigate that latency region. It is this writer's opinion that testing the function of the brainstem auditory regions will gain clinical popularity as electrocochleography becomes more widely accepted and used as a clinical tool.

G. Suggestions for Further Research

Of the four auditory evoked cortical components to be discussed in this chapter, the brainstem component or early response is perhaps understood the least. Questions regarding this response are many. What is the neural origin, or origins, of this response? What are the effects on the response pattern of changes in stimulus parameters (frequency, rise–fall time, waveform, intensity, duration)? What are the effects on the response during different subject states, and what relationship does the response threshold have to behavioral audiometric thresholds? One example of the necessity for establishing normative data in some of the areas just mentioned was discussed briefly before. Namely, can measurement of the brainstem response in persons with suspected brainstem lesions give useful diagnostic information about the presence of such lesions? In order to answer this question, we might first need to know the normal stimulus rate versus response latency function before being able to note some type of breakdown in this function.

Caution should be emphasized regarding the interpretation of research findings with this response component, as well as with any of the responses to be discussed. It is most important to consider all of the instrumentation used, with particular reference to the filtering characteristics of the response measuring apparatus. Much apparent controversy and interreport variability can probably be attributed to the varying instrumentation used and the varying filter characteristics used in this array of instrumentation (Mendel and Goldstein, 1969a). If one laboratory or clinic uses a filter bandpass in its response analysis system which does not filter out any energy in the response component of interest, and another laboratory or clinic uses a bandpass that does filter out some energy in the response, then different response waveforms will result in the two different locations.

III. FAST OR MIDDLE RESPONSE

A. Nature of the Response

There has been much controversy over the origin of the fast or middle component of the auditory evoked cortical potential. The term "middle response" will be used here to distinguish this component from the truly early response described in the preceding section of this chapter. This component occurs between about 8 and 60 msec after the onset of an auditory stimulus (see Figure 2). The several peaks and troughs of this component were first described by Geisler et al. (1958), who believed that this component was generated neurally rather than by musculature beneath the surface of the electrodes. The musculature hypothesis was reported by those who found that the response waveform changed greatly or disappeared altogether when neck and head muscle tonus was systematically varied (Bickford et al., 1964; Mast, 1963, 1965). Geisler (1964) felt that only the amplitude of this response was affected by muscle tonus and that the basis of the response was neural. Ruhm et al. (1967) clearly demonstrated that, with electrodes placed directly on the surface of the cortex, the middle response was present. This is clear evidence that most of the electrical potential seen in this component is neural in origin but that, when electrodes are placed over scalp mus-

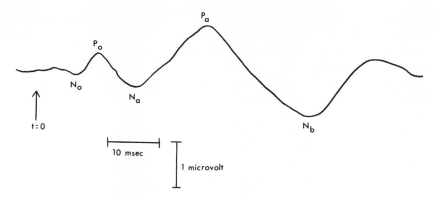

Figure 2 Fast or middle response illustrating typical negative troughs (N_o, N_a, N_b) and positive peaks (P_o and P_a). Positive is up, as suggested by Mendel and Goldstein (1969a); $t = 0$ indicates the onset of the stimulus.

culature, very large electrical potentials associated with muscle contraction tend to obliterate or alter the neural potentials also present at the same time.

If the peaks and troughs of the middle response are neural in origin, where in the auditory system are they generated? Goldstein (1970) feels that they may be generated in subcortical regions involved in alerting more cortical areas that "something is going to happen." Perhaps the reticular formation activity contributes to a portion of this component.

B. Types of Response Measurement and Analysis

The middle response is most easily recorded by using a vertex electrode referred either to a mastoid or to an earlobe electrode, with a ground electrode placed in some convenient location. Due to the very small amplitudes encountered with this response, it is necessary to average responses from as many as 500 to 1000 stimuli before obtaining a clear writeout. Analysis filter bandpass should be between about 3 and 100 Hz (Mendel and Goldstein, 1969a).

Amplitudes may range from a few tenths to several microvolts. The middle response consists of a series of relatively fast waves in the frequency range of 5 to greater than 100 Hz (Goldstein, 1969). Its waveform has been described by several researchers as consisting of two major positive peaks and three major negative troughs (Goldstein, 1969; Lowell, 1965; Ruhm et al., 1967). The two positive peaks are labeled P_o with a latency of 12 msec, and P_a with a latency of 32 msec. The three negative troughs N_o, N_a, and N_b occur at 8, 18, and 52 msec, respectively.

Latencies are expressed as the time in milliseconds from the onset of the auditory stimulus to the peak or trough to be measured. Amplitudes are measured from peak to trough and should always specify which peak and which trough is used in the measurement.

In most of the literature, negative voltages are depicted as *upward* deflections and positive voltages as *downward* deflections; however, a few researchers have displayed data just the opposite way (Figure 2). Usage of two methods for showing voltages only adds to the confusion among newcomers to the field of ECRA, and this writer suggests that negative be *up* and positive *down*.

C. Effect of Stimulus Parameters

1. Repetition Rate. Lowell *et al.* (1960) reported that, as stimulus (click) rate decreased from 1/63 msec to 1/100 msec, the amplitude of the middle response increased. Presentation of stimuli at rates slower than 10 per sec does not appear to produce larger amplitude responses. Mendel (1973) suggested a stimulus repetition rate of 10 per sec as the best for clinical measurement of the middle response.

2. Intensity. In general, there is a direct relationship between stimulus intensity and response amplitude, i.e., as stimulus intensity decreases, so does response amplitude. The latency of the middle response appears to be quite stable with changes in intensity, but Goldstein and Rodman (1967) observed that the peaks of the response were less well-defined and that there was an overall reduction in the number of definable peaks as the intensity of the stimulus approached the behavioral threshold intensity for a given stimulus.

3. Frequency. There have been no studies demonstrating any clear effect of test frequency on the middle response. This is probably due to the stimulus envelope constraints demanded by the fast repetition rates used to elicit this averaged response and by the apparent finding that tonal stimuli are not particularly effective in eliciting a middle response. Filtered clicks or tone pips have been used to elicit this response, but interpretation of frequency information is difficult with such stimuli.

4. Stimulus Waveform. Clicks or tone pips are known to be the most effective stimuli to elicit the middle response. A fast rise time appears to be the main factor in producing a response since Skinner and Antinoro (1969) found that rise times greater than 25 msec are not effective in eliciting this response. Stimulus durations are definitely limited by the fast repetition rates used. This response is mainly elicited by the *onset* of the stimulus, i.e., it is an on-response.

D. Effect of Subject State

If measurement of this response is to become a clinically useful tool, then understanding the effects of the use of sedation on elicitation of this response is mandatory. This is particularly true for testing a pediatric population, members of which are quite often not willing to sit still long enough for a complete test.

1. Awake or Asleep. The middle response latency and amplitude appear to be very stable over at least three awake adult subject states (Mendel and Goldstein, 1969a): (*1*) sitting in the dark with the eyes closed, (*2*) sitting quietly in the light with the eyes open, and (*3*) reading. The response waveform characteristics are, as well, quite stable through the various stages of sleep, whether it be natural sleep (Mendel and Goldstein, 1969b) or sleep obtained by using secobarbitol (Mendel, 1973).

2. Stress. Hypoxia, hyperventilation, and body acceleration through space all have the effect of increasing the latency of the middle response and lowering the amplitude in comparison to a quiescent state (Freeman, 1965). It is interesting to note that, while these changes in the waveform of the middle response took place during stress, there was no noticeable change in the ongoing EEG. Changes in the waveform of the middle response are then more sensitive indicators of increased stress than is the EEG. There is as yet no clear explanation for this finding.

E. Purpose of Testing for This Response

Perhaps the strongest proponent for clinical use of the fast or middle response is Goldstein (1969). For a number of years, he has been examining the middle response to obtain clinical estimates of auditory sensitivity with both adults and children. More recently, Davis (1972) has described the middle response, which he considers to emanate from the medial geniculate and primary cortical projection areas, as being "inadequately exploited."

With the finding of close (usually within 5 or 10 dB) agreement between middle response thresholds and behavioral thresholds for the same stimuli, it seems logical to use the middle response threshold as an electrophysiologic indicator of auditory sensitivity (Geisler *et al.*, 1958; Goldstein and Rodman, 1967; Lowell *et al.*, 1960; Mast, 1965). It is best to view the middle response in proper perspective, that is, as occurring after the cochlear and brainstem response and before the late response and the contingent negative variation (CNV). The middle response then probably gives us information regarding the integrity of subcortical areas of the human auditory mechanism.

F. Discussion

It seems unfortunate that this stable, easy-to-elicit response whose threshold bears a close relationship to behavioral thresholds has, for at least 10 years, been neglected by a great many clinics as a useful clinical audiological tool. Once more information becomes available concerning the effects of different stimuli and the effects of various sedations on this response, the clinical usefulness of measuring this response will increase.

With the measurement of the middle response, we have been able to measure at least as high in the auditory system as the primary projection areas or perhaps the medial geniculate and still remain capable of minimizing, as a variable, the state of the patient during the test. As we will see with the late response, to be discussed next, it becomes difficult, if not impossible at times, to analyze data obtained while a subject undergoes changes in state, both from awake to asleep and from stage to stage of sleep.

It should be noted that some of the earlier papers dealing with the middle response show the earliest component to be N_0, with a latency of about 8 msec. In more recent literature, less mention is made of this particular component, which apparently becomes less distinct as behavioral threshold is approached. N_0 may be related to the brainstem or early response previously discussed. Perhaps the filtering necessary to obtain a good middle response makes N_0 less visible than the filtering required for a good brainstem response. Whatever the cause, the brainstem response is stable, and the N_0 peak of the middle response appears not to be as reliable.

G. Suggestions for Further Research

Research with the middle response should focus in at least the following areas to resolve questions about the origin of the response, both with reference to the ratio of neural to muscular contribution to the response, and with reference to the site of generation of the neural component of this response. Some research has been done in this area (Bickford *et al.*, 1964; Mast, 1963, 1965), but more needs to be done. The effect of sedation on the middle response has only begun to be researched. This is particularly true with regard to the testing of preschool children. The problem of using clicks and tone pips needs to be overcome with assurance that the tonality of the stimulus plays a role in determining the response.

IV. LATE OR SLOW RESPONSE

A. Nature of the Response

The late or slow component of the auditory evoked cortical response was first described in 1964 (Davis, 1964; Davis *et al.*, 1964; Derbyshire and McCandless, 1964; McCandless and Best, 1964; Walter, 1964). It consists of major peaks and troughs occurring between about 50 to 80 msec and 300 msec after the onset of the stimulus. The neurogenicity of this particular component of the auditory evoked cortical response is widely accepted. It is a diffuse response that is easily recordable from nearly anywhere on the scalp, but it has its largest amplitude when recorded from the vertex (Davis, 1939). This response can be elicited by auditory, visual, or tactile stimulation, but the response to auditory stimulation generally shows the largest amplitude with the earliest latencies. Late response waveforms differ, depending on the type of stimulus used (Walter, 1964).

The late response has been described as a slow, variable, on- or off-response (Davis, 1972) with most of its energy in the 5 to 10 Hz range (Appleby, 1965; Scott, 1965). Since the electrical potential of the late component described here is, of course, a portion of the EEG, and since the EEG is a highly variable electrophysiological potential, changes in the EEG pattern create changes in the response waveform of the late response.

While much work was done during the 1950s and early 1960s on analysis of raw EEG (Dawson, 1954) to detect changes in that record associated with presentation of a stimulus, e.g., K-complex, on-effect, off-effect (Davis, 1969), only computer-averaged late responses are discussed in this chapter. Averaged responses are generally easier to detect and measure than responses buried in ongoing EEG.

B. Types of Response Measurement and Analysis

The late response is best described as a polyphasic waveform with several prominent peaks and troughs, as shown in Figure 3. When the vertex electrode is referred to an earlobe (C_z-A_1 or C_z-A_2, Jasper, 1958), prominent negative peaks occur at about 90 (N_1) and 260 (N_2) msec after the stimulus. Positive troughs occur with a latency around 50 (P_1)

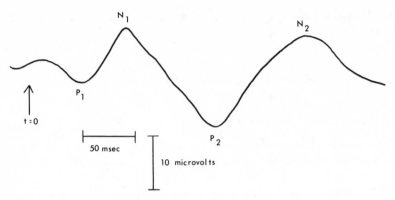

Figure 3 Slow or late response illustrating the two negative peaks (N_1 and N_2) and the two positive troughs (P_1 and P_2). Negative is up, as is the convention for this particular response; $t = 0$ indicates the onset of the stimulus.

and 170 (P_2) msec after the stimulus (Price *et al.*, 1966). There are earlier components of the late response, but they are not often seen, since their amplitudes are small relative to these major components. The amplitude of the late response is usually given as the voltage (peak to trough) between the N_1 peak and the P_2 trough. On the average, the N_1–P_2 amplitude will be several (5 to 20) microvolts. The N_1–P_2 amplitude is the easiest to measure and, in older children and adults, is the most stable portion of the response.

1. Instrumentation. There are several commercially available units to record late response to auditory stimulation—for example, Princeton Applied Research, Grason–Stadler, and Amplaid, to mention a few. All of these units are designed to generate stimuli and give some form of graphic display of the averaged results. Various degrees of averaging resolution are available, with the minimum number of averaging points, or bins, usually being around 50. One thousand to 4000 points may be optionally available to improve resolution, though for most clinical applications of the late response, 50 to 100 points is quite sufficient. An analysis bandpass of 3 to 15 Hz is fine for children, and 1.5 to 30 Hz for testing adults.

While it has been standard procedure for a number of years to look at response waveform with respect to latency and amplitude, some investigators include some measure of the amplitude variability for each point, or bin in their analyses (Derbyshire, 1973; Salomon, 1971). More recently, Whitton (1973) has included a form of the *t*-test, testing whether each data point is significantly different from either 0 voltage or a known response. Whether or not this additional analysis is helpful in looking at the auditory mechanism is not yet known, but the analysis is done in an attempt to eliminate as much tester bias as possible in interpretation. The nature of objectivity in evoked cortical response audiometry will be discussed later.

C. Effect of Stimulus Parameters

The effect of the stimulus parameters on the late response has been examined at length. The main effects of response change to stimulus parameters include repetition rate, intensity, frequency, and stimulus waveform.

1. Repetition Rate. If 10 sec or more are allowed between successive stimuli, the late response assumes its largest N_1–P_2 amplitude. If the interstimulus interval is only 1 sec, the amplitude is approximately 75% smaller than for the 10-sec interstimulus interval (Davis and Zerlin, 1966). For clinical purposes, a stimulus repetition rate of 1 per sec for a total of 50 to 60 stimuli gives the largest or greatest potential in the least amount of time.

2. Intensity. While there is a great deal of inter- and intrasubject variability in response amplitude (N_1–P_2), there is a clear, direct relationship between the intensity of the stimulus and the amplitude of the response. Amplitudes for fairly loud clicks (50- to 70-dB SL) range from 10 to 20 μvolts and get quite small as behavioral threshold is approached (Davis, 1965).

Tonal stimuli exhibit an inverse relationship between stimulus intensity and response latency. Rapin *et al.* (1965) found that, for tone bursts, the latency of the N_1 peak increased from about 110 msec at 50-dB SL to about 170 msec at 5 dB. In contrast, the N_1 latency to click stimuli from 70- to 5-dB SLs remained quite constant at about 95 msec.

The relationship between growth of loudness sensation and growth of N_1–P_2 amplitude has been investigated by several writers (Davis *et al.,* 1966, 1968; Keidel and Spreng, 1965; Tempest and Bryan, 1966). It was hoped that the N_1–P_2 amplitude growth would be a good predictor of loudness growth so that one might objectively look at the loudness growth function in, for example, an uncooperative adult or child. Such information might have been helpful in the recommending of hearing aids for children for whom loudness growth information is most often impossible to obtain. As well, research in this area hopefully would have told us more about the nature of the late response. No close relationship was found, however, between growth of loudness and growth of the late response amplitude.

3. Frequency. Several writers (Antinoro *et al.,* 1969; Evans and

Deatherage, 1969; Henderson, 1972; Rothman and Davis, 1970) have reported that the amplitude of the late response decreases as test frequency goes above 1000 Hz. Henderson (1972) reported that the late response thresholds were within 10 dB of behavioral thresholds at 250 and 500 Hz while, at 4000 and 6000 Hz, late response thresholds were about 20 dB poorer than behavioral thresholds.

Using a *change* in test frequency as the stimulus, McCandless and Rose (1970) reported that there was little difference in response amplitude, whether the test tone rose or fell in pitch. Their results also suggest that the late response can be elicited by a change in an ongoing stimulus as well as by the onset or termination of a stimulus.

4. *Stimulus Waveform.* The stimulus parameters of rise time and duration have been carefully examined for the late response (Davis *et al.*, 1966; Onishi and Davis, 1968). These writers found that, as rise time was increased past 30 msec, the N_1–P_2 amplitude decreased and latency tended to increase. Late response amplitudes did not change appreciably as stimulus duration increased from 0 to 300 msec, nor was N_1 latency affected as long as rise time was held constant at 30 msec.

D. Effect of Subject State

Most research-oriented articles on various aspects of the late response have used awake, alert, cooperative, and highly motivated adults. The late response, however, is highly influenced by the age of the subject, the stage of sleep or alertness, and the type of sedation used to obtain sleep with young or uncooperative subjects. By the age of 7 years, the late response appears much like an adult's response (Davis *et al.*, 1967). At younger ages, it is difficult, if not impossible, to use a standard response pattern or template for an evoked cortical late response for a given child. It becomes imperative to use each child as his own control, obtaining either a very clear late response, i.e., repeatable to auditory stimulation, or a visual or tactile response, for comparison with the auditory response data.

In the very young normal-hearing infant (less than 3 months old), thresholds were found to be no lower than 40-dB HL (Appleby, 1965; Suzuki *et al.*, 1966). Two factors might have produced this finding: (1) the lack of a good readable response and (2) the possibility that these infants still had their middle ears filled with amniotic fluid.

When a person attends to an auditory stimulus, his late response to that stimulus may be enhanced considerably (Dunlop *et al.*, 1965; Haider *et al.*, 1964; Mast and Watson, 1968; Satterfield, 1965). This particular attribute of the late response has not been fully explored in the audiology clinic, particularly when testing a suspected pseudohypoacusic.

The waveform of the late response changes considerably, and at times unpredictably, during both natural and sedated sleep. Peak latencies tend to become longer (Skinner and Antinoro, 1969) as sleep gets deeper. It is, therefore, apparent that if the tester does not know what stage of sleep the subject is in, he cannot validly attempt to interpret averaged electroencephalic activity.

The use of sedation to achieve a stable sleep level is far from being standardized. Several laboratories around the world are currently investigating the effects of different sedatives on various age groups. Some commonly used sedatives are pentobarbital sodium, chloral hydrate, nembutal, and valium. Current work on sedation is frequently announced in the publication of the International Electric Response Audiometry Study Group (Allgemeines Krankenhaus der Stadt Wien, 1090 Wien, Alserstrasse 4, East Austria).

E. Purpose of Testing for This Response

Auditory threshold testing is the most common form of test for which the late response is used. Some clinics take the lowest intensity at which a response was visualized as the "threshold" for a given stimulus (Price et al., 1966), while others extrapolate (using latency and amplitude information) from the lowest intensity at which a response is visualized to label a "threshold" (Davis et al., 1967). Most researchers find the late response thresholds to agree within ±20 dB of the behavioral thresholds (Cody et al., 1967; Davis et al., 1967; McCandless and Best, 1964; Price et al., 1966). In a given subject, however, when behavioral thresholds are not known, as is the usual case, the tester does not know how far he is from the true behavioral threshold. Interpretation, even of threshold testing, becomes difficult.

In the mid-1960s, the first packaged evoked response audiometer became available (Princeton Applied Research Evoked Response Audiometer) and many clinics bought the instrument without really being sure how to use or interpret the "responses" obtained from it. Availability of instrumentation does not ensure its proper use or the valid interpretation of results. It is recommended that extreme caution be used in interpreting the results of evoked cortical response audiometry to parents of young children. Many clinicians have had the unhappy experience of discovering, 2 or 3 years after their examination, that a child diagnosed as being deaf actually has normal or near-normal hearing, or vice versa!

Until the reliability of testing for the late response increases markedly, it should be used only as an adjunct to other audiological tests.

F. Discussion

The amount of information available on the late response is immense, but only a portion of this information is currently applied in the clinic. This has probably occurred because, in the mid-1960s, evoked cortical response audiometry was put forth as a truly objective audiometric test for hearing sensitivity. At this same time, there was great interest in early detection of hearing impairment in children. Many clinics then bought evoked response audiometers for testing the hearing sensitivity of children without full knowledge of the uses for, and limitations of, testing for the late response. The use of novel stimulus paradigms, speech, and deliberate modification of the awake subject's state are just a few of many areas that may easily be controlled in the clinical setting and which allow for enhancement of an often elusive response.

G. Suggestions for Further Research

There are several areas that need attention with regard to the late component of the auditory evoked cortical response. We need to investigate the effectiveness of various speech stimuli in eliciting the late response. The effectiveness of sedations in improving the technique of evoked cortical response audiometry needs continuing research. This is particularly true with a pediatric population. Continued attention is needed to determine how much interpretation can be given to the presence of an auditory evoked cortical response. This information is necessary so that more meaningful comments may be made to parents of young children regarding their child's hearing. We need investigation of both the late response and the middle response in various stages of sleep. Sleep stage discriminators have been developed that allow this type of research (Mendel, 1973).

V. CONTINGENT NEGATIVE VARIATION OR VERY LATE RESPONSE

A general discussion of the contingent negative variation (CNV) follows, without specific reference to stimulus parameters or subject state. Walter (1964) and Walter et al., (1964) first described the waveform of this very late DC potential and the stimulus paradigm necessary to evoke it. The diffuse late component of the auditory evoked cortical response which occurs 300 msec or more after a stimulus is sometimes referred to as an "expectancy wave" (EW) or "CNV" (Walter *et al.*, 1964) or a "very slow response" or DC shift (Davis, 1972), and can be observed in awake subjects (see Figure 4).

Walter *et al.* (1964) found that, when two different sensory stimuli are paired, the response to the first stimulus is increased, while the response to the second stimulus is decreased. These effects were labeled "contingent amplification" and "contingent attenuation," respectively. With paired stimuli, the first becomes less probable and the second more probable because it is always preceded by the first. The electro-encephalic effect is a very slow DC potential called the "CNV" or "EW." In order to evoke the CNV, the second stimulus requires either a mental decision or a motor task. The CNV is an indicator of the expectancy of the second or "imperative" stimulus.

The CNV is a long (1 sec or longer) negative potential which may be as large as 20 μvolts in adults. This response is best visualized by averaging the ongoing EEG, using electrodes placed anteriorly on the scalp. Only 10 to 12 stimulus pairs are necessary to evoke this response, and a partial reinforcement schedule (for the imperative stimulus) will maintain the response. If the imperative stimulus is omitted, the response will disappear, and a 100% reinforcement schedule for the imperative stimulus will then be necessary to reinstate the response.

The CNV appears to require cognition to be elicited and, to this end, the amplitude of the response is related to the semantic content or meaningfulness of the second or imperative stimulus. This response may prove

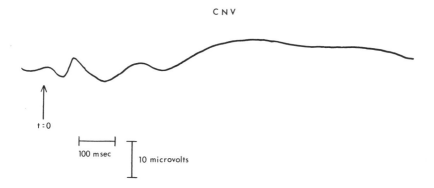

Figure 4 Contingent negative variation. Note the clear DC shift which defines this response component. Negative is up in this figure; $t = 0$ indicates the onset of stimulus.

to be helpful in the future for discovering language problems in children at a very young age, i.e., children for whom speech has little or no semantic content (Cohen and Offner, 1967). With current methodology, however, the response lacks stability in a pediatric population. Perhaps research in this area should focus on various types of speech stimuli for the imperative stimulus as well as on the manner in which the averaging computer is triggered when speech stimuli are used. Basically, the question is, "How does one consistently choose the onset of a speech sample in order to use that time to trigger the averaging computer?"

VI. GENERAL CONSIDERATIONS

A. Methodology

A few comments on methodology are in order, comments which apply to all four of the evoked cortical potentials discussed in this chapter. Good electrode contact with the skin is essential. Many EEG technicians try to have the resistance between pairs of electrodes fall below 5000 ohms. This is easy to do with needle electrodes, but with surface electrodes it is sometimes difficult to attain sufficiently low electrode pair resistance. Most often, electrode pair resistance is checked with an ohm meter. The use of such a meter impresses a small DC voltage across the two electrodes being checked, and some investigators (Salomon, 1971) feel that this polarized condition of the electrodes is detrimental to the recording process. The following procedure is recommended to avoid this polarization: Measure the voltage across a given pair of electrodes with an oscilloscope; insert a variable resistance box in series in the circuit and increase this resistance until the measured voltage across the pair of electrodes, plus the series resistance, is one-half of the voltage measured across the pair of electrodes by themselves; the amount of resistance on the variable resistance box at this point is equal to the resistance present between the pair of electrodes by themselves.

B. Objectivity

Much has been said in the past regarding the objectivity of evoked cortical response audiometry (Goldstein, 1969). It is widely held today that the use of this test is objective only insofar as the patient and instrumentation are involved. Once the tester takes over and has to interpret the negative and positive voltage fluctuations averaged from the ongoing EEG, subjectivity takes over. One of the main reasons for the great surge in interest in evoked cortical response audiometry was the fact that the test was originally thought to be objective with regard to subject, instrumentation, and interpretation. Fortunately, the early claims of "objective audiometry" have quieted considerably in recent years because clinicians noted great discrepancies between cortical evoked response thresholds and behavioral thresholds, particularly in children. These great differences could not, it seems, be fully attributed to subject variability or differences in instrumentation. The fault lay in the basic assumption that the tester, in interpreting the averaged EEG, was completely objective. Most clinicians now realize this, and interpret results of evoked cortical response audiometry with a great deal more caution.

C. Diagnosis

Interpretation of early, middle, and late evoked cortical responses has usually implied that stimulus information has reached the primary auditory projection area of the cortex. The presence of a CNV may also imply that some cognitive process has occurred that is related to the auditory stimulus. Each type of response, taken by itself, informs us of a portion of the auditory mechanism. The brainstem or early response may give information about the functioning of very subcortical regions of the auditory nervous system. The middle, or what used to be called the "early," response may give information about subcortical areas, the primary auditory cortex, and/or the reticular formation. The late response most surely gives information regarding processing in the primary auditory projection areas; the CNV again is a cortex response, but arising primarily from more frontal regions of the cortex.

In the past, specific diagnoses may have been made regarding cortical or subcortical pathology (that may or may not have been present) based on the absence of portions of the late response alone. This writer feels, as do others (Goldstein, 1969; Keidel, 1972), that in order to obtain a more complete picture of the human auditory mechanism, simultaneous recording of early, middle, and late responses as well as cochlear responses is necessary. Only then may comparisons be made between responses at various levels of the auditory system. With appropriate stimulus paradigms and instrumentation, it would be possible to elicit cochlear responses, early responses, middle responses, late responses, and perhaps even CNV with the same stimuli. Further research is needed in this area.

VII. SUMMARY

Four components of the evoked cortical response have been discussed
in this chapter: early response, middle response, late response, and contingent negative variation. Of the four, the late response has been investigated and measured the most and has been used in clinics more
than any of the other three. The early or brainstem response and the
late response clearly give information about specific regions of the auditory nervous system, both cortical and subcortical. For stability and ease
of recording, however, we must turn to the middle response, whose
threshold agrees well with behavioral thresholds for the same stimuli.
The CNV, perhaps the least stable of the four components, may yet offer
the most exciting information about the auditory system, particularly
if novel techniques are devised and stable responses are obtained for
children.

ACKNOWLEDGMENT

Work for this chapter was supported by the Department of Otolaryngology at The
Hospital for Sick Children, Toronto, and the Department of Otolaryngology at the
University of Toronto.

REFERENCES

Antinoro, F., Skinner, P., and Jones, J. (1969). *J. Acoust. Soc. Amer.* **46**, 1433.
Appleby, S. (1965). *Acta Oto-Laryngol. Suppl.* **206**, 146.
Berger, H. (1929). *Arch. Psychiat. Nervenkr.* **87**, 527.
Bickford, R., Jacobson, J., and Cody, D. (1964). *Ann. N.Y. Acad. Sci.* **112**, 204.
Cody, D. T. R., Klass, D. W., and Bickford, R. G. (1967). *Trans. Amer. Acad.
Ophthal. Otolaryngol.* **71**, 81.
Cohen, J., and Offner, F. (1967). *Electroencephalogr. Clin. Neurophysiol.* **22**, 190.
Davis, H. (1964). *Science* **146**, 434.
Davis, H. (1965). *Acta Oto-Laryngol. Suppl.* **206**, 128.
Davis, H. (1969). *Evoked Response Aud.* June.
Davis, H. (1972). Classes of Auditory Evoked Responses. Paper presented before
the *Int. Congr. Audiol., 11th,* Budapest, Hungary.
Davis, H., and Zerlin, S. (1966). *J. Acoust. Soc. Amer.* **39**, 109.
Davis, H., Engebretson, M., Lowell, E. L., Mast, T., Satterfield, J., and Yoshie, N.
(1964). *Ann. N.Y. Acad. Sci.* **112**, 224.
Davis, H., Mast, T., Yoshie, N., and Zerlin, S. (1966). *Electroencephalogr. Clin.
Neurophysiol.* **21**, 105.

Davis, H., Hirsh, S., Shelnutt, J., and Bowers, C. (1967). *J. Speech Hear. Res.* **10**, 717.

Davis, H., Bowers, C., and Hirsh, S. (1968). *J. Acoust. Soc. Amer.* **43**, 431.

Davis, P. A. (1939). *J. Neurophysiol.* **2**, 494.

Dawson, G. A. (1954). *Electroencephalogr. Clin. Neurophysiol.* **6**, 65.

Derbyshire, A. (1973). Personal communication.

Derbyshire, A., Fraser, A., McDermott, M., and Bridge, A. (1956). *Electroencephalogr. Clin. Neurophysiol.* **8**, 467.

Derbyshire, A., and McCandless, G. (1964). *J. Speech Hear. Res.* **7**, 95.

Dunlop, C., Webster, W., and Simons, L. (1965). *Nature (London)* **296**, 1048.

Evans, T., and Deatherage, B. (1969). *Psychonom. Sci.* **15**, 95.

Freeman, J. (1965). Monitoring Psychomotor Response to Stress by Evoked Auditory Responses. USAF School of Aerospace Medicine, Aerospace Med. Div. (AFSC) Rep. #SAM-TR-65-42, Brooks Air Force Base, Texas.

Geisler, C. (1964). *Ann. N.Y. Acad. Sci.* **112**, 218.

Geisler, C., Frishkopf, L., and Rosenblith, W. (1958). *Science* **128**, 1210.

Goldstein, R. (1965). *Acta Oto-Laryngol. Suppl.* **206**, 127.

Goldstein, R. (1969). Use of Averaged Electroencephalic Response (AER) in Evaluating Central Auditory Function. Paper presented before the Amer. Speech and Hearing Ass., Chicago, Illinois.

Goldstein, R. (1970). Personal communication.

Goldstein, R., and Rodman, L. (1967). *J. Speech Hear. Res.* **12**, 697.

Haider, M., Spong, P., and Lindsley, D. (1964). *Science* **145**, 180.

Henderson, D. (1972). *J. Speech Hear. Res.* **15**, 390.

Hood, D. (1971). Central Effects on the Human Peripheral Auditory Mechanism. Doctoral Dissertation, Northwestern Univ., Evanston, Illinois.

Jasper, H. (1958). *Electroencephalogr. Clin. Neurophysiol.* **10**, 371.

Jewett, D., and Williston, J. (1971). *Brain* **94**, 681.

Jewett, D., Romana, M., and Williston, J. (1970). *Science* **167**, 1517.

Keidel, W. (1972). A New Technique for Simultaneous Recording of Auditory Early, Late and dc Evoked Responses in Man. Paper presented before the *Int. Congr. Audiol., 11th,* Budapest, Hungary.

Keidel, W., and Spreng, M. (1965), *J. Acoust. Soc. Amer.* **38**, 191.

Lane, R., Mendel, M., Kupperman, G., Vivion, M., Buchanan, L., and Goldstein, R. (1974) *Arch. Otolaryngol.* **99**, 428.

Lowell, E. (1965). *Acta Oto-Laryngol. Suppl.* **206**, 124.

Lowell, E., Troffer, C., Warburton, E., and Rushford, G. (1960). *J. Speech Hear. Dis.* **25**, 340.

Mast, T. (1963). *Physiologist* **6**, 229.

Mast, T. (1965). *J. Appl. Physiol.* **20**, 725.

Mast, T., and Watson, C. (1968). *Percept. Psychophys.* **4**, 237.

McCandless, G., and Best, L. (1964). *J. Speech Hear. Res.* **7**, 193.

McCandless, G., and Rose, D. (1970). *J. Speech Hear. Res.* **13**, 624.

Mendel, M. (1973). Personal communication.

Mendel, M., and Goldstein, R. (1969a). *J. Speech Hear. Res.* **12**, 344.

Mendel, M., and Goldstein, R. (1969b). *J. Speech Hear. Res.* **12**, 351.

Onishi, S., and Davis, H. (1968). *J. Acoust. Soc. Amer.* **44**, 582.

Price, L., Rosenblut, B., Goldstein, R., and Shepherd, D. (1966). *J. Speech Hear. Res.* **9**, 361.

Rapin, I., Tourk, L., Krasnegor, N., and Schimmel, H. (1965). *Acta Oto-Laryngol. Suppl.* **206**, 113.

Rothman, H., and Davis, H. (1970). *J. Acoust. Soc. Amer.* **47**, 569.

Ruhm, H., Walker, E., and Flanigin, H. (1967). *Laryngoscope* **77**, 806.

Salomon, G. (1971). Personal communication.

Satterfield, J. (1965). *Electroencephalogr. Clin. Neurophysiol.* **19**, 470.

Scott, J. (1965). *Acta Oto-Laryngol. Suppl.* **206**, 155.

Skinner, P., and Antinoro, F. (1969). *J. Speech Hear. Res.* **12**, 394.

Suzuki, T., Tanaka, Y., and Arayama, T. (1966). *Int. Aud.* **5**, 74.

Tempest, W., and Bryan, M. (1966). *J. Acoust. Soc. Amer.* **40**, 914.

Walter, W. (1961). *Electroencephalogr. Clin. Neurophysiol.* **20**, 81.

Walter, W. (1964). *Ann. N.Y. Acad Sci.* **112**, 320.

Walter, W., Cooper, R., McCallum, C., and Cohen, J. (1964). *Electroencephalogr. Clin. Neurophysiol.* **18**, 720.

Whitton, J. (1973). Personal communication.

Author Index

Subject Index

383